What people are saying about *Infertility & Birth Defects:*

"The Ziffs have presented a real eye opener for all to contemplate. Dentistry should take the book's message to heart by demanding that mercury amalgam be outlawed. This is one area that dentistry could really help with in reducing the ever increasing body pollution and all it's attendant ills."
> E.A. Arana, D.D.S.
> President, *American Academy of Biologic Dentistry*.

*****

"An excellent resource for-

1. Patients or clients who want and must learn about their own bodies and the environment to protect themselves.

2. The Clinician - some interesting literature resources not often quoted.

3. For the researcher - a tremendous list of references."
> Mabel C. Brelje, M.D.
> Women's Health Care, Villa Clinic, Lakewood, CO

*****

"Science advances by assessment of known facts, constructing a reasoned hypothesis, and testing this hypothesis in controlled trials.

The Ziffs have done the hard work in their usual thorough fashion. All that is needed now are the relatively simple and inexpensive trials.

Amongst the millions of anxious would-be parents there would be no shortage of volunteers.

Who will accept the challenge"?
> J.G. Levenson, L.D.S., R.C.S.
> President, *The British Dental Society for Clinical Nutrition*

"Do you have mercury amalgam fillings in your mouth? It is not unusual to carry around 10 grams of slowly evaporating mercury when your dentist(s) has filled many of your teeth. This is equivalent to 10 million micrograms. The EPA has a tolerable limit of 1 microgram mercury vapor in each cubic meter of air around you. Your fillings might give off 0.1-0.2 micrograms of mercury vapor each minute (we have measured such values). If you exhale you might poison 1 cubic meter of air in 10 minutes. If you inhale you will poison yourself! You have the capacity to poison 10 million cubic meters of air!

A few years ago I wrote a short paper in the Swedish Midwife Association Journal about teratogenic effects of mercury. I advised already pregnant women to do no dental work during pregnancy; neither to place nor to take out amalgam fillings. I was reported to the Health and Welfare Administration. They sent a letter to the dean of the University of Lund and asked him to retract what I had written. He refused and wrote back that he found the request very strange. Today my advice is official policy in Sweden (no excuses, no thanks).

Do take the information and suggestions in this book seriously! Tomorrow it will be official policy."

Mats Hanson, Ph.D
President, *Scandinavian Dental Patient Organization*
Veberod, Sweden

INFERTILITY
&
BIRTH DEFECTS

IS MERCURY FROM SILVER DENTAL FILLINGS AN UNSUSPECTED CAUSE?

BY

SAM ZIFF
MICHAEL F. ZIFF, D.D.S.

BIO-PROBE, INC.
ORLANDO, FLORIDA

This book is not intended to replace the services of a physician or other licsened health care providers. Any application of the recommendations set forth in this book are at the reader's discretion and sole risk.

Published by:
Bio-Probe, Inc.
P.O. Box 580160
Orlando, FL 32858-0160

Cover Design by George Francuch
Illustrations by Steve Griffin
Text edit by Andy Faulkner

Copyright ©1987 Bio-Probe, Inc.
Library of Congress Catalogue Card No: 87-72238
Cover & Illustrations Copyright ©1987 Bio-Probe, Inc.
ISBN: 0-941011-03-8
Published in December, 1987.

Printed in the United States of America

To order this book and other Bio-Probe books and audio tapes please refer to the information contained in Appendix IV, page 343.

DEDICATED with love
to our devoted and unselfish wives
Helen Ziff and Peggy Ziff.
Thank you for the years of understanding,
support and patience.
December, 1987

DEDICATED also to the millions suffering the indignity, frustration, trauma, and expense of being infertile and realizing that they may never be able to fulfil their dream to have and raise a child. We hope and pray that for some this book may provide an answer to your dilemma!

ACKNOWLEDGMENTS

We are greatful for the excellent suggestions that were made by those individuals who took time from their own busy schedules and lives to review our manuscript in detail. Their efforts have improved and added to the book.

To: Mats Hanson, Ph.D.;
    Patrick Störtebecker, M.D., Ph.D.;
    Mabel C. Brelje, M.D.;
    Jonathon V. Wright, M.D.;
    Sandra C. Denton, M.D.;
    Edward A. Arana, D.D.S;.
    John C. Levenson, LDS, RCS;
    Jeffrey Bland, Ph.D.

    Our heartfelt thanks!

We would also like to acknowledge the special effort and support provided by Hylan B. Ziff and Marley D. Conway.

Whenever a new discovery is reported to the scientific world, they say first, "It is probably not true."

Thereafter, when the truth of the new proposition has been demonstrated beyond question, they say, "Yes it may be true, but it is not important."

Finally, when sufficient time has elapsed to fully evidence its importance they say, "Yes, surely it is important, but it is no longer new."

Montaign
1533-1592

CONTENTS

The implantation of a time-released poison into your teeth -a unique
situation in medical history. Scientific evidence relating this to
chronic mercury poisoning and to the validity of the so-called 'normal'
values of medical tests. Swedish government committee declares
amalgam to be toxic and unsuitable as dental filling material.

It has been said that the decline and fall of the Roman Empire was
caused by chronic exposure to lead from pipes and cookware. Is
modern civilization facing the same crisis from chronic exposure to
mercury?

What the experts have to say about the influence of mercury and other
poisonous metals from the diet on pregnancy and birth defects.

Proof that you are chronically exposed to mercury released from your
'silver' amalgam dental fillings. Signs and symptoms of chronic exposure to mercury and lead.

What is the blood brain barrier and why is it so important?
Evidence that mercury does damage and penetrate this vital barrier.
What does this mean to you and your child? Should you be concerned?

**Chapter 12: THE DIAGNOSIS OF
MERCURY STATUS** 275
Why measurements of mercury in the blood and urine are not valid for
determining the toxic effects of exposure to mercury vapor. Is hair
analysis valid? What are the proper techniques to use? What will it
tell you?

LIST OF FIGURES AND TABLES

FOREWORD
by Jonathan V. Wright, M.D.

There's nothing I can write about the poisonous effects of mercury that hasn't already been written by Sam and Michael Ziff. With meticulous attention to every detail, they've more than amply documented the case against allowing mercury anywhere in our bodies, particularly our teeth.

In this book, they've assembled the special case against mercury as a deadly hazard to human reproduction. Since there's nothing I can add, I'll simply quote a few lines:

Scientific research has demonstrated that mercury, even in small amounts, can damage the brain, heart, lungs, liver, kidneys, thyroid, pituitary, adrenals, blood cells, enzymes, and hormones, and suppresses the body's immune system.

Mercury crosses the placental membrane and is taken up by the fetus.

On May 22, 1987, the Swedish government declared publicly that [mercury] amalgam is toxic and unsuitable as a dental filling material. As a first step amalgam work in pregnant women [was] stopped to prevent damage to the fetus.

As the Ziffs document, all of our children, present and future, Swedish or otherwise, are and will be poisoned to varying degrees by mercury. As parents, can we allow this to continue?

We often cannot control what others do, but we have considerable control over our own behavior, and that of our families. Once you've examined the overwhelming evidence assembled by Sam and Michael Ziff, I'm sure you'll join me in refusing to allow any further mercury poisoning of our own children. Perhaps you'll go further, and have mercury removed when you can. Let "organized" dentistry, medicine, and government argue as long as they will: the decision for you and your children is yours.

Remember "what if they gave a war and nobody came?"

Let's try "what if they recommend mercury but nobody bites?"

The health and even the existence of your children is almost entirely your personal responsibility. Your answers can make all the difference.

Jonathan V. Wright, M.D.

Tahoma Clinic, Kent, Washington

And for all our children whom we no longer allow to be mercury poisoned, thank you, Sam and Michael Ziff.

FOREWORD
by Sandra C. Denton, M.D.

Would it surprise you to learn that your silver dental fillings contain 50% mercury, a known poison? Would it also surprise you to know that mercury leaches out of the filling into the body and can be transformed by bacteria in the mouth and intestinal tract into a more toxic substance, methyl mercury? If you happen to be one of the "one in five" couples in this country who are infertile, would you be surprised to hear that your dental fillings may be the cause? Or if you are an unfortunate parent of a child born with a birth defect (cleft palate, cerebral palsy, tremors, seizures, mental retardation, learning disabilities, behavioral disorders, and many others), would it shock you that mercury has been known to cause each one of these? Do you have any silver/mercury dental fillings in your mouth?

It is known that methyl mercury easily crosses the placental membrane and accumulates in greater concentrations in fetal tissues than maternal. It is also known that fetal excretion of mercury is slower than adult. It is known that developing organs are more sensitive to the effects of mercury. It has been shown with animals and humans that infants may suffer from these toxic effects even though the mothers demonstrate no signs of toxicity. Mercury also passes from the mother to the child during breast feeding.

In the light of this information, it is inconceivable that we continue to place mercury dental fillings in anyone's mouth. And yet we do. Approximately 900,000 fillings are placed every day. An estimated 75% of these are mercury.

Recently the Swedish Social Welfare and Health Administration declared amalgam (a mixture of other metals with mercury) as toxic and unsuitable as a dental filling material. Their recommendation was reported in a Swedish newspaper May 20, 1987. "As a first step in the process to eliminate the use of amalgam in dental fillings, comprehensive amalgam work on pregnant women shall be stopped in order to prevent mercury damage to the fetus."

Sam and Michael Ziff have done an excellent job in presenting evidence incriminating mercury and lead as significant contributors to infertility, miscarriages, stillbirths, and birth defects. It may be difficult to limit our exposure to these substances in our environment. However, one source, mercury dental fillings can be eliminated. There are alternative materials available.

In my practice I have seen many health problems of varying severity and duration dramatically improved or cured upon amalgam removal. Special attention was given to these patients nutritionally to correct many of the biochemical deficits caused by mercury and other metals involved. Questioning what effects mercury might have on learning and behavioral problems in children, I began a search of the literature. I had already collected quite a number of articles when asked to write the foreword to this book. My search has led me to the same conclusion.

After reading this book, I am certain you will not be eager to have another mercury amalgam put in your or your childrens' mouths.

Sandra C. Denton, M.D

Tahoma Clinic
 24030 132nd Ave., S.E.
Kent, WA 98042

PROLOGUE

I received a phone call from a young woman in California who had recently read my book "Silver Dental Fillings - The Toxic Time Bomb." It seems that she and her husband were planning on having a child in the near future, but the book had raised many more questions in her mind concerning their planned pregnancy than it had answered. Both she and her husband had a mouthful of silver mercury dental fillings, and if those fillings had the potential to exert a harmful effect on her unborn child, then she wanted answers to the following questions:

Should she have her silver amalgam fillings replaced with nonmetal fillings prior to conception? If yes, how far in advance of conception should she have it done so as to preclude any harmful effects that may be directly attributable to mercury vapor? If no, why not if mercury is so potentially toxic? Would the chronic release of mercury from her silver amalgam dental fillings during her entire pregnancy present unnecessary hazards to her health and to the health of the fetus? Were there any studies showing that mercury fillings (or any source of mercury) cause metabolic problems with male sperm that could lead to conceptual problems or imperfections in the fetus?

This unknown voice on the phone had focused on what could be the most critical issue of the entire amalgam controversy. The basic controversy is over whether the chronic exposure to low dose mercury vapor released from mercury amalgam dental fillings can ultimately cause physiologic and/or pathologic damage. The critical question of whether such low dose chronic exposure to mercury vapor from mercury amalgam dental fillings can affect the embryo or fetus has received very little attention from the National Institute of Dental Research, the American Dental Association, the scientific community, or academia. Consequently, there is an extremely limited amount of scientific data evaluating or comparing pregnancies between women with mercury amalgam dental fillings and those without any dental fillings. Further, no scientific studies have ever been done investigating this source of mercury as a possible cause of infertility.

In reviewing the scientific information available, it became apparent that there was an important and immediate need to alert women of childbearing age and their mates to the potential harmful effects of mercury, as well as other heavy metals, on parent fertility and the developing child.

A major psychological problem confronting anyone immersed in researching a particular subject is the ease in developing a "mind-set" that relates all of the world's problems to the subject being researched. We hope we have not fallen into that particular trap and that you will find this book to be a fair and impartial presentation of the facts on mercury (and some of the other heavy metals), and their potential toxicity to father-- mother--embryo--fetus--and child.

Sam Ziff

Michael F. Ziff, D.D.S.

1

DO YOU HAVE A POISON IMPLANTED IN YOUR BODY?

It is imperative that the reader consider the data provided in this book in a special frame of reference.

In the chemical world in which we live, we are assaulted "sporadically" by thousands of different chemicals, many of which can be rightfully classified as toxins. These may be present in the air we breathe, the water and other liquids we drink, and in the food we eat. Our exposure to these foreign substances may be brief and fleeting or they may be more intense, such as an eight hour exposure in the work place. Or, as in the case of prescription drugs, some people will be inducing and maintaining a level of one or more foreign chemicals in their blood for years.

However, there is one situation that is unique in the annals of history. Unwittingly, and in the guise of achieving better health, we blindly permit the implantation of a known time-release poison into our body--a time-release poison that, once placed in our body, will start releasing its toxic substance immediately, and thereafter 24 hours a day, 365 days a year, as long as the implant remains. Even after the implant has been removed, the poison it released has the ability to remain in our body throughout our normal life span. That poisonous implant is called a mercury amalgam dental filling and the poison it continuously releases into our body is mercury. We can think of no other situation in the entire history of mankind that parallels this phenomenon.

By definition chronic micromercurialism represents an exposure over a long period of time (chronic) to small (micro) doses of mercury resulting in mercury poisoning (mercurialism). Micromercurialism was first described in 1926 by Alfred Stock, a professor of chemistry at the Kaiser-Wilheim Institute of Germany, on the basis of psychological and physiological changes observed in individuals chronically exposed to very low levels or concentrations of mercury.(1,2) Professor Stock characterized the symptoms of micromercurialism into three groups based on their intensity:

First degree results in lowered working capacity, increased fatigue, light nervous excitability.

Second degree progresses to further weakening of memory, feelings of fear, loss of self-confidence, irritability and headaches. There may also be swelling and inflammation of the mucous membranes of the air passages of the head and throat resulting in upper respiratory discomfort, bleeding gums and other changes in the oral nasal mucosa.

Third degree symptoms approach those of mercury poisoning (mercurialism) but to a somewhat lesser degree. Symptoms that predominate are headaches, general weakness, sleeplessness, decline in intellectual capacity, and depression. There may also be tears, diarrhea, frequent urination, a feeling of pressure in the cardiac region, and shivering.

It was also Professor Stock who first focused scientific attention on the phenomenon of amalgam fillings in teeth giving off mercury vapor and causing psychological and physiological changes. Between the years 1926-1941 Professor Stock wrote and had published many scientific studies on the subject of amalgam fillings and micromercurialism. Although Stock was considered a brilliant chemist and scientist, we found it intriguing that so few of these studies related to amalgam and its instability have been translated into English.

Subsequent to the Stock papers other researchers have attempted to quantify the amount of mercury that disappears from an amalgam filling during its lifetime by measuring the amount of mercury remaining in old fillings. New amalgam fillings have a mercury content of approximately 50%. By measuring the amount of remaining mercury in old amalgam fillings and knowing the number of years it had been in the mouth before extraction, researchers were then able to determine approximately how much mercury per day had escaped from the filling. For example, Phillips and Swartz (1949) analyzed a large number of old amalgam restorations and found that they contained a residual mercury content of approximately 45%.(3) This equated to about a 10% loss in aged amalgams. Radics (1970) did a study on amalgam in extracted teeth and concluded that over a ten-year period individuals with numerous amalgam fillings could have a release of mercury from their fillings amounting to as much as 150 micrograms per day or 1050 micrograms per week.(4)

Vimy and Lorscheider in their 1985 studies wanted to quantify the daily amount of mercury vapor released and inhaled from amalgam fillings by measuring the intraoral mercury vapor concentration after chewing. They concluded that individuals with 12 or more occlusally involved amalgams, estimated to contain 12000 milligrams of mercury, would lose approximately 30 micrograms of mercury per day. Vimy and Lorscheider felt that this was an underestimation of the true loss of mercury from the fillings as they were only measuring intraoral mercury levels and did not take into consideration possible losses from abrasion to corroded amalgams which would result in swallowing of the abraded particles or ions, absorption of mercury by the oral nasal mucosa, and oral habits that might cause greater losses of mercury from amalgam.(5,6)

In still another approach to determining the contribution of amalgams to total mercury body burden the Swedish Department of Health and Safety, in a preliminary study, has determined that the *unstimulated* (no chewing, brushing, etc.) static release of mercury vapor from amalgam fillings would be in the order of 500 micrograms per week.(7) This would tend to support the total weekly loss, from all causes, of 1050 micrograms proposed by Radics.

The projected loss rates outlined above either equal or greatly exceed the World Health Organization (WHO) maximum weekly levels established for food of 200 micrograms methylmercury and 350 micrograms of inorganic mercury respectively. The studies discussed here as well as those covered in Chapter 4 all document the release of mercury vapor from dental amalgam fillings and all of the authors of these studies suggest that this unrecognized source of mercury makes a significant contribution to body burden.

Unfortunately, other scientists doing research on mercury have only viewed the subject in the context of mercurialism and not chronic micromercurialism. As a consequence most toxicological research has neglected amalgam dental fillings as a source of mercury or for contributing to potential mercury poisoning. Recently, however, some studies have started appearing in the literature that do take mercury from dental amalgam fillings into consideration.

Over the years, scientific studies on the distribution of mercury in humans has indicated that mercury tends to collect in certain organs of the body. Other studies indicate that some mercury storage or collection sites will retain mercury for differing periods of time. For example Sugita (1978) showed half-life retention times of mercury in the brain in excess of 20 years (8), and Newton and Fry (1978) indicated a half-life for the kidneys of 60 days.(9) Such determinations have normally been related to industrial exposures and though the subjects in these studies may have had amalgam fillings, this source of mercury was not considered.

In the science of toxicology, knowledge of the distribution, retention and excretion of a toxin is extremely important. In the case of mercury, although their have been many studies reflecting some of this information, nobody had developed a model to account for all the different storage areas and half-life retentions. In 1984 Bernard and Purdue developed a mathematical metabolic model to predict what the distribution, retention, and excretion of a dose of methyl or inorganic mercury would be. Using data from the previous research published since 1960, Bernard and Purdue developed their compartmental models. The use of the term compartment merely means that the body was divided up into 4 different areas or compartments that the research showed accumulated or stored mercury for various lengths of time. These compartments were blood, kidneys, other tissues, and the central nervous system (CNS), with the half-life of mercury in the CNS compartment being 10,000 days (27 years).(10)

Recognizing the potential of Bernard and Purdue's work to finally provide a vehicle for scientifically determining the extent of amalgam's contribution to total mercury body burden and ultimately to micromercurialism, Vimy et al. (1986) set out to develop a simple computer program employing the four compartment model. Using the estimated release rates of mercury vapor from dental amalgam from their 1985 studies permitted them to calculate the potential mercury body burden through use of the computerized four compartment metabolic model. The program permitted the simulation of the cumulative and incremental distribution in each compartment and total body accumulation between one and ten-thousand days for different daily mercury dosages. Applying the 30 micrograms per day dosage derived from their 1985 study, the model predicted that continuous exposure to this dosage for ten-years would result in a total mercury body burden of 5.9 milligrams. The brain concentration of mercury was estimated to be 68 nanograms per gram of wet tissue weight.(11)

What we found so important about the 1986 Vimy et al. study was the fact that it provides a basis for validating the existence of chronic micromercurialism directly attributable to low-dose elemental mercury vapor exposure via inhalation from dental amalgam. Validation will come by utilizing and applying new data derived from studies around the world that bring the presence of amalgam dental fillings into the research protocol. For example, applying the 500 micrograms per week of unstimulated mercury release found in the recent Swedish Department of Health and Safety study to the 210 micrograms per week of stimulated release found by Vimy et al. should produce a three-fold increase in the brain compartment of the metabolic model. Should a new study confirm the 1050 micrograms per week proposed by Radics in his 1970 work, applying the metabolic model should produce a five-fold increase in brain mercury levels, which could also exceed presently established levels for tissue or cellular toxicity.

We feel it is important that every reader understand the importance of Vimy, Luft, and Lorscheider's work to some of the hypotheses we put forth in this book. Some of them represent large leaps in interpretation of existing scientific facts. In those instances where there is no hard scientific data to clearly support our contentions, we hope that our application and combining of existing information into a new concept or hypothesis of how mercury from dental amalgam could be an etiological factor, will be provocative enough to stimulate the research to prove or disprove the theories we are advancing. The important thing to remember as you read our hypotheses on amalgam's possible involvement in endometriosis, cancer, immune dysfunction, other health conditions and nutritional deficiencies is that they simply cannot be dismissed without first conducting valid scientific research to disprove them. Their is sufficient scientific evidence available now to invalidate previous scientifically unsupportable positions claiming that the amount of mercury released from dental amalgam is so small that it presents no health hazard except in people who are allergic to mercury.

Throughout the history of medicine, changes of an accepted precept or concept are painful and agonizingly slow. Nobody likes or enjoys admitting error or negligence in recognition of a problem. Because of this, there seems to be an inherent desire to attack, in defense of what has been accepted and utilized for years. Initially, those who present information or theories in conflict with accepted practices are usually labeled as frauds and subjected to various degrees of ridicule. In some instances, as in the case of those practitioners of alternatives to traditional medicine or dentistry, innovators are maliciously attacked by the guardian angels of these bastions; that is, the societies or associations formed to represent their voluntary membership.

Such is the situation in regard to convincing the dental and medical professions to accept the simple premise that placement of certain kinds of dental fillings may be the cause of serious health problems. The scientific facts are simple and straightforward and cannot be denied or avoided:

1. Mercury and its various compounds are poisons. This fact has been known and documented for over a thousand years.

2. Since 1833, mercury, as an amalgam, has been used as a dental filling material throughout the industrialized world. Whether by design or simple marketing strategy, the dental profession has managed to obscure this fact from the public by calling mercury amalgam "silver amalgam," or just plain "silver fillings."

3. Whatever the name, every silver filling implanted in teeth contains anywhere from 43% to 55% pure elemental mercury. We use the word *implant* because, by definition, an implant is a material that is inserted or grafted into the intact tissues or a body cavity, and teeth are intact living tissue.

4. Various scientific studies, from different parts of the world, have documented the continual release of mercury in vapor form or ionized particles from mercury amalgam dental fillings into the body.

5. Scientific documentation has also demonstrated that there is an absorption rate of 80% or more of inhaled mercury vapor.

6. Science has also documented positive correlations between brain mercury levels and the number and surfaces of mercury amalgam dental fillings implanted in the individual's mouth. (Fillings in posterior teeth can have as many as five different surfaces.)

7. Science has also documented the uptake of inhaled mercury vapor into every physiologically active organ of the human body.

8. Science has also shown that chronic exposure to minute doses of mercury will cause an accumulation of mercury to occur during the lifetime of the organism. This is due to the very slow rate of elimination of mercury from the body.

9. It has been well documented that mercury causes various metabolic and physiologic changes in living tissue and organs, including suppression of immune function.

10. Mercury and its various compounds can cross the placental membrane and be taken up by the embryo and fetus.

11. Significant quantities of mercury can be passed to the nursing child through the mother's milk.

The above list represents irrefutable scientific facts. What has not been documented by science is the relationship and effect of chronic low dose inhalation of mercury vapor from mercury amalgam dental fillings to the etiology of known diseases and syndromes. The lack of investigation of these relationships, however, is certainly not proof that they do not exist.

Medical and pharmaceutical science have devoted their efforts to formulating drugs that will have some type of beneficial effect on signs and symptoms of diseases or syndromes rather than actually correcting the underlying causes. Because of this, very little is known about what causes these dysfunctions in the human organism. In fact, if one carefully reads the traditional medical diagnostic manuals or textbooks, most of the known disease states of man are of unknown cause.

Within this frame of reference, the medical and dental professions, when questioned about the biocompatability and safety of implanting mercury amalgam, a known poison, in the human body, have traditionally responded, "It has been used for over 150 years and with the exception of those few individuals who are allergic to mercury, nobody has died from it."

The sad truth of that statement is that, in over 150 years of implanting a poison in human bodies, only a handful of dedicated researchers have even attempted to evaluate what role this chronic low dose inhalation of mercury vapor might have in the etiology of the myriad of diseases from which people suffer. If a person dies of a tumor of the brain, mortality statistics would reflect that fact. Death would be attributed to the tumor and there would be no further investigation of the cause of the tumor. Suppose, however, that the individual has had a mouthful of amalgams most of his life and that an autopsy study, if performed, revealed a high mercury content of the brain. Is it possible that the mercury was involved in initiation of the tumor? If it was, what should be listed as the true cause of death? Although we are posing a hypothetical question to elaborate on our point that nobody knows how many deaths may have been caused by mercury initiating the metabolic defect, recent autopsy studies in Sweden have shown an increased incidence of brain tumors in dentists. (Svenska Dagbladet 9/10/85) The hypothesis, therefore, does have scientific support for consideration and investigation.

This total indifference to the routine implantation of a devastating poison in the human body manifests itself in some very terrifying medical concepts. Clinical laboratory analysis is a major cornerstone of modern medicine. Individuals going to their physician with a complaint must undergo a battery of laboratory tests evaluating their body fluids. The basic decision of what treatment protocol is to be utilized is normally predicated on these laboratory findings.

However, at least to our knowledge and investigation, not once in the history of medicine have normal laboratory diagnostic values been established for people without mercury amalgam dental fillings or other metals in their teeth/mouths. Think about this fact for a minute:

THERE ARE NO VITAL STATISTICS OF ANY KIND THAT SEPARATE PEOPLE WHO MAY HAVE BEEN SUBJECTED TO A LIFETIME OF CONSTANTLY INHALING A POISON FROM THOSE WHO HAVE NOT BEEN SUBJECTED TO THE KNOWN METABOLIC DISTURBANCES ATTRIBUTABLE TO THIS - MERCURY POISON!

Not only does this mean that you may be subjected to medical treatment based on a set of flawed standards, it even gets more basic than that. The efficacy or contraindications of prescribing a drug have never been considered in the context of how that drug reacts biochemically in the presence of mercury. Clinical human trials of new drugs are accomplished without regard as to whether the recipient has been subjected to the toxic properties of mercury for a lifetime. Does an immune system that may be compromised by mercury respond the same as one that has not?

It is important that the reader not misunderstand our intentions. We are not saying that mercury is the only factor involved in disease or poor health. There are hundreds of chemicals that possess the capability of causing metabolic dysfunctions in humans. We maintain, however, that although you may be exposed to some of these toxic chemicals, none of them have ever been implanted in your body. Only mercury amalgam dental fillings hold that unique distinction. Once they are implanted in your teeth you are continuously subjected to toxic mercury vapor. There is no parallel to this in the entire history of mankind. It is incumbent upon the U.S. government, medicine, and science to develop new criteria for evaluating the effects of this poisonous implant, giving special consideration to these factors:

1. Mortality and morbidity (disease) statistics should be separated according to the presence or absence of mercury amalgam dental fillings. This is critical when viewed in the context of major disease states. Do people with mercury amalgam dental fillings have more heart attacks, get cancer, diabetes, Alzheimer's disease, and other diseases more frequently?

2. What about infertility and birth defects? Do infertile couples have more mercury amalgam dental fillings? Do both parents of children with some type of birth defect have mercury amalgam dental fillings? Or does only one parent have mercury amalgam dental fillings? How many birth defects have been found in children of women receiving dental treatment during pregnancy, which subjected them to the additional body burdens of mercury caused by placement or replacement, or the routine polishing of, mercury amalgam dental fillings?

3. Government dietary surveys that determine deficiencies of nutrients in the population should consider whether or not those exhibiting deficiencies of vitamins or minerals have mercury amalgam dental fillings.

4. New laboratory blood values should be developed that establish "norms" for individuals who have never had mercury amalgam fillings.

There is no question that we all have our own biochemical individuality. This is an established scientific fact. There is a large body of scientific evidence that also demonstrates that the child is a product of maternal nutrition. To our knowledge, nobody has yet compared maternal nutritional status between pregnant women with or without mercury amalgam dental fillings.

There is another aspect to the mercury story that must not be overlooked, the synergistic potential of lead and mercury being present at the same time. Lead, in itself, has been the subject of intense investigation since the 1700s. However, only recently has research started to appear that evaluates the presence of both toxic elements together in mammals. The limited results to date indicate a compounding or more severe metabolic effect when both elements are present (synergism).

The Center for Disease Control (CDC) considers lead poisoning "one of the most prevalent and preventable childhood health problems in the United States today." In this regard, the CDC has lowered the concentration of lead in blood considered to be a danger to children. In the 1960s, blood-lead levels in children of less than 60 micrograms per one-tenth liter of blood were not regarded as a hazard. This has since been revised twice by the CDC and blood-lead levels in children of 25 micrograms per one-tenth liter of blood are now considered cause for concern and monitoring.(12)

Significant considerations of heavy metal poisoning were described in an excellent article on lead written by Dianne Dumanoski which appeared in *The Boston Globe* on July 15, 1985.(12) We would like the reader to visualize the analogy to mercury. The article stated "Today lead seldom kills, but specialists now believe it still represents a significant, though invisible hazard." It was also pointed out that in low-level lead poisoning, a child with no identifiable outward symptoms may suffer subtle neurological damage. Lead may cause serious behavioral and biochemical changes even at blood-lead levels that are considered "low" or "normal" in industrialized societies.

The article noted the work of David Otto, which found that brain wave activity changed as lead increased in a child's body. Changes were evident in children with blood levels of 10 to 15 micrograms. The average blood lead level for kids in the U.S. is 15.

Schwartz, of the EPA, felt that the reductions of lead in gasoline will have a significant public health impact. Using epidemiological calculations, he estimates that the 50 percent reduction in gasoline lead between 1976 and 1980 will result in 50,000 fewer heart attacks, strokes and deaths between 1980 and 1990.

Mercury is considered to be more toxic than lead and has also been shown to cause neurological and intellectual impairment, yet dentists routinely place mercury amalgam dental fillings in children of age two or younger. To date, no scientific studies have been undertaken to determine what, if any, effect this implantation of a poison has on the child's immature physiologic structures or intellectual development. Nor has anyone evaluated what devastating effect this might have on the child who has a blood-lead level of 25 micrograms.

Nobody really knows how many men, women, and children in the United States have mercury amalgam dental fillings and other nonprecious, potentially toxic metals in their mouths. The most conservative estimates would indicate the number to be around 125 million. One hundred twenty five million unsuspecting individuals are living with a potential metabolic time-delay toxic time bomb implanted in their bodies.

In 1981 it was estimated that one of every ten married couples in the United States was infertile.[*] That is a frightening statistic in itself, and it is impossible to quantify the pain, emotional stress, and physical trauma these couples endure.

The other aspect of life reflected in the title of this book is birth defects, a phenomenon that extracts its toll not only in pain, emotional and physical stress, and trauma, but in costs that are truly mind-boggling. It is estimated that the lifetime medical costs of caring and providing for children born with serious birth defects may exceed $1,000,000.00 per child. There are believed to be well over 2000 kinds of human genetic defects or diseases, and the number continues to increase rapidly. More than 120,000 infants with genetic disease are born each year in the United States.(13, p. 542) One million dollars times one hundred twenty thousand equals $1,20,000,000,000.00-one trillion, twenty billion dollars.

ON MAY 22, 1987, AN HISTORIC EVENT TOOK PLACE. ON THAT DATE THE SWEDISH GOVERNMENT HEALTH BOARD DECLARED PUBLICLY THAT AMALGAM WAS TOXIC AND UNSUITABLE AS A DENTAL FILLING MATERIAL. FURTHER, AS A FIRST STEP, AMALGAM WORK IN PREGNANT WOMEN WILL BE STOPPED IN ORDER TO PREVENT DAMAGE TO THE FETUS.(14)

We hope the action taken by the Swedish government and the scientific information presented in this book will stimulate our government and the medical and scientific communities to seriously consider our hypothesis that the implantation of mercury in the human body may well be one

* Page et al. Human Reproduction. W.B.Saunders Co. (3rd ed), page 170, 1981.

of the hidden etiological factors associated with the ever increasing rates of infertility and birth defects. Perhaps more importantly for those infertile couples who have tried everything else without achieving successful conception, this book may provide at least one additional possibility to be explored.

2

HOW MERCURY GETS INTO IN OUR ENVIRONMENT

Mercury is believed to have originated on Earth several billion years ago. Although it is found in many naturally occurring ores, cinnabar is the ore with the highest mercury content. Cinnabar is found on all continents except Antarctica and is the ore that is mined commercially for mercury.(15) When the cinnabar ore is roasted at high temperatures, it gives off elemental mercury in liquid form. Once extracted, mercury remains liquid at ordinary temperatures. It is this quality that is associated with its original identification as hydrargyrum (hydra = water; argyrum = silver), which then translates readily into quicksilver, or liquid silver. The chemical abbreviation of mercury is Hg.(16)

Mercury is also present in the earth's waters. There appears to be a natural migration of a certain amount of mercury from the land into the water. To give you some idea of the mercury content of various categories of water, Professor Alfred Stock did some detailed analytical work of the waters around his native Germany and published the following levels in 1934: (17)

Micrograms per Liter

Sea water 0.03
Rainwater . . . . 0.05 - 0.47
Rhine River 0.10
Spring water . . . . 0.010 - 0.05

Tap water (Berlin) 0.010
Tap water (Karlsruhe) . . . . .0.01 - 0.05

Our atmosphere, the air we breathe, also contains mercury in the form of elemental (metallic) mercury vapor or as an aerosol (a suspension of insoluble particles, or dust). According to a recent Environmental Protection Agency Report "current atmospheric levels of mercury are believed to be 20 ng Hg/m^3," or 20 nanograms (a nanogram is a billionth of a gram), of mercury per cubic meter.(18)

Man, in his infinite wisdom, has managed to impose man-made alterations on the distribution of mercury on the land, in the water, and in the atmosphere. For example, it is estimated that the burning of coal alone releases 6-10 million pounds of mercury into the atmosphere.(19) Collectively, there are approximately 40 million pounds of mercury set free into the environment each year by all human activities, including the production and use of mercury pesticides and fungicides and industrial wastes derived from factories utilizing mercury in their manufacturing processes.(20) These man-made events are all additives to the elemental mercury vapor and dust emitted into the atmosphere by the natural process of degassing from the earth's crust and oceans. In the global cycle of mercury, some of the mercury will stay airborne for months or possibly years, while some, considered as soluble, will be returned to the land and water by precipitation in a matter of days.

Contamination of our water and land introduces the potential for greater quantities of mercury to enter our food chain. Only limited studies have been done on the mercury content of various foodstuffs. Nevertheless, it is obvious that in the routine business of living (eating, breathing, and drinking) we are going to have a daily intake of mercury in various forms.

This may sound like a great deal of mercury and therefore a lot of mercury exposure to humans. However, let us keep in mind that all of that mercury is being distributed in a very large amount of air and water. Human mercury exposure from these sources certainly can't be good. The burning question, however, is the relative danger of a source of mercury directly within the mouths of humans. Another major consideration is the comparative ease by which the various forms of mercury can enter the human body. This leads us to the question, what are the different forms of mercury?

It is generally agreed among most scientists and chemists that there are two basic categories of mercury compounds: inorganic and organic(21) The term *inorganic* refers to elemental metallic mercury and its vapor and ions; mercurous (containing univalent mercury) and mercuric (containing bivalent mercury) salts, and those complexes in which mercuric ions can form reversible bonds to such tissue ligands as thiol groups of protein. The last statement merely means that once inside the body, the mercury can attach itself to sulfur-containing compounds that are part of a protein molecule.

We can absorb inorganic mercury by inhalation of the vapor from elemental mercury or aerosols of mercuric salts. It can enter orally or be absorbed through the skin, mucous membranes and digestive tract. The symbol for elemental mercury vapor is $Hg^{0.}$ The zero indicates that this form of mercury is electrically neutral (does not have an electrical charge). Consequently, this form of mercury is fat soluble and can readily pass through cellular walls and membranes, including those protecting the brain and placenta.

Elemental mercury is also the most volatile form of the metal because it readily gives off vapor when agitated, compressed, heated, or exposed to the air at normal temperature.

Elemental mercury is used in dentistry to make the mercury amalgam dental fillings so euphemistically called "silver fillings." It is also the form of mercury used in barometers, thermometers, and some other medical instruments.

Some authorities classify mercury into three categories, placing elemental mercury in a category by itself because it is not combined with anything else. Elemental mercury consists of the metallic mercury, the uncharged mercury vapor, and the electrically charged ions before combining with any other substance. It is these ions that combine with carbon to form organic mercury compounds or other substances to form inorganic mercury compounds.

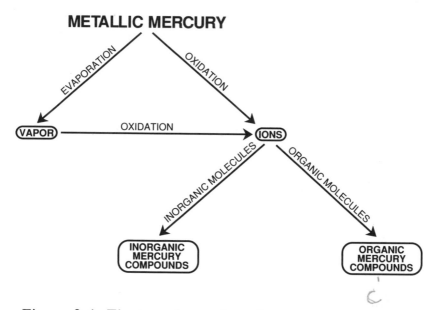

Figure 2-1: The transformation of mercury.

The major problem, once mercury has entered the body or its cells, is the formation of inorganic combinations with numerous substances always present in the body that are required for normal functions. This constitutes the toxic effect of mercury. Mercury vapor (elemental) and methylmercury (organic) are the most toxic forms of mercury simply because of the ease in which they can enter tissues and organs of the body.

Mercurous chloride is the best known of the mercurous compounds. It was also referred to as calomel (not to be confused with calamine) which for years was used as a cathartic. Fortunately, it is not used for that purpose any longer. However, it is still used in some skin creams and cosmetics as an antiseptic. Mercurous iodide was once used as a treatment for syphilis.(22)

Another form of inorganic mercury is yellow mercuric oxide which has been used as a topical antiseptic fungicide in chronic skin conditions, conjunctivitis, and corneal ulcers. In a recent report from Europe, a four-month-old infant had been treated with a yellow mercuric oxide ointment for eczema. Twelve days after the start of treatment, the child was hospitalized and diagnosed as being mercury poisoned and died thirty-two days later. The child had severe combined immunodeficiency disease. There were also high levels of mercury in the cerebrospinal fluid.(23)

Mercuric salts are a very irritating and toxic form of the metal. Mercuric chloride has antibacterial properties and was a popular disinfectant agent. Mercuric chloride is also known as "corrosive sublimate" and is known to cause ulcers of the gastrointestinal tract.

Continued exposure to mercuric salts can cause neurological and behavioral changes. The phrase "He is mad as a hatter" and the character of the Mad Hatter in Lewis Carrol's *Alices's Adventures in Wonderland*, stem from the changes that used to take place in people who worked in the felt hat industry. The use of mercury nitrate in the process of making fur felt for hats was derived from a process introduced in

France in 1685. This use has now been discontinued because of the harmful effects it caused on the workers.

Organic mercury is classified as those mercury compounds in which the mercury is directly linked to a carbon atom by a covalent bond (sharing of electrons). Within this group there are several compounds--such as methylmercury, ethylmercury, and phenylmercury--each with a varying ability to produce toxic effects. Alkylmercury (ethyl, methyl, and so on) salts have been widely used as fungicides. Use as such has led to major incidents of human poisoning from the inadvertent consumption of mercury- treated seed grain. The worst incident occurred in Iraq in 1972. Wheat and barley seed grain that had been treated with methylmercury was distributed for use in planting only. Instead, the grain was ground into flour and made into bread. As a result, approximately 6500 people were hospitalized and 500 died.(24)

Mercurochrome and merthiolate (thimerosal) both contain organic mercury and are used as antiseptics. They are utilized in dilute solutions and are considered to be relatively safe by the medical profession. This opinion is likely to change because of recent developments. The FDA has recently published an advisory concerning the death of a child whose physician was treating the child's ear infection with merthiolate.(25)

The ingestion of fish containing greater than normal concentrations of methylmercury was the cause of a Japanese catastrophe. Residents of Minamata, Japan, who consumed fish as a large portion of their diet, were poisoned. The fish were taken from Minamata Bay, where a major chemical plant emptied its wastes (effluent) from a manufacturing process that used inorganic mercury as the catalyst. Microorganisms in the bay converted the inorganic mercury to methylmercury, where it was then taken up by the plankton algae that the fish ate. Approximately forty-six people died from Minamata Disease.(26) This unfortunate circumstance also occurred at Niigata, Japan, and in the Great Lakes region of the United States.

Phenyl mercuric propionate is used as an antimildew additive. It is incorporated in many of the water-based paints used on exteriors and interiors. It is a potentially dangerous source of toxic mercury vapor. Cases have been reported of children being poisoned by mercury vapors released from wall paint in their rooms.

It is obvious from the preceding information that all forms of mercury present significant toxicity potential.

3

DIETARY INTAKE OF MERCURY AND OTHER HEAVY METALS

In July 1977 a meeting was held in Stockholm, Sweden, to investigate "Factors Influencing Metabolism and Toxicity of Metals." The purpose of the meeting was to examine relationships between different metals and other factors which could modify the toxic manifestations of metals. This particular consideration was deemed necessary due to the fact that human beings are exposed to a number of toxic elements and existing data indicated that interactions of possible health significance do occur.(27) The Task Group defined several aspects regarding the types of interactions:

Synergism "This occurs when the effect or response of the combined exposure is greater than additive. An example involving metals is the greatly increased teratogenic (capable of causing birth defects) effect seen in animals from the combined injection of cadmium and lead in relation to the effects of the same type of administration of each of the metals separately."(27) In other words, exposure to lead and cadmium together has a greater capacity to cause birth defects than exposure to each metal separately. Different types of synergism occur. For example, it is possible that the combination of two metals will result in a deficiency of another essential metal.

Antagonism "This occurs when one factor reduces the effect of another."(27) In our discussion of selenium in Chapter 11, we point out how selenium reacts with mercury to reduce its toxicity. In effect, the selenium is antagonistic to mercury. Drugs used therapeutically would also fit into this category, as they usually work by inhibiting the function of some other factor to achieve their effect.

Another factor is the interaction resulting from suboptimal intake or absorption of essential substances: "So far, when discussing the various types of joint actions it has been assumed that there is an optimal supply of nutrients. However, a suboptimal supply of nutrients, not in itself sufficient to cause a deficiency, may influence the metabolism and toxicity of a metal. There are numerous examples of this type of interactive joint action, one being the effect of low intakes of calcium and iron on lead metabolism and toxicity."(27) Another example would be the effect of mercury on an individual who is deficient in selenium.(28)

The Task Group went on to emphasize the fact that although the potential significance of many of these factors had been suspected for years, they had not really been documented. Consequently, and perhaps more importantly, the scientific recognition of the potential adverse effects of many of these factors may have been obscured or avoided through routine application of general hygiene and preventive medicine principles.

In animal studies, during the neonatal period, there is a high, nonspecific rate of intestinal absorption of a great number of metals which appears to diminish with age during the entire prepubertal period. In the case of lead and mercury, this could be of significance because these metals can be excreted in mothers' milk and passed to their children. In this regard, during the Iraqi episode, where there had been widespread poisoning caused by eating bread made from grain treated with a methylmercury fungicide, breast-fed children of mothers who had eaten the bread had increased - concentrations of blood mercury. It was also reported that methylmercury blood levels of newborn children were significantly higher than the mothers' blood mercury levels. Apparently, the intestinal absorption processes of children at that age are not able to distinguish between toxic metals and essential trace elements that may be present in the mother's milk.(27)

Because there is an increased demand for essential nutrients by the mother during pregnancy and lactation, any marginal deficiencies might cause increased absorption and retention of toxic elements. When mother's milk is the only source of food, this could also increase the child's body burden of toxic metals. Furthermore, toxic metals compete with essential elements which might also cause significant deficiencies in neonatal uptake of essential minerals.

The Task Group stated that "Based on these data, pregnancy and lactation are usually considered as periods when exposure to toxic metals should be avoided because of the possible adverse effects on the embryo, fetus and the neonate."(27) Of course, current data on the release of elemental mercury vapor from dental fillings did not start appearing in the literature until one year after the Task Group Report was published. Therefore, there was no identification of this as an additional maternal exposure to a toxic metal during the critical periods prior to pregnancy, as well as during pregnancy and lactation.

There was a section in the Task Group Report that dealt with the effects of other nutrients, including vitamin intake. Many different studies were cited in this section, establishing that there were many instances where published research indicated that these factors could have a significant impact on the absorption of toxic metals and their subsequent pathological effect. This section concluded with the following statement: "The real significance of these observations in the occurrence and frequency of increased metal toxicity for human populations has never been documented. However, the participation of these factors in the reported lead poisoning for population groups with suboptimal dietary intakes of various nutrients has been repeatedly discussed."(27)

Our food and water supply contains a myriad of metals and other contaminants, many of which are considered to be toxic. Moreover, it has been shown that mercury and lead are synergistic, thereby amplifying the toxic effects of both metals.

Research into the hazards of mercury in the food chain during the 1960s occurred predominantly in Japan, Sweden, and Finland. The United States had not embarked on a serious evaluation of this particular hazard. To rectify this situation, a study group on mercury hazards was convened by the Secretary of Health, Education, and Welfare (HEW) as an adjunct to the HEW Secretary's Pesticide Advisory Committee. The study group, after visiting Sweden and Finland in August 1970, completed a report to the committee in November 1970. That report was published in 1971.(29)

In 1970, the Swedish Commission on Evaluating the Toxicity of Mercury in Fish released its recommendations on Allowable Daily Intakes (ADI) of methylmercury. The recommended ADI was based on the lowest whole-blood concentrations for toxic symptoms of 0.2 micrograms per gram, on the basis of a steady intake. (A daily intake of 0.3 milligrams for a 150-pound individual should produce a blood level of 0.2 micrograms per gram, and a hair mercury level of 60 micrograms per gram.) Using this data, the commission then applied a safety factor of 10 in defining the ADIs, giving the following safe levels: for blood, 0.02 micrograms per gram; for hair, 0.06 micrograms per gram, and for ADI, 0.03 milligrams/70 kilograms, or 0.4

micrograms per kilogram of body weight (150 lb individual). The HEW Study Group felt that the current U.S. Food and Drug Administration (FDA) interim standard for mercury in fish and seafood of 0.5 micrograms per gram, or 0.5 parts per million, was adequate for protection. However, they also felt that the margin of safety might not be large.(29)

Some of the other conclusions and recommendations of The Study Group were:

-- to develop and to apply more sensitive diagnostic techniques to identify possible subclinical and late mercury toxicity;

-- to eliminate or reduce all controllable sources of mercury contamination;

-- to terminate the use of all alkylmercury pesticides and restrict the usage of all other mercurial pesticides on a basis of demonstrated need only;

-- to seek safe substitutes for remaining mercurial pesticides not now possible to eliminate;

-- to identify and bring under control other sources of mercury contamination or exposure (e.g., discarded electrical equipment, chemicals, paints, cosmetics, pharmaceuticals, sewage, and fossil fuels).(29)

Determining the heavy metal residues contained in foods is a difficult, time consuming, and expensive task. Consequently, most scientists attempting to use available data normally tend to utilize a combined value indicating the approximate daily intake from food and water. This fact notwithstanding, since 1964 the U.S. Department of Health and Human Services, through the FDA, has used "The Total Diet Study" to monitor the diets of adults. They have also started including data on infant and toddler diets. The program monitors the diets of the participants, as well as their dietary intakes of residues of pesticides, other chemicals, and six heavy metals: arsenic, lead, selenium, zinc, cadmium, and mercury.

"The adult-market basket samples, which represent the basic two-week diet of a 16-19-year-old male, were collected within four different geographical areas of the United States, i.e., South, Northeast, North Central and West, with the specific diet of each region determining the composition of the market basket." After August 1, 1974, ten of the thirty market-basket samples normally collected were reformulated to represent the diets of the infant (six month old) and the toddler (two year old).(30-33) Tables 3-1, 3-2, and 3-3 have been derived from references 30-33.

TABLE 3-1
DIETARY INTAKES OF METALS IN ADULT TOTAL DIET

Studies-FY 1977 vs, FY 1978
Intake (micrograms/day)

Metal	FY 77	FY 78
Arsenic[a]	1.6	59.1
Cadmium	36.9	30.9
Lead	79.3	95.1
Mercury	6.3	3.4
Selenium	110.7	156.2
Zinc[b]	18.0	16.8

a = arsenic trioxide (As2O3)
b = milligrams/day

TABLE 3-2

**DIETARY INTAKES OF METALS IN INFANT AND TODDLER
TOTAL DIETS**
Studies-FY 1976 vs. 1977 vs. 1978
Intake in micrograms per day

Metal	Infant			Toddler		
	FY 76	FY 77	FY 78	FY 76	FY 77	FY78
Arsenic[a]	0.4	4.6	2.0	12.3	24.7	18.0
Cadmium	12.3	5.8	6.0	14.2	7.7	11.0
Lead	26.9	22.1	25.0	30.1	27.8	35.0
Mercury	0.6	1.0	0.2	0.8	1.1	0.7
Selenium	10.8	15.1	18.0	45.0	46.3	52.0
Zinc[b]	8.2	4.3	5.0	9.5	7.8	9.0

a = arsenic trioxide
b = milligrams per day

The market baskets from which the data is derived were made up of food items from twelve different food classes. In 1977 for example, the arsenic, lead, and mercury content of the different food classes was found to be:

TABLE 3-3
MARKET BASKET FOOD CLASSES

Food Class	Adult Intake (micrograms/day)		
	Arsenic[a]	Lead	Mercury
Dairy products	0.0	7.16	0.45
Meat, fish and poultry	62.8	6.28	4.62
Grain and cereal products	8.2	12.2	0.37
Potatoes	0.13	6.09	0.29
Leafy vegetables	0.0	1.09	0.01
Legume vegetables	0.0	13.0	0.03
Root vegetables	0.07	1.58	0.07
Garden Fruits	0.0	10.4	0.05
Fruits	0.17	9.67	0.16
Oils, fats and shortening	0.18	1.14	0.18
Sugar and adjuncts	0.0	2.32	0.09
Beverages(includes drinking water)	0.0	8.32	0.0
Total	71.6	79.3	6.32

a = arsenic trioxide.

In 1983, Bouchet and his colleagues in Belgium did a duplicate meal analysis of nine different metals. Daily meals were taken from a hospital in Brussels, and persons living in the Brussels, Liege, and Charleroi areas. The authors brought out some of the difficulties inherent in analyzing trace elements in food: their normally low concentrations; the variable matrix effect of the different food items; the method of sample preparation suitable for one metal is not necessarily applicable to another element. Consequently, they checked the recovery and the variability of each metal analysis. They also confirmed that freeze-drying the samples did not cause trace element losses. (34)

One hundred and twenty-four daily meals were analyzed. The following median values for 24-hour intakes were found: cadmium, 15 micrograms; lead, 95.7 micrograms; manganese, 2.6 milligrams; copper, 1.3 milligrams; chromium, 0.24 milligams; mercury, 6.5 micrograms; calcium, 541 milligrams; zinc, 13.2 milligrams; arsenic, 11.5 micrograms. The distributions of the individual results suggested that about 1-2% of the daily meals sampled had mercury and cadmium contents that exceed the tolerable level proposed by the World Health Organization (WHO) of cadmium 70 micrograms/day, and mercury 5 micrograms/kilograms body weight per day. In the case of lead, the WHO provisional standard of 3 milligrams/week was exceeded by 10% of the sample meals tested. Over half the meals that exceeded the lead standard came from the hospital kitchen.(34)

Mykkanen et al. (1986) studied the dietary intakes of mercury, lead, cadmium, and arsenic in 1768 Finnish children ranging in age from 3 to 18 years. Their data showed that the intake of heavy metals increased with age. In the case of lead and mercury, lead increased from 49 micrograms/day at age 3 to 61 micrograms/day at age 15, and mercury fluctuated, from between 3.2 micrograms/day for 6 year olds to 4.4 micrograms/day at age 15.(35)

Cereals, potatoes and other vegetables, and milk products were the main sources of the four heavy metals investigated. This appeared logical as over 50% of the daily energy of Finnish children comes from cereals, milk, and milk products.

In their discussion, Mykkanen et al. refer to a German study which clearly indicated that exposure of German children to heavy metals in the diet was twice that of Finnish children and adolescents. They also referred to a 1983 study of pre-school children in the United States that indicated ingestion of twice as much lead as the 3- and 6-year-old Finnish children.

Another major conclusion of Mykkanen and his colleagues was that most existing standards--that is, maximum allowable intakes--which are expressed as milligrams per kilogram of body weight, are really not applicable to data on children. Their conclusion was based on the fact that intakes in proportion to body weight were seven-fold greater in the younger age groups. They felt that this indicated that the risk of undue heavy metal exposure via diet is highest in the youngest children.(35)

A startling fact, revealed in a 1986 study by Johnson and Shubert, was that the algae-based product Spirulina contained high levels of lead (9.1 to 24.4 micrograms per gram), organic mercury (2.6 to 12.4 micrograms per gram), and manganese (13.0 to 205.0 micrograms per gram). The report concluded that: "Concentrations of mercury in Spirulina are higher than 'prudent' intakes recommended by the USA Food and Drug Administration and WHO/FAO."(36)

In a recent report, Schreiber (1983) did a compilation of available data on the mercury content of various species of fish.(37) We have extracted just a few that would relate to fish or fish products consumed in the U.S. (data given in total mercury per kilogram of wet weight):

Herring	0.07-0.1		
	0.025	(mean)	Canned
Pollack	0.038-0.370		
	0.02-0.17		Canned
Mackerel	0.027-0.26		
	0.04	(mean)	Canned
Redfish	0.2	(mean)	
Tuna (albacore)	0.54	(mean)	
Tuna (albacore)	0.3	(mean)	Canned
Tuna (yellowfin)	0.54	(mean)	Canned
Tuna (bonito)	0.25	(mean)	Canned
Hake	0.11	(mean)	
Cod	0.1-0.38		
Sardine	0.015	(mean)	Canned
Greenland halibut	0.15	(mean)	
Shrimp	0.06	(mean)	

Methylmercury was the predominant type of mercury identified in all of the fish analyzed.(37)

Although the main focus of this book is on mercury vapor released from amalgam dental fillings the information provided in this chapter is intended to give you a better insight into the contribution that diet can make to total body burden of mercury, lead and other heavy metals. The dietary intake of heavy metals is a subject that should not be treated lightly by anyone who is serious about maintaining or achieving good health.

History has shown that dietary intake of toxic metals can cause a myriad of health problems, including infertility and birth defects. Although these events were catastrophic in nature, the everyday ingestion of heavy metals in the beverages we drink or the foods we eat is no less important. This is especially true for the individual whose health is fragile and who is more susceptible than normal to the effects of stress and environmental contaminants.

4

MERCURY AMALGAM FILLINGS
AND ENVIRONMENTAL LEAD:
A HAZARDOUS COMBINATION

The term *silver amalgam fillings* is really misleading because the main ingredient of amalgam, approximately 45-50%, is mercury. Not many trusting parents know that the term amalgam means a combination of mercury with other metals. Silver only accounts for about 33% of the finished amalgam. The balance of the ingredients can be made up of varying percentages of zinc, copper, and tin.

[NOTE: For reasons of clarity, whenever we refer to this dental material in the balance of the book, it will be called mercury amalgam.]

MERCURY AMALGAM FILLINGS

Although it was clearly demonstrated in 1926 that mercury vapor was released from mercury amalgam dental fillings, the dental profession chose to ignore this fact.(38) Dentists have always been taught to believe that once mercury has been combined into the filling material, it remains "locked in" and can't come out. In fact, in January 1984, the American Dental Association (ADA) was publishing information that stated, "When mercury is combined with the metals used in dental amalgam, its toxic properties are made harmless."(38) This statement was subsequently modified in September 1986 to read "its toxic properties are made *virtually h*armless.(39) The sad fact is that no scientific research exists to support either statement. In making such statements the ADA might be found to be negligent, since the scientific documentation directly contradicts the ADA position.

Until recently, most dentists believed what they were taught in school and what the ADA said about mercury staying "locked in." Now, however, there is scientific evidence proving that the mercury does not stay "locked in" and that its toxic properties are not made harmless. Starting in 1979 (Gay et al.) scientific research has again been published indicating the release of mercury vapor from mercury amalgam dental fillings.(40) Since that date there have been an ever-increasing number of scientific studies confirming this release of mercury vapor under varying conditions.

In 1981 Svare et al., at the University of Iowa, expanded on the 1979 findings of Gay et al. The Svare study evaluated forty persons with mercury amalgam dental fillings and eight without any fillings. The purpose of the study was to determine if the normal function of chewing caused any added release of mercury from mercury amalgam dental fillings. Test subjects were required to exhale into a plastic bag and the air within the bag was assayed for the amount of mercury in the sample. Readings were taken before chewing gum and after chewing gum for ten minutes. These researchers found that before chewing gum, the group with mercury amalgam fillings had more mercury in their expired air than the group without any fillings. After chewing gum, the forty with mercury amalgam fillings had a 15.6-fold increase of mercury vapor in their expired air. The test participants without any fillings, however, HAD NO CHANGE IN THE MERCURY CONTENT OF THEIR EXPIRED AIR. Finally, the researchers concluded that the magnitude of the increase in mercury vapor appears to be related to the number of mercury amalgam dental fillings present. Another observation made by Svare and his associates was that persons with badly corroded and pitted mercury amalgam fillings had the highest pre- and post-chewing breath levels of mercury.(41)

Taking a slightly different approach to the overall problem of mercury vapor release from dental fillings, Emler and-Cardone (1984) of Oral Roberts University, set up a study to determine whether the Svare group findings would also be true with children and to also examine whether the type of dental filling made a difference. Mouth-air mercury levels were measured at rest and after chewing in a group of twenty children who had no dental fillings but who needed to have restorative work done on one or more teeth. Ten of the patients received mercury amalgam dental fillings and ten received nonmetal (composite) dental fillings.(42)

The mouth-air mercury levels were measured in these children prior to, immediately after the dental work was done, and one week later. As might be expected, those children who received composite fillings had no change in their mercury levels from preoperative levels. Such was not the case with the children who had received the mercury amalgam fillings. The mouth-air mercury levels in this group were raised significantly immediately after placement. An extremely interesting finding was that when the mouth-air mercury levels were taken one week after placement, the resting (prechewing) levels were the same as their preoperative levels; however, after chewing, the mouth-air mercury levels were significantly higher than the preoperative levels in the children with mercury amalgam fillings. In other words, the mercury release was not temporary. Putting mercury amalgam fillings in these children placed them at greater health risk because of their increased exposure to mercury vapor.

In another part of the world, Patterson et al. (1985) in New Zealand took yet another approach in confirming the finding that mercury amalgam dental fillings were unstable and released mercury when stimulated. In this case, the stimulation was the routine task of brushing teeth. Breath samples were taken from a total of 167 adults with mercury amalgam dental fillings and from three adults and two children who had no amalgam fillings. (43)

The test subjects were required to brush their teeth for one minute with a soft toothbrush and a commercial toothpaste. Breath samples were collected before and after brushing. The researchers recorded large increases in breath-mercury concentrations after brushing. Some of these increases exceeded probable safe exposure limits and appeared to be high enough to represent a chronic toxicological hazard for some people. Another very interesting finding that emerged from this study was the fact that once the amalgam filling was stimulated by brushing, it continued to release mercury vapor and it took about an hour for the mercury levels to drop to one-third of their peak values. The Patterson group concluded that any mild abrasion of the mercury amalgam filling surface, either by eating a meal, chewing gum, or brushing, would result in the release of mercury vapor.

There was another bit of data collected by Patterson and his colleagues that is considered very significant, although they did not elaborate on it. When patients exhaled through the mouth their breath contained 13-40 micrograms of mercury per cubic meter of air. However, if the air was exhaled through the nose it contained only 0.2-0.3 micrograms of mercury per cubic meter of air. Where did the rest of the mercury go? Some, of course, entered the blood via lung absorption. However, there is another explanation of this phenomenon. Mercury vapor released by mercury amalgam fillings is taken up by the oral and nasal mucosa. From there, mercury can be further transported directly to the brain and the pituitary gland, via open venous pathways and by the olfactory nerves.

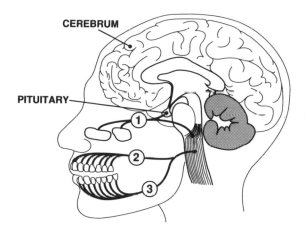

Figure 4-1: Direct pathways from mouth and nose to brain.
(1) Nerves from nasal cavity directly to brain.
(2) Nerves from upper teeth.
(3) Nerves from lower teeth.
NOTE: Veins in this region have no valves thus allowing direct passage from the oronasal cavity to the brain.

In 1936, Stock discovered this phenomenon during experiments he conducted on himself. After inhaling through his *nose* a few breaths containing about 25 micrograms of mercury, Stock soon experienced dizziness, headache, and an inflammation of the mucous membranes of the nose. It took several days for his symptoms to disappear. Some weeks later Stock repeated his self-experiment, but this time he inhaled the mercury vapor through his mouth. To his astonishment Stock found that by breathing through his *mouth* he could inhale ten times the mercury vapor (approximately 250 micrograms of mercury) without getting any of the symptoms of mercury intoxication that he had gotten when he had inhaled the mercury vapor through his nose.(16,44,45) Dr. Patrick Störtebecker clarified the pathways associated with this phenomenon through his "Principle of the Shortest Pathway," showing how mercury from the oral cavity could enter the brain through the trigeminal nerve and oronasal pathways, thus bypassing the blood brain barrier.(16,46,47)

The preceding studies utilized exhaled air to measure breath mercury vapor levels. Did this actually relate to intra-oral (within the oral cavity) mercury vapor levels and the amount of mercury actually being inhaled? Answers to these questions were provided by researchers in Calgary, Canada, in 1985. Doctors M.J. Vimy and F.L. Lorscheider set out to determine the magnitude of the problem. Forty-six subjects were involved in this project; thirty-five had mercury amalgam fillings and eleven had no amalgam fillings. In the group with mercury amalgam fillings, all of the fillings were over one year old. To ensure that they were getting accurate data, the study testing protocol required that the test subjects could not eat, drink, smoke, chew, or place anything intra-orally for one hour prior to testing. (5)

Readings were taken prior to stimulation. Subjects were then given sugarless gum to chew continuously for a ten-minute period, at the end of which a second intra-oral mercury reading was taken. To eliminate any bias concerning exhaled air, the subjects were required to breathe through their nose while the intra-oral mercury reading was being taken. The people with mercury amalgam fillings had unstimulated mercury vapor readings that were nine times greater than the base levels in control subjects with no amalgam fillings. Chewing stimulation in subjects with amalgam fillings increased their intra-oral mercury levels six-fold over their unstimulated mercury levels. This represented a fifty-

four-fold increase over levels observed in the control subjects without amalgam fillings. The researchers also determined that there was a significant correlation between the
mercury vapor released into intra-oral air after chewing
stimulation and the numbers and types of amalgam fillings
present in the person's mouth.

In a follow-up study using the same test subjects, Vimy
and Lorscheider set out to determine if it was possible to estimate the daily dose of mercury vapor that would be attributable to a person's mercury amalgam dental fillings. To
simulate the normal pattern of eating, test subjects chewed
sugarless gum for thirty minutes. During this time, intra-oral
mercury vapor readings were taken every five minutes. At
the end of thirty minutes, the gum was removed and readings were again taken every five minutes for an additional
thirty minutes. In all, thirteen separate mercury vapor readings were taken in series on each subject. (6)

By plotting their data and applying statistical analysis,
Vimy and Lorscheider were able to determine that the increased release of mercury vapor from amalgam fillings continued for approximately ninety minutes after chewing had
stopped. In effect, during the time a person with mercury
amalgam dental fillings would be eating a meal, they would
have elevated intra-oral mercury vapor levels. This elevated
intra-oral level of mercury vapor would decline slowly during
the next ninety minutes after chewing had stopped. These
researchers also found that subjects with twelve or more
occlusal amalgam surfaces (an occlusal amalgam filling is
on the chewing surface of the tooth) were receiving an estimated daily dose of 29 micrograms of mercury. These mercury dosages from mercury amalgam dental fillings were as
much as eighteen-fold the allowable daily limits established
by some countries for mercury exposure from all sources in
the environment. The U.S. Environmental Protection Agen-

cy (EPA) allows 30 micrograms per day of intake of all forms of mercury from all sources for the 154-pound person, and 20 micrograms per day of all forms of mercury from all sources other than food.(18) Vimy and Lorscheider concluded that mercury from dental amalgam fillings makes a major contribution to the total daily dose of mercury a person receives.(6) In a recent study done in Sweden, researchers found that an increased release of mercury vapor from mercury amalgam dental fillings could be accomplished by drinking hot fluids.(48)

At the August 1987 Scandinavian Occupational Hygiene Meeting held in Iceland, Ingvar Skare of Sweden's National Board of Occupational Safety and Health presented data from that organization's study of mercury exposure from amalgam. Currently, the Board is discussing a reduction of the maximum allowable concentration (MAC) of mercury vapor in air and is also exploring the introduction of biological threshold levels. To do this the Board is evaluating background levels of mercury in air and biological material that could be caused by factors other than occupational exposure.

Some of their initial findings are very significant. They have observed that amalgam carriers often have mercury levels in their exhaled air that are above the occupational MAC levels, and that during chewing, the release of mercury vapor increases 3-4 times. Further, preliminary results have shown that the nonstimulated base level emission of mercury vapor from amalgam can be the equivalent of 500 micrograms per week, which would exceed the WHO maximum allowable weekly intake levels in food.

The presentation conclusion was that "The emission of mercury vapor from amalgam is not insignificant and must be considered during evaluations of occupational exposures, especially if the permissible levels will be reduced. The fact that amalgam emission has so far been neglected might partly explain why correlations between air measurements and measurements of biological samples have been weaker for the lower ranges of external exposures. Amalgam exposure is very likely the largest source of non-occupationally exposed persons' "normal values"--extreme consumers of fish from inland lakes excluded."(7)

What all of these researchers have done is establish irrefutable scientific evidence that mercury vapor is released from mercury amalgam dental fillings, especially when they are stimulated by chewing, brushing, hot fluids, and so on. Is this an important point? Based on the scientific evidence, we say it is extremely important. However, the ADA does not consider the amount of mercury vapor released by amalgam dental fillings to be of sufficient magnitude to cause any health problems, unless of course you happen to be hypersensitive (allergic) to mercury. They have taken this position even though the U.S. Environmental Protection Agency, World Health Organization, and world experts in mercury toxicology have stated that they have been unable to define a harmless level for mercury vapor exposure.

Furthermore, the ADA has stated categorically that no credible scientific evidence exists to show that mercury in amalgam used in nonallergic patients is related to the cause or effect of any specific disease or malady. They have taken this position even though they are aware of the fact that thousands of people who have had their mercury amalgam fillings replaced with nonmercury fillings have experienced remarkable improvements or total cures of health problems existent for years. They and the medical community can ignore such information because it is anecdotal, merely stories of patients claiming to have been cured by having their fillings replaced, without having all the data recorded and evaluated scientifically.

We, as well as other anti-amalgam individuals, dentists, physicians, and scientists all over the world, are greatly troubled by the above statements. On the surface, they sound very official and convincing. However, when one examines them closely they take on more of the character of a cleverly contrived ploy, a "red herring" if you will, designed to cloud the real issue and facts. The truth of the matter is that there is a disease that can be caused by exposure to mercury vapor. It is called mercury poisoning. That is the real issue and that is what the ADA should be investigating. There is absolutely no difference between the elemental mercury vapor released from mercury amalgam dental fillings and the elemental mercury vapor inhaled by employees working in factories that use elemental mercury in their manufacturing processes. Nowhere in toxicology, emergency medicine, or diagnostic textbooks are the physicians told that elemental mercury vapor is the cause of any disease. What they do tell the physician is that the primary way to diagnose mercury poisoning is by the signs and symptoms displayed or voiced by the patient and determining the degree and form of mercury the patient was exposed to. They then go on to list all the various signs and symptoms that can be caused by mercury. In fact, the emergency medicine textbooks state that if a patient displays the signs or symptoms of mercury intoxication, they should be hospitalized and treated for mercury poisoning. If after treatment the signs and symptoms previously displayed by the patient have ameliorated or disappeared, the disease the physician treated would be listed on the patient's chart as "mercury poisoning."

Unfortunately, at this time at least, the medical profession is not aware of the scientific research demonstrating the significant release of mercury vapor from mercury amalgam dental fillings and therefore does not consider it as a source and/or cause of mercury poisoning. This leaves the task of recognizing it up to you. Only you can make the decision as to the significance and importance of the phenomenon to your health and to that of your children. Scientific research has demonstrated that mercury, even in small amounts, can damage the brain, heart, lungs, liver, kidneys, thyroid gland, pituitary gland, adrenal glands, blood cells, enzymes and hormones, and also suppresses the body's immune (defense) system. In addition, mercury has been shown to pass the blood brain barrier and placental membrane, and cause permanent damage to the brain of a developing baby. To give you a better understanding of the insidious nature of mercury poisoning, let's look at the symptoms of mercury toxicity contained in the medical literature and textbooks and summarized in Tables 4-1 and 4-2.

TABLE 4-1 SIGNS AND SYMPTOMS OF ELEMENTAL MERCURY VAPOR EXPOSURE

1. PSYCHOLOGICAL DISTURBANCES (ERETHISM)

Irritability
Nervousness
Shyness or timidity
Lack of attention
Loss of self-confidence
Decline of intellect
Lack of self control
Fits of anger
Depression
Anxiety

Drowsiness
Insomnia
Agony
Confusion

2. ORAL CAVITY DISORDERS

Bleeding gums
Alveolar bone loss
Loosening of teeth
Excessive salivation
Foul breath
Metallic taste
Leukoplakia (white patches)
Stomatitis (inflammation of the gums)
Ulceration of gingiva, palate, tongue
Burning sensation in mouth or throat
Tissue pigmentation

3. GASTROINTESTINAL EFFECTS

Abdominal cramps
Gastrointestinal problems, colitis
Diarrhea

4. SYSTEMIC EFFECTS

CARDIOVASCULAR
Irregular heartbeat (tachycardia, bradycardia)
Feeble and irregular pulse
Alterations in blood pressure
Pain or pressure in chest

NEUROLOGIC
Chronic or frequent headaches
Dizziness
Ringing or noises in ears
Fine tremors (hands, feet, lips, eyelids, tongue)
Shaky handwriting

RESPIRATORY
Persistent cough
Emphysema
Shallow and irregular respiration

IMMUNOLOGICAL
Allergies
Asthma
Rhinitis
Sinusitis
Lymphadenopathy, especially cervical

ENDOCRINE
Subnormal temperature
Cold, clammy skin, especially hands and feet
Excessive perspiration
Pale skin or uncontrolled blushing

OCULAR
Optic neuritis
Mercurialentis (colored reflex, lens of the eye)
Constricted visual fields

OTHER
Muscle weakness
Fatigue
Anemia
Hypoxia

Edema
Loss of appetite (anorexia)
Loss of weight
Joint pains
Irregular menstruation
Miscarriage
Hesitant, stuttering speech

5. SEVERE CASES

Hallucinations
Manic-depression

****

TABLE 4-2
SYMPTOMS OF ORGANIC MERCURY EXPOSURE

1. EARLIEST SYMPTOMS

Fatigue
Headache
Forgetfulness
Inability to concentrate
Apathy
Depression
Outbursts of anger
Decline in intellect

2. LATER FINDINGS

Numbness and tingling of hands, feet, lips
Muscle weakness progressing to paralysis
Dim or restricted vision

Hearing difficulty
Speech disorders
Loss of memory
Incoordination
Emotional instability
Dermatitis
Renal damage
General CNS dysfunctions

Symptoms for Tables 4-1 and 4-2 were extracted from the following references:
--Goodman and Gilman's The Pharmacological Basis of Therapeutics (6th ed). Macmillan Publishing Co.,Inc. NY, 1980.
--National Institute for Occupational Health and Safety (NIOSH). Occupational Exposure to Mercury: A Criteria for a Recommended Standard, 1973
--Oettingen, W.F.von. Poisoning A Guide to Clinical Diagnosis and Treatment. W.B. Saunders Co., Philadelphia 1958.
--Casarett and Doull's Toxicology, The Science of Poisons (3rd ed). Macmillan Publishing Co., Inc., NY, 1986.
--Report of an international committee: Maximum allowable concentrations of mercury compounds.(MAC Values). Arch Environ Health. 19:891-905, 1969.
--Environmental Health Criteria 1, Mercury. WHO, Geneva, 1976.

****

All the symptoms listed in Tables 4-1 and 4-2 were derived from evaluating people who had suffered from industrial exposure or ecological exposure to mercury. The study of micromercurialism (low level mercury exposure) has been very limited in scientific literature. However, there is sufficient evidence to suggest that continual exposure to small doses of mercury over long periods of time can produce most of the same signs and symptoms. After all, the same biochemical pathways in the human physiology that, when affected by larger doses of mercury result in clinically observable symptoms, are also affected by low, continuous mercury exposure regardless of the source.

Mercury is so toxic to the human organism that there can be cell death or irreversible chemical damage long before the appearance of clinically observable symptoms indicating that something is wrong. Further, you could be experiencing some of the symptoms of the mercury released from mercury amalgam dental fillings, but since the mercury exposure is so gradual and because the time between placement of the fillings and the onset of the symptoms can vary so dramatically (from days to years, based on your own biochemical makeup and sensitivity), it may not be readily apparent or identifiable as being associated with dental mercury. Under these conditions your physician would have extreme difficulty in relating subclinical symptoms (not readily apparent or identifiable as being associated with a particular disease or health problem) to mercury toxicity.(49,50)

ENVIRONMENTAL LEAD

Lead exposure has been so extensively studied and publicized over the years that most people are aware of the fact that it is a health hazard, especially to children. Because of the addition of tetraethyl lead to our fuels, lead is in the air, water, soil, and, consequently, in our food chain. The exposure to lead from automobile exhaust fumes has decreased substantially over the years, due to the introduction of unleaded fuels and the government requirement that all automobile manufacturers produce cars utilizing only unleaded fuels.

Still, we inhale about 40 micrograms of lead daily. Scientists estimate that about 15 micrograms are retained and absorbed by the lungs. Daily dietary intake can vary dramatically, but it is estimated that an additional 25 micrograms is the average amount absorbed in the gastrointestinal tract. After absorption, inorganic lead is deposited in the kidneys, bone, teeth, and hair, with small quantities accumulating in the grey matter of the brain. Because of the high dietary intake of meat and soft drinks, most people also have a high dietary phosphate intake, which seems to cause lead to be deposited in bone. As a result, 95% of the total body burden of lead is concentrated in the bones.(22) The signs and symptoms of chronic lead poisoning are similar in many ways to those of chronic mercury poisoning as shown in Table 4-1.

Table 4-3   SYMPTOMS OF LEAD EXPOSURE

1. PSYCHOLOGICAL DISTURBANCES

Irritability
Restlessness
Hyperkinesia
Agressive behavior
Insomnia

2. ORAL CAVITY EFFECTS

Metallic taste
Lead line on the gingival margin

3. GASTROINTESTINAL EFFECTS

Constipation
Diarrhea occasionally
Intestinal spasm with abdominal pain (lead colic)
Vomiting

4. SYSTEMIC EFFECTS

NEUROLOGIC
Headache
Palsy
Vertigo
Ataxia
Falling
Mental deterioration
Cerebral involvement
Subtle CNS involvement
Loss of sensory perception

BLOOD
Microcytic hypochromic anemia
Decreased synthesis of heme

OCULAR
Visual disturbances
Retinal stippling

OTHER
Inhibition of sulfhydryl enzymes
Renal injury
Malaise
Fatigue
Weakness
Ashen color of face
Pallor of the lips
Premature aging

Outside of adult exposure in the work place--primarily lead smelters and storage-battery factories--medical concern is generally directed toward children, who appear to be more vulnerable. Children are exposed chronically to low levels of lead through their diets, in the air they breathe, the dirt and dust of play areas, and in the water they drink. Because of this chronic exposure and new research on the effects of this kind of exposure, permissible lead-blood levels have been revised downward several times. In fact, science at this point is not exactly sure what level of lead in the blood constitutes a health hazard.

In this same vein, a recent report indicated that nearly 40 million Americans could be getting excessive amounts of lead in their drinking water. As a result, the EPA is reducing acceptable levels in drinking water from about 50 parts per billion to 20 parts per billion by June 1988. (51)

Scientific research is emerging showing the toxic effects to be greater when both lead and mercury are present in the body at the same time. There is no escaping the presence of both metals in our bodies because both are present in the air we breath, the food we eat, and the water we drink. A major variable exists, however. Those individuals who have mercury amalgam dental fillings will have a greater exposure to mercury vapor than those people without this poison in their mouths. Therefore, those individuals with mercury amalgam dental fillings could be at greater risk to the combined effects of mercury and lead.

5

THE BLOOD-BRAIN BARRIER

In Chapters 1 and 4 we briefly discussed some of the studies showing that mercury enters the brain, and that there is scientific evidence showing a positive correlation between numbers and surfaces of amalgam fillings and mercury brain content. Consequently, we feel it is important for the reader to have some appreciation of the normal mechanism that is supposed to restrict the entry of substances into the brain.

The transfer of substances such as nutrients, waste products, oxygen and carbon dioxide, hormones, and poisons in and out of the cells of the body is accomplished through the smallest of blood vessels, the capillaries. Since the cells of the brain are so vital and cannot be replaced, the capillaries of the brain have a special structural design to provide extra protection for the critical brain cells. Unlike capillaries elsewhere in the body, the cells lining the brain capillaries are overlapped and less porous. This special structural design is called *the blood-brain barrier*. It prevents many substances from passing into or out of the brain that would easily pass to and from other body cells.(52)

Substances that can dissolve in fats (lipids) readily penetrate the membranes of cells, as these membranes have large amounts of fat-containing molecules. Elemental mercury vapor and methylmercury are fat soluble substances and therefore easily penetrate cell membranes, including those of the placenta and the blood-brain barrier. Water soluble substances, especially those of large molecular size, do not readily penetrate the blood-brain barrier. This barrier does, however, selectively allow passage of certain smaller water soluble substances necessary to the brain, such as glucose and essential amino acids.(53)

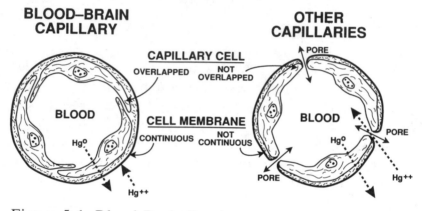

Figure 5-1: Blood-Brain Barrier.
Cell membranes are made of fat molecules. Mercury vapor and methylmercury are fat soluble, and thus penetrate through all capillary cells, including those of the blood-brain barrier. Once inside the brain tissues the mercury is oxidized to ionic form, is no longer fat soluble, and is therefore hard to remove.

The blood-brain barrier is of special significance to the issue of mercury released from amalgam dental fillings. The mercury released from these fillings is primarily in the form of elemental mercury vapor, which readily and thoroughly enters the body via inhalation and passes rapidly into the blood.(22) In 1966, Berlin and associates (54) exposed mice to equal amounts of radioactive mercury vapor and intravenously injected radioactive inorganic mercury salt. The amount of mercury in the animals was measured by whole-body scintillation counting for a period of up to thirty two days after exposure. The animals were sacrificed at different times after exposure and the distribution of mercury in the bodies was studied by whole-body section, autoradiography, and organ assay. The authors found that the mercury-vapor-exposed animals had ten times more mercury in their brains than those animals injected with inorganic mercury salt. This study clearly demonstrated that, although inorganic mercury will penetrate the blood-brain barrier, mercury vapor will enter the brain far more readily. This has been explained by the fact that mercury vapor has no electrical charge (is non-ionic) and is fat soluble. This ease of entering the body and its fat soluble cells account for the extremely potent toxicity of mercury in its elemental vapor form. The rapid and easy penetration of the blood-brain barrier by mercury vapor has been confirmed by a number of other investigators, including Magos (55) and Cutright and associates (56). Passage into the fetal brain has also been shown by Magos (57) and Clarkson (58).

More than fifty years ago the discovery was made by Professor Alfred Stock that mercury vapor released from mercury amalgam dental fillings could enter the brain via a route that completely bypassed the blood-brain barrier.(44,59) In Sweden, Dr. Patrick Stortebecker, a neurologist, has done concentrated studies from 1954 to 1982 on the various pathways in which toxins move from the oral nasal cavity directly to the brain. Dr. Stortebecker considers this distribution route for mercury vapor released by mercury amalgam dental fillings to be the most dangerous and damaging.(16)

Once mercury vapor has entered the body and/or body cells it becomes oxidized to the ionic form of mercury (containing an electrical charge). The oxidation of mercury vapor occurs in the blood and in the body cells. Ionic mercury is the harmful form of mercury because it is now chemically active and can readily combine with body substances, exerting its toxic influence in that manner.(60)

In 1977, Gerstner and Huff (61) pointed out that elemental mercury vapor, after entering the blood stream, is oxidized through the mercurous into the mercuric ion. They stated: "Completion of these reactions requires several minutes; because of this delay, elemental mercury exists in the blood for a sufficiently long time to reach all tissues and organs. This fact has serious consequences. In its elemental form, mercury easily penetrates the blood-brain barrier and infiltrates nerve cells, where final oxidation proceeds. Such an ease of penetration-- which is well documented for the blood-brain barrier--also applies presumably to the placental barrier, as indicated by a few observations during human pregnancies. By overcoming the two critical barriers, elemental mercury is particularly dangerous during long-term or chronic exposures, representing a potentially serious hazard in many occupations." One is compelled to wonder what Gerstner and Huff would say if they were aware of the chronic exposure to mercury vapor from dental amalgam fillings, especially regarding women of childbearing age.

Once mercury has penetrated the blood-brain barrier its oxidation to the ionic form is completed. This ionic mercury now has an electrical charge and is no longer fat soluble. Ionic mercury is very active chemically and readily combines with body substances, thereby exerting its toxic effect. Moreover, this ionic mercury can no longer easily penetrate the blood-brain barrier and is very resistant to removal from the brain. Studies by Sugita (8) and Bernard and Purdue (10) have clearly shown that mercury is retained in brain tissue for extremely long periods of time. In addition, autopsy studies by Schiele et al. (62) and Friberg and associates (63) have demonstrated a definite correlation between levels of mercury found in the brain and the number and surfaces of dental amalgam fillings present. There is absolutely no doubt that mercury from dental amalgam fillings ends up in the brains of patients.

It is clear that inhalation of mercury vapor results in transient blood levels of elemental mercury vapor, some of which is being oxidized in the blood but most of which is passing rapidly into body cells, including those of the brain. Moreover, some of the mercury released from dental amalgam fillings is mixed with saliva and food, being swallowed, and enters the body as ionic mercury. Ionic mercury has also been traced directly from the fillings into the body through the tooth structure and soft tissues of the mouth. Therefore, some of the dental amalgam mercury has been found within the blood in ionic form. The effect of this ionic mercury on the blood-brain barrier is also vitally important.

Steinwall (64) investigated the toxic effects of mercury and other materials on the blood-brain barrier in 1977. He stated that "certain heavy metals, and particularly mercuric ions, are highly injurious to the barrier. Organic mercurials, e.g., methyl mercury ions, showed comparable damaging potency." He found that extremely small amounts of mercury ions damaged the blood-brain barrier, much smaller amounts than were required for the other materials known to damage the barrier.

In 1977, Chang reviewed the scientific knowledge of the neurotoxic effects of mercury. Chang stated: "Mercury was found to penetrate and damage the blood-brain barrier very rapidly, leading to a dysfunction of the blood-brain barrier system." Chang pointed out that the research of himself and co-workers "demonstrated that when mercury ions are absorbed into the bloodstream, though of minute amounts (less than 1.0 part per million), they are capable of impairing the blood-brain system within hours, leading to an extravasation of normally barred plasma solutes."(49) This means that even very small amounts of mercury ions will rapidly damage the blood-brain barrier, allowing passage into the brain of harmful substances from the blood that otherwise would be denied entry. In other words, mercury will not only damage the brain but it will also increase exposure of the brain to other harmful substances in the blood. Considering the variety of environmental pollutants contemporary society is exposed to, the importance of this influence could be of great significance. Chang also went on to state:

The blood-brain barrier acts by no means merely as a physical barrier. It acts also as an active site for the regulation of the uptake of biological metabolites from blood to the nervous system. It is conceivable, therefore, that the impairment of the blood-brain barrier, together with the possible inhibition of certain associated enzymes by the mercury, is probably responsible for the great reduction of the uptake of amino acids and other metabolites by the nervous system after mercury administration.(49)

Amino acids are the building blocks of proteins which, of course, are the materials used to construct the cells of the body, as well as enzymes and hormones. In the human brain, there is no scientific evidence that brain cells can be regenerated. This is why mercury damage to the brain is permanent and irreversible.

In a 1984 study, Khayat and Dencker also demonstrated the accumulation of inhaled mercury vapor in the whole respiratory tract (nasal mucosa, trachea, and bronchi), as well as the brain.(65) The same authors, in an earlier 1983 study, had also demonstrated the accumulation of inhaled mercury vapor in the cerebral spinal fluid and the spinal ganglia.(66)

The developing fetus gets its blood supply from the mother. Since mercury vapor readily traverses the placental membrane, the oxidation of mercury vapor in the fetal blood or at the fetal blood-brain barrier itself no doubt results in damage to the fetal blood-brain barrier. The unoxidized elemental mercury entering the fetal brain tissue may be one source of harm, but the damage to the fetal blood-brain barrier may be even more important, preventing the uptake of vital amino acids for the construction of the irreplaceable brain cells.

Considerable scientific attention has been devoted to the prenatal effects of exposure to organic mercury (primarily methylmercury) in pregnant women. A number of studies have described the effects on infants of prenatal exposure to methylmercury while the exposed pregnant mothers exhibited little or no observable signs or symptoms from exposure. The neurological effects on these infants were as severe as cerebral palsy and even death, but less easily recognizable symptoms were more common. For example, Amin-Zaki and associates (67) studied thirty-two infants exposed prenatally to methylmercury in the Iraq epidemic. Ten of the infants had cerebral palsy. Nine of the infants died within three years, representing a mortality rate of 28% compared to the rate of 6% in the control group. Of the twenty-three surviving infants, 52% had delayed mental development, 78% had delayed speech development, and 70% had delayed motor development. Other studies have demonstrated learning deficits in infants exposed to methylmercury while in utero.

There is absolutely no doubt that exposure to methylmercury in pregnant women presents a serious threat to the fetus. The only question is how relevant this information is to the effects of exposure to elemental mercury vapor for the unborn child. In 1969, the International Committee for MAC Values for Mercury Compounds (68) reported that studies in animals and humans indicate that methylmercury easily penetrates to the fetus via the placenta. Ware and associates, in 1974, demonstrated that methylmercury damaged the blood-brain barrier within 4-6 hours after administration, and that the blood-brain barrier dysfunction was caused by mercury ions.(69) Friberg and Vostal (60) have stated that "studies involving human fetuses have revealed that elemental mercury passes the placental barrier easier than the other forms of mercury, and can be detected in stillborn babies of mothers treated with injections of mercury."

The World Health Organization, in their comprehensive reports on mercury stated: "The most hazardous forms of mercury to human health are elemental mercury vapor and the short-chain alkylmercurials (70)," and, "The primary biochemical lesions associated with mercury poisoning have not been established. Virtually nothing is known of the biochemical disturbances associated with exposure to metallic mercury vapor."(71)

The information that we have presented obviously indicates that exposure to elemental mercury vapor poses no less of a threat to the unborn child than does exposure to methylmercury. In spite of the wealth of information strongly demonstrating the potential risk of elemental mercury vapor to the unborn child, the scientific community has not yet seen fit to responsibly investigate this awesome question.

A few feeble attempts have been made to look at the relation of mercury vapor exposure to "birth defects" that were readily noticeable at birth. The absence of evidence showing that prenatal exposure to mercury vapor causes an increase in visible birth defects in no way proves that exposure is harmless to the unborn child. The major influence of mercury vapor on the fetus is not the promotion of birth defects, but rather the toxic effect on the body cells, particularly those of the brain

It has been scientifically established that prenatal exposure to mercury will result in learning defects, as well as delayed development in speech and muscular function. It has also been established that mercury will damage the blood-brain barrier, resulting in a decrease in the substances needed to build the vital, irreplaceable brain cells. These are the areas that should be investigated by the scientific and professional communities. To continue to ignore these potentials is nothing less than irresponsible, for they have a profound influence on the quality of life of our children.

6

THE PLACENTA

During pregnancy the placenta joins mother and offspring, providing endocrine secretion and selective exchange of soluble blood-borne substances. The placenta is connected to the umbilical cord, through which the developing fetus gets nourishment and discharges waste products and carbon dioxide. The placenta also produces hormones that regulate the course of the pregnancy. Few mammalian tissues change as dramatically as the placenta during its short life span.(52,72) Moreover, the placenta is fetal tissue and most of the factors that affect fetal growth also affect placental growth.(73)

The circulatory systems of the mother and fetus are separated by a very thin membrane in the placenta. The purpose of this membrane is to ensure that there is no actual mixing of maternal blood with the fetal blood. This placental membrane was formerly called the placental barrier. Its function was assumed to be one of protecting the fetus from possible damage from any of the potentially toxic drugs or substances that might be present in the mother's blood. The Thalidomide disaster in 1961 demonstrated that the passage of toxic substances from mother to fetus did occur and could result in tragic birth defects and deformities. As a result, there emerged a new science and discipline within the scientific and medical communities devoted to investigating xenobiotic substances (a chemical foreign to the biological system). Primary concern at this time is focused on the effects of often-prescribed pharmaceuticals and the basic question of whether they can be safely administered during pregnancy. Although there are many xenobiotics that can affect birth weight and size of the child as well as nutritional and environmental factors, there is also scientific data from both human and animal studies showing mercury can affect birth weight and size. Based on these facts and the study that follows, the possible effect of mercury from dental amalgam on birth weight should be a subject of some priority for investigation. It is certainly a subject that bears intense scrutiny in women of child bearing age who have 12 or more occlusally involved mercury amalgam dental fillings.

Recently, Naeye (1987) published a study titled "Do Placental Weights Have Clinical Significance?" Based on the standardized evaluation of 38,351 placentas, Dr. Naeye developed the following relationships: "Findings of the present study show that placental weight can have clinical significance. Relatively low weights were associated with high hemoglobin levels in neonates and lower-that-expected body size at 7 years of age, whereas overweight placentas were associated with consequences of acute antenatal hypoxia, including neonatal death and long-term neurologic abnormalities." Interestingly, the report also found that approximately one-third of the children who had neonatal neurologic abnormalities still had them at seven years of age.(73)

Another very interesting aspect of the study was the conclusion that for those women who smoked during pregnancy, the placentas were normal sized. However, Dr. Naeye felt that the reason for this was that the placenta compensates for the smoking-induced fetal hypoxia (lack of oxygen) by increasing its size, as long as the hypoxia was not accompanied by a deficiency of nutrients as occurs with sustained, low uteroplacental blood flow. Three aspects of that conclusion are considered of great importance in regard to mercury: (1) Mercury reduces the blood's ability to carry oxygen and, although fetal blood flow might be normal, the reduced oxygen content of the blood would parallel the hypoxic condition. (2) As brought out in Chapter 11 of this book, mercury has the ability to affect the balance or status of most of the body's essential nutrients. (3) To our knowledge, no scientific study has ever addressed the relationship between chronic mercury exposure and placental weight/birth weight.

There appears to be an ever-increasing number of children born with either mental or physical impairment, or both. From the time of fertilization until birth, the offspring is dependent upon maternal sources for all nutrition. There are four major areas that are considered to be critical or determinants in the outcome of fetal development: (1) the mother's nutritional status; (2) the structural and functional quality of the placenta; (3) the genetic makeup of the offspring; and (4) the presence of physical, chemical, or mechanical insults to mother and child during pregnancy.(52) When one considers the toxicity of mercury and the potential it possesses to disrupt normal biochemical functions, it is quite apparent that mercury could also affect or have an impact on the satisfactory outcome of fetal development in all four of the aforementioned factors or areas of concern.

As a preface to the discussion of the scientific data, we would like to quote from a scientific study by Goodman et al. published in 1983: "The mechanisms of action of mercury and cadmium-induced fetotoxicity--whether directly on the differentiating embryonic tissue, indirectly through action on the maternal and placental tissues, or a combination of both--remain to be elucidated. A possible contributory factor in cadmium and mercury fetotoxicity may be an effect on the transmembrane transport of nutrients, such as amino acids, across the placenta to the fetus. An inhibition of nutrient transport may cause fetal death, congenital malformations, or growth retardation."(74)

While the authors state very little is known about how cadmium and mercury cause damage to the fetus, they are suggesting that the toxic effects may be occurring in the placenta where the presence of these metals might be preventing the passage of required nutrients to the embryo/fetus.

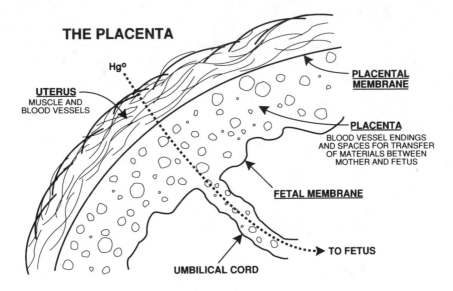

THE PLACENTA

Hg⁰

PLACENTAL
MEMBRANE

UTERUS
MUSCLE AND
BLOOD VESSELS

PLACENTA
BLOOD VESSEL ENDINGS
AND SPACES FOR TRANSFER
OF MATERIALS BETWEEN
MOTHER AND FETUS

FETAL MEMBRANE

TO FETUS

UMBILICAL CORD

Fgure 6-1: The placental membrane will stop many substances. However, it is made of fat molecules, mercury vapor and methylmercury, being fat soluble will penetrate the membrane.

The thoughts expressed by Goodman et al. were confirmed in a 1984 study by Danielsson et al. when they investigated the effect of placental mercury and cadmium on fetal mouse uptake of four nutrients. Their findings, after maternal administration of labeled (radioactive) nutrients, were: mercury caused a dose-dependent decrease in fetal uptake of vitamin B_{12} within four hours; cadmium caused a greater decrease of B_{12} uptake; mercury caused a greater decrease in fetal uptake of a-aminobutyric acid than did cadmium; both elements caused a decrease in fetal uptake of zinc; and the fetal uptake of deoxyglucose was largely unaffected. The authors concluded that although cadmium may cause fetotoxicity mediated mainly through the placenta, mercury probably causes more direct damage to the fetus.(75)

Some of the evaluations made by Danielsson et al. regarding the various causes involved in the decreased fetal uptakes were very significant.For example, their finding that zinc in high doses could prevent the inhibiting effect of placental mercury on fetal uptake of vitamin B_{12}, as well as their feeling that the general depression of mouse fetal growth caused by a direct effect of mercury on the fetal tissues could be related to lower demands in the fetus for placental transport of nutrients.(75)

The lack of knowledge concerning the mechanisms of mercury toxicity as they relate to the human reproductive cycle brought up by Dr. Goodman and his associates is compounded further by the scarcity of scientific studies investigating the effects of mercury vapor. The majority of scientific studies on mercury have dealt with methylmercury or inorganic mercury. Another very disturbing aspect concerning existing research is that very little attention has been paid to the threat posed by low-level chronic exposures to toxic metals. A great deal of the available scientific data was derived from acute exposures where a large single injection of the toxic metal being investigated was administered and the results examined. Be that as it may, it is important that as much scientific data as is available be brought to the readers attention, regardless of the form of mercury or the testing protocol used. The fact is that mercury is mercury once it reaches the body's cells, and mercury vapor enters the body and its cells far more readily than most other forms of mercury.

In 1974, Baglan and his colleagues (76) investigated whether the human placenta could be used as a possible indicator of environmental exposure to various trace elements. The researchers measured eight trace elements--including mercury, lead, and cadmium--in the placenta (over 1,000 placenta samples were utilized), maternal blood, and fetal blood. The trace element levels for the various tissues were then correlated against one another. For four of the elements (mercury, selenium, rubidium, and cobalt), the concentrations in the placenta correlated against the levels in maternal and fetal blood. The authors concluded that a determination of the elemental levels in the placenta would therefore reflect the elemental concentrations in the mother and the infant.

In the case of mercury alone, similar results pertaining to the placenta and the infant had been published in 1973 by Mansour et al.(77) These researchers found that the placental transfer of mercury varied with the chemical form of mercury; that is, methylmercury was more readily transferable than mercuric nitrate. Another important conclusion reached was that the mercury concentrations in the placenta and the infant's hair are directly related to the infant's body burden of mercury.

What about the presence of several different metals in the placenta? Does the combination result in different effects in the placenta and the offspring when compared to the effects of exposure to a single metal? Can certain combinations of metals reduce or increase the toxicity normally associated with a single particular metal? What quantities of toxic metals have to be accumulated in the placenta before there is an adverse effect on the embryo or fetus? As you can see, there is an endless list of questions that need to be answered. Scientists are beginning to provide some data, but when it comes to mercury vapor, there are gigantic gaps in present knowledge.

Karp and Robertson (1977) published a study in which they investigated whether the trace elements found in the placenta could alter placental enzyme activities. Moreover, the researchers wanted to see if there was a difference between different geographical locations. Fifty-eight placentas were collected from hospitals in Charlotte, North Carolina, Birmingham Alabama, and Augusta, Georgia, and tested for different enzyme activity and metal content. One of the findings was that the enzyme isocitric dehydrogenase (ICD) was depressed by mercury, but there was a variance between the different cities. The researchers felt that they had found significant correlations among trace metal levels and placental activities of three enzymes and felt that this suggested that there was an effect of the metals on enzyme activity.(78) Isocitric dehydrogenase is involved in one of the energy producing functions called the citric acid cycle.

Five hundred and three pregnant women participated in a 1975-1976 study done in Belgium by Lauwerys et al.(79) The purpose of the study was to evaluate the extent of exposure to heavy metals (lead, mercury, cadmium) during fetal life. The women ranged in age from 16 to 43 with a median of 26 years. An interesting observation of this study was that all three metals are transferred from the mother to the fetus, but the barrier role of the placenta was different for the three metals. They found that while there was no barrier preventing the transfer of mercury, there was a slight barrier to the transfer of lead, and that the greatest barrier was to the transfer of cadmium. With regard to mercury, the researchers found a significant correlation between maternal mercury-blood levels and mercury-blood levels in the newborn infant. It is unfortunate indeed that Lauwerys and his associates did not take into consideration whether the study participants had amalgam fillings, as elemental mercury vapor readily passes the placental membrane.

Orlando et al. (1978) published the results of investigations into the concentrations of trace metals in twenty-eight term placentas in Italy. The researchers found that cadmium and chrome concentrations were higher than those reflected in the literature, and they felt that the mercury and lead concentrations were indicative of an appreciable exposure to these trace elements. The report also reflected some rather interesting findings concerning other relationships: (1) a moderate positive correlation between zinc and lead; (2) no significant difference of cadmium concentrations between smokers and nonsmokers; (3) no significant difference between lead concentrations and residential district; (4) and no relationship between mercury and fish product consumption.(80) Here again, it is truly unfortunate that the researchers did not take into consideration the relationships between subjects with amalgams and those without amalgams. It would have been extremely interesting in view of their findings that there was no relationship between mercury content and fish consumption.

In one of the few animal studies, Greenwood et al. (1972) used rats to investigate the transfer of metallic mercury vapor (the same kind released by mercury amalgam fillings) from mother to fetus. Two groups of animals were used. One group inhaled radioactive metallic mercury vapor and the other group was given radioactive mercuric chloride by injection. The animals were sacrificed 2-1/2 minutes after exposure. In the animals injected with ionized mercuric chloride, the amount of mercury in the blood was twenty-five times greater than in the animals that inhaled metallic mercury vapor. The researchers assumed this vast difference in blood levels to be related to the fact that metallic mercury vapor rapidly diffuses from the blood into tissues (remember, metallic mercury vapor has no electrical charge and can therefore penetrate tissues with ease).(81)

Of much greater significance, Greenwood and his associates found that despite the great difference in blood levels, the amount of mercury actually passing through the placenta and being taken up by the fetus was about the same. They also found that in the animals that had inhaled metallic mercury vapor, nearly 50% of the mercury taken up by the placenta passed through the placenta into the fetus compared with a 1% pass-through in the group that had been injected with inorganic mercury. The researchers concluded: "These results indicate a potential for damage to the fetus in situations of exposure to mercury vapor."(81)

As stated previously, the placenta will trap or accumulate more inorganic mercury than organic mercury. In rats and mice, as much as seventy-five times more radioactive inorganic mercury per unit weight is found in placentas than in fetuses (77,82-84). Conversely, with methylmercury (organic mercury) similar amounts are absorbed by placental and fetal tissues (77,82,84,85).

Further confirmation of this was published in 1977 by Kelman. Using guinea pigs and a protocol that was able to separate fetal uptake from placental transport, Kelman demonstrated that the placental clearance of organic mercury was more than twelve times that of inorganic mercury. The author concludes his report with the following statement: "Elucidation of the relationship between the movements of inorganic and organic forms of mercury across the placenta should be of value in understanding the risk of exposure incurred by the fetus from each form of mercury when both are present in mercury-polluted environments."(86)

Another major factor, not actively evaluated in most of the studies reviewed, is that the presence of selenium in the placenta can modify and greatly reduce the transplacental passage of mercury to the embryo/fetus. Consequently, as with the failure to consider amalgams as a chronic source of mercury, failure to consider maternal and placental levels of selenium might be a confounding factor bringing into question study results that categorically state fetotoxicity of mercury is not a major problem.(87)

In context with the above, a 1977 study done in Athens, Greece by Alexiou et al. evaluated the trace element content of zinc, cobalt, selenium, rubidium, bromine, and gold in eighteen human placentas and in the liver of six infants who had died at birth. The authors found that the concentrations of essential trace elements such as zinc, cobalt, and selenium were present in significantly higher concentrations in the liver than in the placenta. The nonessential trace elements of bromine, rubidium, and gold were higher in the placenta than in the liver. Dr. Alexiou and his colleagues commented: "The observed difference in the distribution pattern of the studied trace elements in placenta and liver tissues should be extended to other essential and nonessential trace elements. It would also be interesting to study the distribution pattern of trace elements in various pathologic conditions of the fetus."(88)

We consider the last sentence of the preceding paragraph to be an extremely dynamic statement that focuses on a tremendously important issue. For example, rubidium combines vigorously with mercury.(89) Is this why inorganic mercury is trapped more readily in the placenta? To our knowledge, nobody has ever investigated this relationship or the possible biochemical consequences. Certainly the hypothesis that there is a relationship between the distribution patterns of trace elements and the ever-increasing number of birth defects and malformations demands the most serious and mature consideration of the medical and scientific communities all over the world.

In 1984, Tsuchiya and his colleagues investigated the interrelationship of heavy metals and their influence on the next generation. Total mercury and methylmercury, lead, cadmium, manganese, copper, zinc, and iron were determined in the maternal blood, placenta, umbilical cord, and umbilical cord blood. Samples were collected at delivery from 231 pregnant women who were living in the city of Nagoya, Japan, during 1974 and 1978. Total mercury and methylmercury, cadmium, and iron were higher in cord blood than in maternal blood, whereas copper and zinc were lower. Significant positive correlations were observed between maternal and cord blood with regard to total mercury and methylmercury, lead, cadmium, and manganese contents. Significant correlations were also observed between many pairs of metals, particularly in the umbilical cord and its blood. The last sentence of their summary reads: "These results suggest a more serious and complicated influence of heavy metals on infants than their mothers."(90)

A 1985 study by Nakano, using human placental tissues, investigated the transplacental movement of inorganic and organic mercury. Inorganic and organic mercury determinations were made using forty-one paired samples of maternal blood, placental blood and umbilical cord blood from women who had no particular exposure to mercury compounds in their history. The ratio between placental concentration and maternal blood concentration of the two mercury forms was significantly higher in the inorganic than in the organic form, indicating that inorganic mercury does preferentially accumulate in the placental tissues. Nakano's data also indicated there was a preferential transfer of the organic mercury across the placenta. Nakano felt that his data suggested that the placenta is less permeable to inorganic mercury and that the organic mercury reaching the fetus through the transplacental route may be metabolized into an inorganic form.(91)

Nakano's conclusion was confirmed in experiments performed by Suzuki et al. in 1984. The researchers wanted to clarify the normal metabolism of mercurials in the human feto-placental system. They obtained the following samples to be utilized in their study from pregnant women just after delivery: maternal blood, umbilical cord blood, chorionic tissues of the placenta (the outermost extraembryonic cellular membrane from which the placenta develops), and placenta blood vessels. They also obtained tissue samples of fetal liver and brain from induced abortion cases.(92)

Suzuki and his associates found that organic mercury was commonly detected in all four maternal samples, with slightly more elevated values in the umbilical cord blood and chorionic tissues of the placenta than in the maternal blood. Inorganic mercury however, was detected only in the chorionic tissues of the placenta and placenta blood vessels, and not in maternal blood or umbilical cord blood. In the fetal liver, 27-60% of the mercury was in the form of inorganic mercury. However, in four of the five fetal brain samples, inorganic mercury was not detected. The researchers studied the capability of the fetal liver to change (demethylate) organic mercury to inorganic mercury. Their results indicated that the fetal liver demethylated approximately 1% of the methylmercury in a 24-hour period.(92) It is not understood why inorganic mercury in the fetal brain was not detected, as this is contrary to other studies which showed large increases of brain mercury after inhalation of mercury vapor.

In a 1982 study, Khayat and Dencker studied the effects of ethanol (alcohol) and aminotriazole (a chemical that causes the inhibition of oxidation of mercury vapor) on the fetal uptake and distribution of metallic mercury vapor in the mouse. The results of their experiments were extremely revealing. They found that in normal animals and in ethanol-treated ones, the corpora lutea of the ovaries accumulated mercury, which could interfere with normal pregnancy by changing the progesterone production. (The corpus luteum secretes progesterone.) They also found that ethanol caused an increased accumulation of mercury in the liver and the thyroid after mercury vapor inhalation, both in the mother and in the fetus.(93)

The researchers ended their paper as follows: "In conclusion, this study showed that even though the fetus as a whole will not get as high doses of mercury vapor as many maternal organs, certain cells or organs may be at risk due to higher concentrations in these particular areas. Furthermore, environmental chemicals, such as the herbicide aminotriazole or ethanol intentionally taken into the body, may considerably increase the fetal body burden of mercury and its concentration in certain tissues like the liver or thyroid, after mercury vapor inhalation."(93)

Outside of the very few who have conducted experiments with mercury vapor, most scientists and researchers are ignoring elemental mercury vapor in their research and in their recommendations for future research areas considered critical. It appears that most of these researchers have forgotten the scientific data demonstrating that once in the blood, elemental mercury vapor remains in its elemental form for minutes, during which time it can penetrate most tissues without difficulty. It is this capability that permits it to also readily move through the placenta to the embryo or fetus, as does organic mercury. This fact has been established by the research studies noted above. Consequently, when researchers state their concerns about inorganic and organic mercury in our mercury-polluted environment, they are failing to account for, or take into consideration, the contribution of mercury vapor being released from mercury amalgam dental fillings that has been scientifically documented since 1926.

In their failure to pay adequate notice to this phenomenon, researchers are also failing to comprehend that once elemental mercury vapor from amalgam dental fillings passes through the placenta and moves into the embryo/fetus, it will oxidize into the inorganic form of mercury. At this point, there is no chemical difference between it and the methylmercury from fish that may have been demethylated to the inorganic form after transplacental passage into the embryo/fetus.

Most of the published research has assumed that the only exposure to elemental mercury vapor is from a minute amount contained in the atmosphere. Most research therefore has only focused on probable exposure from dietary mercury, which is usually in the form of organic methylmercury. However, it would appear that a glaring omission has been made by not considering the exposure to elemental mercury vapor from mercury amalgam dental fillings. A woman contemplating pregnancy, or who is presently pregnant, has to ask how the medical profession can make intelligent decisions concerning pregnancy if the statistical data utilized to formulate those decisions and treatment protocols did not differentiate between women without amalgam dental fillings and those with amalgam dental fillings.

SUMMARY

1. The placental membrane will selectively retard the passage of certain chemical substances to the embryo/fetus.

2. Organic mercury and metallic mercury vapor readily pass through the placenta and are taken up by the embryo or fetus where an unknown percentage will be oxidized to inorganic mercury.

3. Transport of cadmium through the placenta appears to be restricted.

4. Lead appears to be only slightly restricted in its passage through the placenta into the embryo and fetus.

5. Xenobiotics: Starting with Thalidomide, science now knows that most drugs will readily pass the placenta and can be taken up by the embryo or fetus.

6. Very little is known regarding the synergism of lead and mercury when both are present at the same time. The limited research that is available indicates that the combined toxic effects of both metals is greater than each of them separately.

7. The maternal nutriture can have a great bearing on how the body's natural protective systems will respond to foreign chemicals.

8. Scientific evidence suggests that the presence of mercury, lead, and other heavy metals in the placenta, umbilical cord, and cord blood may produce a more serious and complicated influence on infants than their mothers.

9. Alcohol will cause an increased uptake of mercury vapor by the maternal thyroid and the fetal thyroid and liver.

7

EFFECTS OF MERCURY ON IMMUNE FUNCTION AND ON PREGNANCY

In this chapter we will present information on the immune system, and how mercury and lead can suppress or alter it. We will also bring out some unique aspects of how mercury vapor is handled by the body and why this leads to accumulations of mercury in the brain. Finally, we will relate available scientific data on the possible effects of mercury vapor on pregnancy.

Most everyone has heard the terms *allergy* and *immune system*. However, few people really understand what the terms mean. Simply put, your immune system is your body's natural defense system. If your immune system is functioning correctly, you are usually protected against and are able to fight off any type of foreign element (antigen) that gets into your body. Whether it be a bacteria, virus, drug, chemical, or altered body cell, your body's immune system routinely neutralizes, destroys, or rejects it without overreacting.

On the other hand, when your immune system is not functioning properly, you get an obvious reaction to the foreign substance which could be anything from a stuffy nose to asthma. This is commonly called an *allergic reaction*. A major aspect of the controversy surrounding the use of mercury amalgam in dentistry deals with the number of people who may be allergic to their mercury amalgam dental fillings.

ALLERGY TO MERCURY/AMALGAM

In 1983, the ADA, in a published policy statement, addressed the issue of sensitivity to mercury by stating, "The Association wishes to emphasize that except in individuals sensitive to mercury, there is no reason why a patient should seek at this time to have amalgam restorations (silver fillings) removed."(94) In 1984, the ADA elaborated on this theme further by stating, "Although cases of allergy to mercury have been reported in the literature, the prevalence of mercury allergy is estimated to be less than 1%."(95)

The preceding statements form one of the cornerstones of the ADA and National Institute of Dental Research (NIDR) position that amalgam is safe. The information that follows should provide a better understanding of the ADA and NIDR position and what little, if any, scientific data there is to support their statements.

First, let's look at the ADA statement that only a few people are allergic or hypersensitive to mercury amalgam dental fillings. In 1984, the ADA hosted an international "Workshop on the Biocompatibility of Metals in Dentistry" sponsored by the NIDR. (Appendix 2 contains the Recommendations of the Workshop, which list four recommendations related to determining what the incidence of hypersensitivity to mercury/metal alloys really is). In a question and answer session following one the presentations, the statement was made that "less than 1% of the population is allergic to amalgam." There was no scientific data or documentation presented to support this conclusion, which was based on a search of the literature that revealed only a few published case histories dealing with actual allergic reactions to amalgam dental fillings.

Although some of the persons in attendance at the Workshop cited published scientific studies demonstrating allergic reactions ranging from 5% to 26%, this information was totally ignored. As is the case with most "rumors," when repeated enough times it appears to become fact. Therefore, the official position espoused by various ADA spokespersons as a scientific fact is "the incidence of allergic reaction to dental amalgam fillings is less than 1%." ONE PERCENT OF THE U.S. POPULATION WOULD REPRESENT MORE THAN TWO MILLION PEOPLE WHO MAY BE ALLERGIC TO THEIR DENTAL FILLINGS.

What, exactly, is meant by an allergic reaction, and how do you test for it? One of the standard methods utilized by the medical profession to determine hypersensitivity is the use of skin testing. Dilute concentrations of the suspected allergen (the substance causing the reaction) are applied to the skin by use of a patch (held on by tape) or injected just below the surface of the skin. There is considerable controversy concerning the use of the mercury patch test procedure. One potential problem encountered is that the patch test itself could greatly exacerbate your symptoms and reaction if you are already hypersensitive to mercury. Another is that the patch test could end up making you hypersensitive to mercury.

Still another problem stems from the difference of opinion among medical allergists as to what type of mercury to test with and how dilute to make the solutions. The biggest controversy seems to be over the kinds of responses that constitute a positive (allergic) reaction. Some say you are positive if the skin turns red and wheals (burns, itches, swells). Others say that there are systemic manifestations, such as changes in blood pressure, temperature, and pulse.

Based on limited anecdotal and scientific information, it appears that individuals who may have any of the following health conditions should not allow themselves to be mercury patch tested: pregnant women, diagnosed cases of systemic lupus erythematosus, multiple sclerosis, leukemia, mental illness (especially manic depression) and acrodynia. In fact, if you have any question at all about taking the test, ask your physician if a mercury patch test presents any risk to you.

Now let's look at some of the scientific studies that have been published around the world dealing with hypersensitivity to mercury.

1. In 1969, Djerassi and Berova found that 16.1% of their test subjects exhibited a positive reaction to amalgam and its components. What is unique about the Djerassi and Berova study is that they used sixty controls who did not have any amalgam fillings. The controls were subjected to the same series of patch tests that the 180 other test subjects were given. NONE OF THE CONTROL GROUP--THOSE WITHOUT AMALGAM FILLINGS--HAD ANY POSITIVE REACTION TO THE PATCH TESTS. Conversely, 16.1% of all the other patients in the study had a positive reaction. Did age of the amalgam fillings have a bearing? Of the study patients whose amalgam fillings were more than five years old, 22.5% had a positive reaction. The greater percentage of reactions in patients with fillings five or more years old would appear to be further proof that mercury is escaping from these fillings and that a great many people are unable to accommodate the added burden of this poison.(96)

2. A 1973 study by the North American Contact Dermatitis Group involving 1,200 subjects, demonstrated that 5% had a positive reaction to a 1% solution of ammoniated mercury and 8% had a positive reaction to Thimerosal (merthiolate that contains mercury).(97) It should be noted that thimerosal is also the chemical preservative that was used in many contact lens solutions.

3. In 1975, Brun published the results of a study in which 1,000 patients with contact dermatitis were tested for hypersensitivity to mercury; 11.3% of the patients tested positive to the mercury patch test. The authors also provided a comparison of their results with those published by the World Health Organization, showing similar results.(98)

4. Nebenfuhrer et al. (1983) tested 1,530 in-patients--780 men and 750 women--with a routine allergy series that included mercury. Mercury allergy was found in 9.6% of those tested (91 women and 57 men).(99)

5. Mobacken et al. (1984) reported that 16% of a group of 67 patients with oral lichen planus (an inflammatory disease of the oral mucosa) reacted to a mercury patch test. They found that most reactions were caused by elemental mercury.(100)

6. Miller et al. (1987) published results of a study performed at Baylor College of Dentistry in Dallas, Texas. This study utilized 171 volunteer dental students who were patch tested for hypersensitivity to mercuric chloride. Students exhibiting an allergic reaction had an average of 9.5 amalgam restorations. Those students in the negative-reaction group had an average of 7.7 amalgam restorations. Students with amalgam restorations that were at least five years or older had a mercury hypersensitivity rate of 31.6% and those with ten or more amalgam restorations had a 44.3% mercury hypersensitivity reaction. Dr. Miller and his associates stated that the results of their study indicated that the number of amalgam restorations was more important than the age of the amalgam restorations, in the development of hypersensitivity to mercuric chloride.(101)

We consider the data provided by Dr. Miller and his associates to be the most important information on the subject of mercury hypersensitivity ever published in the United States. For example, of the 171 students in their study, 31.5% had an average of 9.5 amalgam fillings. If you apply that percentage to the 125 million Americans with amalgam fillings, it would mean that approximately 39 million people should have an average of 9.5 amalgam fillings in their mouth. Of the 39 million, 44.3% or about 17 million people, should be hypersensitive to mercury.

It would appear from the preceding data that there could be anywhere from two million to seventeen million people in the United States who may be allergic to mercury. In the context of this book, this places a great many women in the increased risk category. The preceding data also indicates that the ADA has grossly misrepresented the potential incidence of allergic reactions that may be directly attributable to the presence of mercury amalgam dental fillings.

MERCURY AND THE IMMUNE SYSTEM

The scientific documentation has firmly established that mercury causes dysfunction of the immune system as well as autoimmune disease itself. There are many scientific papers detailing the fact that mercury alters and/or suppresses the immune system. There have been two papers published that show *amalgam* can modify the immune system. The first paper by Verschaeve et al. in 1976 showed that study subjects exposed to low dose mercury from amalgam had lymphocyte chromosome aberrations. This, in effect, means that it is possible for mercury vapor from amalgam to induce genetic damage.(113)

The body's defense against agents that are harmful or alien is through an extremely complex system of cells and chemicals. There are two basic systems that make up the total immune system. One is a nonspecific system and is not dependent on the presence of an antigen to react. Immune reaction to an inflammation would be a nonspecific type of reaction. The other system is called either "specific" or "acquired" and involves antigen-dependent reactions of classes of lymphocytes called T cells and B cells. In our discussion, we will deal primarily with the acquired system. The cellular elements of the body's defenses are the white blood cells (leukocytes). Some of these leukocytes engulf (phagocytize) or chemically destroy harmful materials. The body must be able to identify these alien or harmful materials, distinguish them from the normal cells and chemicals of the body, and initiate defensive actions when needed. This is accomplished by other white blood cells called lymphocytes.

Some lymphocytes, called B cells, produce specific defense chemicals called antibodies. B cells are considered part of the humoral immune response. Humoral pertains to bodily fluids--such as the blood, lymph, saliva, tears, and the secretions of the mucous membranes in the nose, vaginal tract, and small intestine--and represents the immune response associated with circulating antibody. Antibodies are immunoglobulins, which are a protein produced by plasma cells usually having antibody activity. Each immunoglobulin is composed of one or more molecules, linked by disulfide bonds.(Disulfide means there are two sulfur atoms present that bond other components of the immunoglobulin together.) Immunoglobulins are further identified by class or category as IgG, IgM, IgE, IgD, or IgA (Ig stands for immunoglobulin and the letters A-G indentifiy a particular category of immunoglobulin that performs a particular function in the immune system.)(102,103) Although we have not seen any specific research showing mercury and lead binding to the disulfide fragments of immunoglobulin, it certainly doesn't rule it out as a possibility because both ions have a demonstrated affinity for the sulphur atom.

The cellular immune response takes place inside the cell or on the outside surface of the cell and involves other lymphocytes called T cells. T cells identify foreign materials, distinguish them from normal body constituents, initiate and aid the cellular and chemical defense response (called helper, or T-4 cells), and end the response when the foreign substance has been rejected (called suppressor, or T-8 cells).(5102,103)

The process of distinguishing normal body constituents from harmful elements is obviously critical. It is accomplished by the recognition of certain chemicals on the surfaces of cells by the T cells. There are several mechanisms by which the immune response, if unfavorably altered, will fail to identify or treat body substances as being "self." (103) Moreover, should a foreign chemical attach to a normal body constituent (such as mercury attaching to the sulfur atom of a body protein), the resulting product will no longer be recognized as self by the immune system. This may result in a hypersensitive (allergic) reaction or even autoimmune disease if the insult persists over time.

The prefix "auto" denotes a relationship to self, and autoimmunity relates to a specific immune response against your own tissues. In effect, tissues of your own body appear to be foreign to your immune system so it tries to attack and destroy them. Sometimes this condition is called "autoallergy." Some of the features commonly found in autoimmune diseases are (1) antibodies directed against T-cell and B-cell lymphocytes; (2) antinuclear antibodies (ANA) directed against DNA or its segments; (3) elevated blood levels of certain antibodies, especially in the IgM and IgG categories;

and (4) the proliferation of antibodies against numerous self
antigens (autoantigens) by the B cells, which is called
"polyclonal B-cell activation." If the antibody is specific or
derived from one cell type, it is called a *monoclonal antibody.(103)*

AUTOIMMUNITY AND MERCURY

Table 7-1: The major cells of the body's defenses

WHITE BLOOD CELLS [Leukocytes]		
NON SPECIFIC [Phagocitize (Engulf) or destroy chemically]	SPECIFIC [React to antigens]	
Neutrophil Eosinophil Basophil Monocyte	LYMPHOCYTES	
	T-Cell Lymphocytes	B-Cell Lymphocytes
	T-4 (Helper) T-8 (Suppressor) T-Cytotoxic	Plasma Cells (Produce Antibodies)

In 1970, Caron and associates demonstrated that low doses
of inorganic and organic mercury caused an alteration of
lymphocytes from humans that were allergic to mercury.(104) Weening and associates (1980) found that 90%
of rats exposed to low doses of inorganic mercury had mer-

cury-induced antinuclear antibodies (Anti means against and nuclear means the nucleus or within the cell itself. Therefore, an antinuclear antibody would be one that attacked the nucleus of a cell).The mercury exposed rats also had a significant decrease of mitogenic stimulation of lymphocytes (mitogenic means the the division or duplication of cells), an increased production of migration inhibitory factor (migration means the passage or movement of leukocytes or white blood cells through the vessel and inhibition means to stop. Therefore, an increase would mean less lymphocytes would be available to respond to an immune challenge), and an immune complex kidney disease (circulating antigen-antibody complexes cause blood vessel injury within the kidney) with accumulation of IgG complexes. (105)

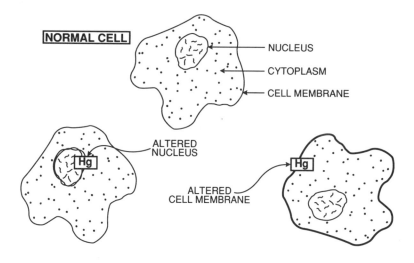

Figure 7-1: How cells may be altered by mercury. Once altered the body may not recognize these cells as "self" and thus form antibodies against them. (Antinuclear Antibodies if the nucleus has been altered.

Druet et al. (1982) noted that the immune disease caused by mercury was not limited to the kidneys; lesions were also found in the spleen, intestine, liver, lung, and heart. They also pointed out that numerous forms of mercury could cause the disease, regardless of the route of administration, be it inhalation, oral, intravenous, subcutaneous, or percutaneous.(106) In another report that same year, Druet stated: "Data presented strongly suggest that mercury modifies immune homeostasis in BN [Brown-Norway] rats and that, as a consequence of immune dysregulation, autoantibodies are produced, some of which are of pathogenic significance."(107) Andres, in 1984, found that oral administration of mercuric chloride caused autoimmune lesions in the small and large intestines with local IgA reactivity, as well as circulating IgG in the blood that was reactive to the kidney tissue.(108)

In 1986, Robinson and associates found that mercuric chloride induced antinuclear antibodies in various strains of mice. They concluded that the chemical toxicity of mercury resulted in the release of nuclear components of DNA that were antigenic and capable of inducing an antinuclear antibody response.(109) A two-part study appeared in the *Journal of Immunology* in May of 1986. The first part, by Hirsch et al., found that mercuric chloride induced a polyclonal B-cell activation in Brown-Norway rats, resulting in autoimmune disease. The second part of the study found that the autoimmune disease resulted in specific (monoclonal) antibodies in the IgM and IgE categories. (110,111)

Also in 1986, Pelletier and associates determined that mercuric chloride induced an autoimmune disease due to a T-cell- dependent polyclonal activation of B cells in Brown-Norway rats. The authors stated that "these experiments demonstrate that mercuric chloride induces autoreactive

T cells and suggest that these cells may be responsible for the autoimmune disease."(112)

In a 1984 paper, Dr. David W. Eggleston described a simple scientific experiment involving three patients.(114) He assayed the blood levels of his patients for the T-lymphocyte percent of total lymphocytes before and after the insertion and removal of dental amalgam and or replacement of restorations. Two of the patients had amalgam fillings and one patient had one pin-retained composite resin restoration, without any other dental restorations present. The amalgam fillings of the two patients were removed and replaced with either provisional acrylic or gold restorations. The pin-retained composite was removed and replaced with a porcelain-fused-to-nickel alloy crown. Blood assays for T-lymphocyte percentages of total lymphocytes were again taken. The replacement of the amalgam caused an increase in the number of T-lymphocytes. Placing of the nickel alloy caused a suppression of the number of T-lymphocytes.(114)

To confirm the effects of amalgam and nickel on the lymphocytes, amalgams were again placed in one of the two patients that originally had them, and the nickel alloy was replaced with a porcelain-fused-to-gold crown. Blood assays of T-lymphocytes were taken again. In the patient who had amalgams reinstalled, there was a decrease in the number of T-lymphocytes. In the patient that had the nickel replaced with porcelain/gold, there was an increase in the T-lymphocytes. The amalgams were then removed for a final time and replaced with permanent gold restorations, and again the T-lymphocytes increased.(114)

What Dr. Eggleston demonstrated with his experiment was that amalgam and nickel were able to change and impair an important immune function indicator known as the T-4/T-8 ratio. Two major components of the immune system are the lymphocyte white blood cells, normally referred to as T cells, and B cells. Within the T cell family there are several types, two of which have been labeled T4 and T8. Proper immune system function is dependent upon a delicate balance of the T4/T8 ratio. A low T4/T8 ratio can predispose you to autoimmune diseases such as systemic lupus erythematosus, hemolytic anemia, multiple sclerosis, severe atopic eczema, inflammatory bowel disease, and glomerulonephritis (kidney disease).(114)

Based on the scientific data presented thus far it is obvious that the statements being publicly made by the ADA, indicating that the amount of mercury being released from mercury amalgam dental fillings does not present a health hazard except in those individuals who are allergic, are incomplete and have not evaluated all of the available scientific facts.

We feel it is truly unfortunate that medical researchers have paidso little attention to the effects of chronic low dose inhalation of mercury vapor, from mercury amalgam dental fillings, on the immune system.Scientific data demonstrating that mercury suppresses immune function has been available for years. For example, Trahktenberg, in her monograph on mercury in 1969, cites her primary research, which clearly indicates immune dysfunction from exposure to mercury.(2) The concluding paragraphs, on page 224, of the section in her monograph treating the immune system state:

Thus prolonged action of low mercury concentrations on mammals leads to changes in a number of immunological indicators: agglutinin titers, active leucocyte percent, phagocytic number, complement activity of blood serum. The dynamics arising under the influence of toxic effects of immunological shifts is characterized by two periods: an initial short-term stimulation of immunological response, and by its subsequent stronger suppression. There is a significant decrease in the preventive properties of the blood obtained from immunized animals subjected to chronic action of mercury.

***

Our experiments on protein resynthesis in animals affected by mercury suggest that in micromercurialism, there is a suppression of this resynthesis and a decreased capability of the organism to form antibodies under antigenic stimulation and that these two are closely connected.

***

Immunity indicators, especially agglutinin formation, change under prolonged exposure to low mercury concentrations and reflect general physiological relationships.

Our data confirm opinions that changes in immunological indicators as a rule appear significantly earlier than many other signs of latent toxic effects even in the very earliest stages of toxic aggression.

***

Table 7-2
Mercury and the Immune System

Effect	Researcher	Reference #
Lymphocyte Alteration	Caron et al.	104
Antinuclear Antibodies	Weening et al.	105
Decreased mitogenic stimulation	Weening et al.	105
Increased migration inhibitory factor	Weening et al.	105
Immune complex kidney disease	Weening et al.	105
Immune lesions in spleen, intestine, liver, lung, heart	Druet et al.	106
Autoantibodies	Druet et al.	107
Autoimmune lesions - intestines, circulating anti-kidney IgG	Andres	108
Antinuclear Antibodies	Robinson et al.	109
Polyclonal B-cell activation	Hirsch et al., Pelletier et al.	110,112
Autoimmune disease	Hirsch et al., Pelletier et al.	110,111,112
Monoclonal antibodies	Hirsch et al.	111
Lymphocyte chromosomal aberrations	Verscheave et al.	113
T-cell suppression	Eggleston	114
Immune dysfunction	Trahktenberg	2
Antibody production	Trahktenberg	2

Table 7-2: Some scientific documentation of the harmful effects of mercury on the immune system.

Subsequently, there have been many scientific articles expanding on the effects of mercury on the immune system. The same can also be said for the effects of lead on immune function. As you will see in Chapter 11, these two toxic metals have the potential to create biochemical, physiological, and pathological havoc in the body. With regard to infertility and birth defects, research must be funded to determine exactly what effects mercury's suppression of the maternal immune system may have. Further information on this subject is contained in Chapters 8 and 9.

Of an even more immediate nature is the need to fund research to determine if the chronic low dose inhalation of mercury vapor emanating from mercury amalgam dental fillings may be a factor in the susceptibility to AIDS (Acquired Immune Deficiency Syndrome) of persons living in industrialized nations.

Scientific data demonstrates also that immunocompetance can be easily compromised through dietary deficiencies of critical nutrients.(237) Even in this country of plenty, U.S. government studies show that large percentages of the U.S. population suffer from various nutritional deficiencies. If a person, because of life style and diet, has in fact experienced some imbalance in immune function, the presence of a mouthful of mercury amalgam dental fillings may ultimately be the cause of sufficient *additional* suppression to render the immune system ineffective in coping with the AIDS virus.

POSSIBLE SYSTEMIC AND PREGNANCY EFFECTS

"On October 10, 1986, Lars Friberg, one of the world experts on mercury, made the following statements in the Swedish newspaper *Skaraborgs Lans Allehande:*(115) "Even if the risks are small, dental fillings with mercury and amalgam can be dangerous for sensitive persons, and pregnant women should not do any extensive amalgam repairs during pregnancy....There are always persons who are more sensitive than others and we have to protect them. If you add all persons who are very sensitive towards amalgam, you could end up with a considerable number." Dr. Friberg is a professor at the National Institute of Environmental Medicine in Stockholm, Sweden, and is also a member of the expert commission appointed by Sweden's Medical and Social Welfare Board to study the question of amalgam toxicity.

In 1985 the Swedish Health Board appointed an expert commission to investigate the controversial question of the risk of mercury poisoning from amalgam. The findings of the expert commission, which were endorsed by the Health Board, were released at a press conference. A Swedish newspaper, Svenska Dagbladet, featured the story on the front page of their May 20, 1987 issue. (14) The headline read: "SOCIALSTYRELSEN STOPS AMALGAM USE" (The Socialstyrelsen is the Swedish Social Welfare and Health Administration). The article went on to say that

> amalgam is an unsuitable and toxic dental filling material which shall be discontinued as soon as suitable replacement materials are produced....As a first step in the process to eliminate the use of amalgam in dental fillings, comprehensive amalgam work on pregnant women shall be stopped in order to prevent mercury damage to the fetus....We realize now that we have previously made an error in our judgement on this question. Patients have suffered unnecessarily and we will now rectify our mistakes and in different ways try to solve the problem. "It means no less than to give patients the best possible treatment," explained Viking Falk from the Socialstyrelsen when the report was presented. This is an unusual test of the country's leading medical authority and their responsibility, espe-

cially against a background that the Socialstyrelsen's dental experts have for many years worked firmly against researchers and patients who have tried to warn of the toxic risk with amalgam.

It is important to point out that we will not know the degree of implementation of the expert commission findings until the Health Board publishes their directives on the subject.

The U.S. government has not as yet deemed it necessary to appoint a commission of medical experts to investigate the potential toxicities of mercury amalgam dental fillings. Their existing position is therefore in stark contrast to the one taken by the Swedish government.

As indicated in the allergy section of this chapter, a percentage of the population is going to have an adverse health effect--in this instance, allergic-type reactions--from mercury amalgam dental fillings. A good question at this point might be; Is it possible that mercury vapor being inhaled from my mercury amalgam dental fillings might be causing other "systemic" problems not manifested by outward, observable signs such as allergic reactions?

To even begin to answer that question, we have to have some knowledge of what happens to that small dose of mercury vapor we take in each time we inhale. Research has shown that there is an approximate absorption through the lungs of 80% of each dose inhaled. When we use the word *absorption* in this context we mean that 80% of the mercury vapor inhaled passes from the lung into the bloodstream. Remember, we are talking about elemental mercury that has a neutral electrical status, permitting it to readily cross or penetrate cell and organ membranes until such time as it is oxidized into the ionized form of mercury. Once ionized, it has an electrical charge and therefore has much more difficulty in passing into or out of cells.(61,116)

It takes approximately 4-5 minutes for elemental mercury to be oxidized after entering the blood. It takes approximately one minute for blood to completely circulate through the entire body. Therefore, each dose of elemental mercury vapor entering the blood exists in its non-ionic form long enough to reach all tissues and organs. What happens next will be covered in subsequent chapters. The important point to remember is that the blood circulating throughout our body provides an extremely efficient mercury transportation system, capable of rapidly exchanging chemical substances between various tissues and organs.(61)

A study was done in Japan in 1977 by Suzuki and his colleagues, investigating mercury content of amniotic fluid. There were fifty-seven Japanese women with a gestational age of four months to term involved in the study. Women in the early or middle stage of pregnancy (4-7 months) were undergoing a termination of pregnancy for various reasons. The amniotic fluid was sampled mostly by amniocentesis. Using a method established by Magos(118), the researchers determined both the inorganic and organic mercury content of the amniotic fluid. Inorganic mercury was detected in all but two samples, while organic mercury was found in only thirty of the samples. They also found that inorganic mercury levels were significantly higher than the organic mercury levels. Both inorganic and organic mercury levels were highest in the seventh month of pregnancy. This study provides evidence that the fetus is exposed to inorganic mercury, because the fetus swallows amniotic fluid.(117)

In a different approach, but with the same theme, Bara and his associates (1985) studied the effects of metal pollutants (lead, cadmium, mercury, arsenic) on total electrical conductance using human amnion isolated from the placental zone. (Amnion is the membrane that contains the fetus and the amniotic fluid around it.) The total conductance through the isolated amnion was decreased on the fetal side by lead and arsenic and on the maternal side by cadmium, mercury, and arsenic. What is so important about this study is it showed that lead, mercury, and cadmium inhibited magnesium. When magnesium was added, the electrical conductance increased significantly.(119)

Although the authors did not elaborate on the possible consequences resulting from the inhibition of magnesium by these toxic metals, magnesium is an essential element and is critical to the functioning of several hundred enzymes in the body. Consequently, we now know that mercury and lead are in the amnion and, as demonstrated by Suzuki, mercury is also present in the amniotic fluid. It is also apparent that both lead and mercury can affect availability of magnesium, as well as electrical conductance. Therefore, it seems plausible to conclude that there has to be some diminished metabolic effect on both maternal and fetal organisms.(119)

The reader should bear in mind that after oxidation, elemental mercury vapor is in the ionized form and indistinguishable from other forms of inorganic mercury in the body. Just as elemental mercury vapor is converted to inorganic mercury, there is also scientific evidence suggesting that some portion of methylmercury may also be converted to inorganic mercury in the body. It would have been valuable if Suzuki et al. had determined the numbers and surfaces of amalgam fillings present in these women because the authors were puzzled by the excess of inorganic mercury present in the amniotic fluid and where it might have come from.

In 1982, Kuntz et al. published a very important study dealing with this very point. These researchers set out to determine maternal and cord-blood mercury levels from an urban population sample; changes, if any, in maternal blood mercury levels during pregnancy; and correlation of any changes with potential sources of mercury exposure.(120)

The study followed fifty-seven prenatal patients, with no known exposure to the element mercury or any of its compounds. Changes in whole blood total mercury concentration from the initial prenatal clinic examination through delivery and postpartum hospitalization were monitored. On hospital admission for labor and delivery, whole blood total mercury averaged 1.16 parts per billion (ppb), compared to 0.79 ppb from the first prenatal clinic visit. These levels represent a 46% increase and significant difference in maternal concentration of a substance previously recognized for its peculiar ease at crossing the placental barrier. The authors concluded: "Previous stillbirths, as well as history of birth defects, exhibited significant positive correlation with background mercury levels." The authors also searched the literature of the last 5 years and found no other report of cohort heavy metal surveillance throughout pregnancy.

In their conclusions, the authors stated that patients with large numbers of dental fillings exhibited a tendency to higher maternal blood-mercury levels.(120)

In a study published in 1984 by Dr. Abraham and his associates, additional information was provided regarding the association between blood-mercury levels and amalgam dental fillings. Forty-seven male medical students with mercury amalgam dental fillings and four medical students and ten graduate students without mercury amalgam dental fillings participated in the study.(121) The purpose of the study was to investigate if there was any relationship between numbers and surfaces of amalgam dental fillings, mercury levels in mouth air, and mercury levels in blood. Baseline data on mercury levels in the blood and in mouth air were taken before any stimulation by chewing, drinking, and so on. Then stimulated blood and air samples were taken between 7:15 and 9:15 each morning for three weeks. (Participants had not eaten or taken anything to drink after midnight of the previous night.) Stimulation was accomplished by having each participant chew a stick of sugarless gum for three minutes at the rate of 120 beats per minute by following the beat of a metronome.(121) The researchers found that "Pre- and post-chewing mouth air mercury levels in subjects with amalgams were higher than in those without amalgams. Within the amalgam group, the mean post-chewing mouth air mercury levels were higher than the pre-chewing levels." Within the group that had no amalgams THERE WAS NO CHANGE IN MOUTH AIR MERCURY LEVELS AFTER CHEWING.

They also found that "blood-mercury concentrations were also higher in subjects with amalgams than in those without. As with mouth air mercury levels, the differences in blood mercury concentrations may be attributed to the presence of dental amalgams. A feasible explanation for this is that the mercury volatilized from the amalgam surfaces is inhaled and reaches the blood via pulmonary absorption."(121)

What is interesting about comparing the study done by Abraham et al. and the one by Kuntz et al. is that the average blood-mercury levels in the Abraham group of forty-seven male medical students with amalgams was the same as the blood-mercury levels in the Kuntz group of fifty-seven pregnant women with amalgams. Bear in mind that in the Kuntz et al. study, a significant correlation was found between the history of stillbirths and mercury levels in both maternal and cord blood. Kuntz et al. also found that the occurrence of malformed infants in previous births correlated significantly with prenatal blood-mercury levels.

None of the histories of the participants in either of the two studies reflected any possible exposure to mercury except for that related to the presence of mercury amalgam dental fillings. Abraham et al. conclude their report with the following statement: "Given these facts, the small increase in blood mercury levels that is statistically associated with dental amalgam restorations should be a matter of concern for dentists as well as for the recipients of these restorations."

We would also like to point out some personal observations regarding the Abraham and Kuntz studies. The participants in the Abraham et al. study were only required to chew gum for three minutes. Subsequent work by Vimy and Lorscheider in 1985 (6) demonstrated that increased release of mercury vapor from amalgam fillings upon stimulation does not reach its highest level or peak until ten minutes of stimulation. It would have been interesting to see what the mouth air mercury levels were after an additional seven minutes of chewing.

Prior to the work of Abraham et al. and Kuntz et al., two studies done in Germany--Kroncke et al. (1980) and Ott and Kroncke, 1981(122,123)--had failed to show a correlation between blood mercury concentrations and the number of amalgam fillings. However, there is some reasonable doubt concerning whether the patients tested in these studies had any external exposures to mercury other than their amalgam fillings. Also, neither of the studies attempted to account for cigarette smoking or alcohol consumption in the test participants, which could have also influenced the results (both the Kuntz and Abraham studies took all of these factors into consideration).

Another important aspect of both the Kuntz and Abraham studies is the fact that the unstimulated mercury levels were all higher than the controls. This means that increased blood-mercury levels were not solely related to stimulated release of mercury vapor from the dental fillings. Rather, it was a combination of the stimulated release and the chronic un-stimulated release of mercury vapor from amalgam dental fillings, 24 hours a day, 365 days a year that caused an increase in blood mercury levels.

In 1986, another study was published by Snapp et al. corroborating the causal relationship between the presence of mercury amalgam dental fillings and elevated blood-mercury levels. There were five subjects in the study, all of whom had amalgam dental fillings. Initial baseline blood-mercury levels were taken. A minimum of four weekly blood determinations were made to obtain the baseline blood-mercury levels.(124) Exposure to external sources of mercury vapor and tobacco and alcohol consumption were also monitored throughout the study.

Once valid baseline blood-mercury levels were established, all dental amalgams were removed at one appointment and replaced with either composite or gold restorations. During amalgam removal every effort was made to minimize mercury exposure to the patient by using water spray on the drill bit, and additional water spray and high-speed suction utilized by the assistant. After removal of the amalgams, blood-mercury levels were then monitored for 60-90 days. The mean post-amalgam-removal blood mercury levels were then determined for each subject and this was compared to pre-amalgam-removal blood levels. "In all five subjects, there was a statistically significant reduction in blood-mercury levels....This study showed there was a reduction in blood-mercury levels when existing dental amalgam restorations were removed and replaced with a nonmercury-containing restorative material."(124)

In a recent study by Olstad et al. (June 1987), urine-mercury concentrations in seventy-three Norwegian school children with a mean age of twelve years were determined. A significant positive correlation was found between urine-mercury and the extent of mercury amalgam dental fillings. The researchers found no correlation between urine-mercury levels and allergy or absence from school. However, they appeared concerned enough to comment that, although they saw no need for an "immediate" re-evaluation on the continued use of amalgam as a dental filling material, the results of their study were considered unfavorable for amalgam when its pros and cons are balanced against those of alternative materials.(125)

There have been two other studies that are raising the level of concern about mercury vapor being released from mercury amalgam dental fillings. The first study was done by Schiele et al. in 1984. Autopsy studies of the brains and kidneys were done on forty-four people who had died accidental deaths. There were twenty-five male and nineteen female accident victims between sixteen and fifty-seven years of age who were analyzed. Collectively there were less than ten teeth missing, and the number of amalgam fillings per individual ranged between three and thirty-one.(62)

The statistical analysis showed a clear correlation between the number and surfaces of amalgam fillings and the mercury content of the brain and kidneys. In addition, there was a correlation between age of the subject and mercury content in the brain.(62)

The second study is being done at the Karolinska Institute in Stockholm, Sweden, which is one of the premiere scientific research facilities in the world. The study is still in progress and the researchers, Friberg et al., are continuing to develop new data and explore the issue further, although the initial major report was published in the Swedish Medical Journal in 1986.(63)

As in the Schiele et al. study, autopsy studies were done, this time on seventeen victims of accidental deaths. The Swedish researchers also found that mercury in the central nervous system was related to the number of amalgam fillings. Tissue from various areas of the brain were analyzed for total mercury content. The analysis showed, on average, a higher concentration of mercury when the number of amalgam fillings was large compared to when the number was lower. One important difference between the two studies is that the Swedish team was able to also determine the inorganic mercury percentage of the total mercury value. At the time of publication, only six cases had been analyzed for inorganic mercury content of the brain tissues; however, the researchers found a high percentage of inorganic mercury. It is possible, of course, that the methylmercury derived from dietary sources could have been converted to inorganic mercury. This possibility, however, does not detract from the fact that the researchers found a clear correlation between the numbers and surfaces of amalgam fillings and the mercury content of the brain.(63)

Dr. Magnus Nylander, a member of the Swedish team, in a letter to the editor of *Lancet* (the premiere British medical journal), presented the observation that three of the subjects analyzed were dentists and all of them had very high levels of mercury in their pituitary glands in comparison to the other autopsy cases in the study.(126) Dr. Nylander went on to bring out a very important aspect of mercury vapor transport: "Mercury from the vapor of dental amalgam may have been absorbed by the nasal mucosa and directly transported to the cranial cavity and pituitary. Fifty years ago the German chemist Alfred Stock described direct transport of mercury via mucosa from the nasal cavity to the brain and Störtebecker discusses direct transport of mercury from nasal cavity via the cranial venous system and the olfactory nerves." Dr. Nylander concluded his letter with the statement: "These data suggest that patients with several amalgam fillings may have increased levels of mercury in their pituitary glands and that dentists should handle amalgam carefully."

Thus far, the following scientific points have been made:

1. Mercury is an extremely dangerous poison and environmental pollutant.

2. Mercury amalgam dental fillings release mercury vapor and abraded ions during the life of the fillings, the amounts of which dramatically increase whenever the fillings are stimulated.

3. Mercury amalgam dental fillings can cause a variety of allergic-type reactions in up to 22% of the recipients.

4. The presence of mercury amalgam dental fillings in the oral cavity can cause an increase in blood mercury levels.

5. In schoolchildren, there was a positive correlation between the number of mercury amalgam fillings and the amount of mercury concentrated in the urine.

6. There is some evidence that mercury can cause abortions, stillbirths, and birth defects.

7. Mercury vapor released from amalgam dental fillings can cause an increased burden of mercury to accumulate in the brain.

8. Amniotic fluid contains greater quantities of inorganic than organic mercury.

9. The amnion itself contains mercury, lead, cadmium, and arsenic, and the presence of these metals depresses metabo-

lic functions of magnesium and reduces electrical conductance.

10. Pregnant women, who had no external exposure to mercury during their pregnancy except for their amalgam fillings, had a significant increase in mercury blood levels from conception to delivery.

11. There is evidence indicating that mercury vapor released from amalgam dental fillings can cause a modification and/or suppression of the immune system.

12. There is also evidence that various forms of mercury as well as lead, derived from dietary or atmospheric sources can cause immune system dysfunction.

8

INFERTILITY

A fascinating report was presented on the NBC evening news on March 19, 1987. The report was entitled "Infertility" and presented some statistical data and personal vignettes outlining the magnitude of the problem. Three points brought out in the report were particularly impressive:

1. The number of infertile couples is increasing each year, with the total number already over one million. Approximately one out of every five couples n the United States is considered to be infertile.

2. Over 50% of the problem is related to some problem with the man's sperm, the predominant condition being one of reduced sperm motility. The reporter also stated that very little could be done about this aspect of the infertility problem.

3. Infertility has become a specialty within the medical profession and is extremely complicated and expensive. In vitro fertilization usually costs well over $5,000 for each attempt, without any guarantees of a full-term pregnancy.

Of course, we have been equally fascinated for some time by the hypothesis that heavy metal pollutants are a major cause of the infertility problems in all industrialized countries. Although other elements may be involved, this chapter will focus primarily on the scientific data dealing with the relationship of mercury to the overall problem of infertility. We also provide limited data on lead and infertility. There are some studies that indicate exposure at low levels are without any effect on fertility. This may well be true in relation to the report and research protocol that was employed. However, remember that when you are speaking of the toxic effects of mercury, that (1) it can take upwards of twenty years after being exposed, in some instances, for the toxic effects to manifest themselves; (2) very little consideration, if any, has been given to chronic exposure in individuals who may have a sensitivity to mercury; (3) human data and statistics on the possible causes of infertility have never considered chronic exposure to mercury vapor released from amalgam dental fillings; and (4) to our knowledge, no consideration has ever been given to the possible synergistic effects of lead and mercury, which are both present in the male reproductive organs. Therefore, in the epidemiology of infertility, no thought has ever been given to evaluating this group, male and female, on the basis of those with toxic metals in their mouth and those without.

THE MALE REPRODUCTIVE SYSTEM

In the male, the testes and prostate seem to have an affinity for various essential and nonessential elements. The distribution of these elements in the testes and prostate appears to be fairly constant.(127) Maintenance of the normal balance between the various essential elements is considered critical to the proper function of these organs, just as it is in most other organs and glands of the body. Therefore, when required essential elements are low or deficient, the organ may not be capable of functioning properly. On the other hand, if there is an overabundance of the essential elements, this could lead to toxicity. The fact that there are nonessential minerals such as aluminum, lead, chromium, antimony, nickel, cadmium, gold, and mercury present leaves one to wonder why they are there. Can they affect normal function? Can they bind to essential elements and render them ineffective? Can they cause enzyme dysfunction? The answers to these questions are not readily available since there hasn't been enough research done investigating the effect of heavy metals on the male reproduction system.

A recent (1986) German study entitled "The distribution of heavy metals in human ejaculate. A histochemical study," the authors evaluated the sperm, ejaculate fluid, and the spermatogonic cells of men. *Histochemical* means the identification of chemical components in cells and tissues. The spermatozoa cell is the germ cell of the male that ultimately impregnates the ovum.(128)

The researchers demonstrated the presence of heavy metals in the sperm, the ejaculate fluid, and the spermatogonic cells. The heavy metals were localized in the sperm. The sperm with a lower motility index often did not show the presence of any heavy metals. The authors speculated that the absence of essential heavy metals such as zinc, copper, iron, or manganese may lead to the inhibition of enzyme systems in the sperm which are deemed essential for motility.(128)

If scientists were evaluating a male to determine the cause of reduced sperm motility and were looking for mercury specifically, they may or may not find it. However, it is known that the presence of mercury can inhibit zinc and manganese. So the question becomes one of is it a zinc deficiency causing the problem, or is it the presence of mercury in the testes or prostate that is inhibiting essential heavy metals?

Pursuing the same thought further, a 1984 study by Skandhan and Abraham performed a spectroscopic analysis of seventeen normal and pathological semen samples to determine the different elements present. The instrument used had a sensitivity of one microgram per gram. The elements observed were sodium, calcium, potassium, magnesium, phosphorus, iron, manganese, zinc, copper, boron, silicon, thallium, vanadium, aluminum, mercury, and gold. The authors stated that this was the richest source of gold reported in biological materials. They also determined that the gold was coming from the caput epididymis (the upper part of the cordlike structure within the testis in which spermatozoa are stored). Their study also revealed mercury, silver, boron, thallium, and vanadium were present in high concentrations (one microgram per gram) in seminal plasma.(129)

In a 1975 study by Lee and Dixon, the authors investigated the reproductive effects of methylmercury hydroxide and mercuric chloride on spermatogenesis in male mice. They also wanted to determine the half-life of mercury compounds in the testes. They found that the uptake of methylmercury into the testes was approximately four times greater than that of inorganic mercury, and the half-life of methylmercury in the testes was 3.43 days, whereas that for inorganic mercury was 55.5 days. The authors speculated that the faster uptake of methylmercury into the testes was related in part to its fat solubility, which permits easy penetration of cellular structures. Elemental mercury vapor from amalgam dental fillings has the same fat solubility as methylmercury and would therefore be readily taken up by the testes during the initial five minutes when it is circulating in the blood in its elemental state prior to being ionized.(130)

Lee and Dixon then did serial mating studies with the mice. After first administering mercury to the male mice, the mice were then allowed to mate, under very controlled conditions, to assess the effects of the mercury on fertility. Their statistical analysis indicated significant antifertility effects. They also found that the mercury ion-induced antifertility effects at the dosage used in the experiments were reversible. These results suggest spermatogenic effects of fat soluble forms of mercury having important health consequences in men.(130)

Perhaps a more effective way of clearly bringing out the antifertility effects of mercury is to talk of its use as a contraceptive. Beginning in 1938, evidence was presented about a new contraceptive product, the active ingredient of which was phenylmercuric acetate. Experimental evidence demonstrated that phenylmercuric acetate and phenylmercuric nitrate were the most effective spermicides known.(131) The product was marketed in England under the tradename "Volpar," and preliminary reports of clinical trials indicated it to be highly effective.

In 1944, Eastman and Scott (132) set out to confirm the efficacy of the mercury compounds as contraceptives. The results of their experiments confirmed the earlier published reports on the very high spermicidal potency of both phenylmercuric acetate and nitrate. In 100 fertile women who used the phenylmercuric acetate jelly for one year, in conjunction with an occlusive diaphragm, only one pregnancy resulted that could be regarded as a failure of the method. The researchers also concluded that the toxicity of the phenylmercuric acetate jelly was low.

One of the problems in investigating the toxic effects of chemicals on sperm has always been the laboratory protocol used. Some of the methods used to determine sperm motility have been cinematography (133,134) and multiple exposure photography (135). Both of these procedures and protocols are time-consuming and by their very nature can only measure a small number of spermatozoa. A recent paper by Mohamed and his associates (1986) outlined a new laboratory technique using the laser light-scattering technique to evaluate sperm motility. The authors utilized this new method to determine the in vitro dose-effect relationship of methylmercury on sperm motility utilizing semen samples from normal male monkeys.(136)

The authors concluded their paper with the following: "In conclusion, methylmercury decreased sperm swimming speed and the percentage of motile spermatozoa in a dose-related pattern in vitro. Further investigations are required to elucidate the mechanism of action of methylmercury." The authors felt that their study demonstrated the usefulness of the laser light-scattering technique in testing the toxic effect of chemicals on sperm motility. They also felt that another important application of this method could be to biologically monitor the effect of chemicals on sperm motility in the work place. They stated "This would be very important if the effect on sperm motility proves to be the 'critical effect' that is reversible and that appears before other deleterious effects of toxic chemicals."(136)

One other aspect of the effect of mercurials on sperm involves research indicating that both inorganic mercury and organic mercury can inhibit the synthesis of DNA (deoxyribonucleic acid) in spermatogonia.(130) As DNA is the carrier of genetic information, it is apparent that if mercury can inhibit the ability of DNA to multiply or replicate, the consequences on reproduction could be significant. This aspect of the effect of mercury on the spermatogonia is also in agreement with the work of Sakai and Takeuchi (1972).(137) Other published studies have shown the inhibition of both DNA and RNA synthesis (138), as well as meiotic cell arrests.(139) Lehninger stated: "The nucleic acids, DNA and RNA, have the same universal functions in all cells, to participate in the storage, transmission, and translation of genetic information. DNA serves as the repository of genetic information, whereas different kinds of RNAs help translate this information into protein structure."(13)

We don't mean to imply that all the research published on mercury's effects on fertility has indicated that either inorganic or organic mercury have categorically caused lethal or mutagenic effects on male sperm. There are several studies that show it had no or minimal effect on subsequent serial mating experiments. It would take a team of impartial scientists to evaluate the validity and correctness of the protocols utilized in the various studies and then compare them to each other.

Our intent is merely to show that there is sufficient scientific evidence to warrant the most serious consideration of the hypothesis that the chronic release of mercury vapor from mercury amalgam dental fillings may be a major etiological factor in male reproductive dysfunction. It would certainly appear that the state-of-the-art laboratory techniques are adequate to determine whether heavy metals per se are a factor in those males who have already been medically diagnosed as having a reproductive dysfunction related to sperm motility. It would also appear to be a rather inexpensive study to then determine epidemiologically, within this same group of dysfunctional males, those individuals with toxic metals in their mouths. It would certainly go a long way toward providing acceptable scientific data clarifying the hypothesis.

You probably wonder why we occasionally use the term "heavy metals." The term is used because there are other metals that can also impact or affect the same biological systems that mercury does. An excellent review of this subject entitled "Environmental metals and male reproduction" has been presented by I.P. Lee in a 1983 book.(127) Dr. Lee, in his review on the effects of lead, cites published research that indicates: (1) 94% of testicular samples contained a median lead concentration of 12 micrograms per gram and 88% of the prostate samples contained 10 micrograms per gram of lead; (2) lead was found in the tail of the spermatozoa; (3) in animal studies when blood levels were greater than 30 micrograms per 100 milliliters, there was a twofold increase in the size of prostate glands due to prostatic hyperplasia, and the sperm were less mobile.

Dr. Lee, in his discussion of multigeneration studies of male rats exposed to oral lead intake where fertility decreased to 65% of the control level, brings out a very important consideration. He stated: "These results suggest that potential risk may be realized eventually by human offspring born from fathers occupationally exposed to significant concentrations of lead." Dr. Lee then cites research suggesting that the prevalence of sterile marriages, abortions, and stillbirths is thought to be related to toxic effects of lead on the testes of male lead workers.(127)

In an earlier study on lead by Lancranjan et al. (1975), the reproductive ability of 150 men occupationally exposed to lead was studied by clinical and toxicological analysis. The findings of this study revealed that: (1) lead poisoning, as well as moderate increased absorption of lead, decreased the fertile ability of men. The researchers found low sperm counts, a reduction in the vitality of the sperm, and malformed sperm; (2) slight increases in lead absorption did not significantly influence the fertile ability; and (3) hypofertility induced by lead is probably due to its direct toxic effect on the gonads, as no interference with the hypothalamo-pituitary axis was evident.(140)

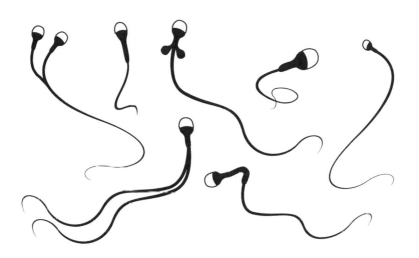

Figure 8-1: Normal and abnormal sperm. Different forms of sperm abnormality. Clinically, a man is considered sterile if more than 25% of his sperm are abnormal.

We would also like to point out that lead has many of the same biochemical pathways in the human body as does mercury, including a similar affinity for sulfur-containing protein molecules. Research is just beginning to appear examining the toxicological effects of lead and mercury present at the same time. Preliminary evidence seems to indicate that the sum of the two is more toxic than either individually.

The body is provided with some safety systems to take care of, or accommodate, toxic chemicals. One of these systems centers around the mineral selenium. Selenium has the ability to bind with the mercury molecule, forming a complex that is not considered to be toxic. In the process, of course, the selenium itself is rendered ineffective to perform its normal biological functions.

Recent animal studies have indicated that selenium is involved in the processes of the male reproductive system, and that selenium accumulated in the testes, where it was sub-sequently incorporated into developing spermatozoa.(141) Other studies demonstrated that rats that had been fed selenium-deficient diets over a long period of time produced sperm that had motility dysfunction and also pathologic damage.(142) It also seemed that a regulatory mechanism existed giving priority to the testes for selenium supplies at the expense of other tissues.(141) The implication in some of these findings indicates that selenium may be necessary for normal development of spermatozoa.(143) Based on the applicability of animal data to humans, it would seem reasonable to assume that chronic exposure to mercury, which also has an affinity for the testes, would bind with a great deal of the available selenium, in effect causing a deficiency of this essential element. Here again, we are only pointing out the complexity of the problem.

Although not directly related as a cause of infertility, the following study does bring out the fact that mercury has many deleterious effects on the body, not the least of which may be impotence. McFarland and Reigel (1978) (144) have described the loss of libido in six men (with no known previous exposure) poisoned by a single eight-hour exposure to metallic mercury vapor that resulted from an industrial accident. Nine men on the work shift were exposed to the vapor. Six of the nine were subsequently hospitalized with symptoms of acute mercury poisoning. All six men were followed medically for a number of years. All six complained of nervousness, irritability, lack of ambition, and loss of sexual desire. The authors suggested that the persistence of these symptoms following a brief exposure to mercury vapor indicates chronic mercury poisoning.

The authors' suggestion that the men had chronic mercury poisoning would be very easy to explain if it had been ascertained that the men all had amalgam fillings in their teeth.

This is explained by the fact that there are three phases involved in the elimination of mercury from the body, the last of which is a very slow phase. This slowest phase has a half-life in the body of 100 days.(145) This means it would take more than 100 days for half of a single dose of mercury to be eliminated from the body. Consequently, if you have amalgam fillings releasing mercury vapor, the slowest phase of each dose inhaled would have a half-life of at least 100 days. You would be accumulating mercury, in various storage depots in the body, over the lifetime of the amalgam fillings as long as they were present in the mouth.

THE FEMALE REPRODUCTIVE SYSTEM

There is practically no data available on the possible impact of elemental mercury vapor on female fertility. Of course, defining the cause of female infertility is much more complicated than investigating the effect of mercury on male sperm. To our knowledge only one study has investigated the effect of elemental mercury vapor and the female reproductive function. It was done in 1973 by Baranski and Symczyk.(146) The researchers exposed twenty-four female rats to elemental mercury vapor for 6-8 weeks before mating. The animals were exposed six hours a day to a concentration of 0.3 parts per million. There were twenty-four control female rats that were not exposed to any mercury vapor.

There were twenty-four rats in each group at the start of the experiment. However, the authors only state that eighteen of the exposed group mated and became pregnant, whereas twenty-three of the nonexposed group mated and became pregnant, indicating that 25% of the exposed group became infertile.

Their findings indicated that exposure to mercury vapor had a major effect on postnatal mortality. In the first four days after birth, 26% of the offspring from the mercury vapor exposed group died, compared with only 1% of the nonexposed control offspring. The mercury vapor did not appear to have any effect on the total number in the litter or the numbers alive at birth but autopsy evaluations done at two months of age indicated the females from the mercury-exposed group had much lower kidney and liver weights and significantly higher ovary weights than their counterparts in the control group. There also was a considerable reduction in female fertility within the exposed group and a significant increase in the estrus cycle of the exposed females (the period of sexual receptivity).

In other studies, Lamperti and Prinz (147,148) injected hamsters with inorganic mercury (mercuric chloride). They used radiolabeled mercury and radioautography to determine the transport and deposition of the mercury after injection. In studying the ovaries they found that there was a concentration in the corpora lutea rather than the follicles, which inhibited ovulation. They also found mercury in the hypothalamus and anterior pituitary and concluded from the series of experiments that the primary effect of mercury is at the hypothalamic and/or pituitary levels. In other words, it is an indirect effect. Mercury affected the hypothalamus and/or the pituitary, which in turn did not provide the right chemical hormonal signal to the ovaries, thereby diminishing their reproductive function.

In the sexually mature female, fertility is dependent on the functional integration of the hypothalamus, pituitary, ovary, and uterus. It all begins with the secretion of a hormone (gonadotropin releasing hormone), which then stimulates the pituitary to release two of its hormones (follicle stimulating hormone and luteinizing hormone). The latter hormones stimulate production of estrogen which, through a feedback mechanism to the pituitary, increases the release of luteinizing hormone. The surge of luteinizing hormone, in turn, starts a series of events culminating with the release of the egg selected to ovulate.(149-151) In a 1983 book on reproductive toxicology, Smith suggests that interruption of these hormonal pathways by xenobiotics will disrupt the female reproductive function.(152)

There is some indication in the literature that female menstrual cycle disturbances may be involved as a cause factor in infertility. We therefore felt that it would be appropriate to include in this chapter those studies indicating an increase in menstrual cycle disturbances for women who are occupationally exposed to mercury vapor.

Mikhailova et al. (1971) reported menstrual disturbances in 26.8% of women working in an atmosphere polluted with mercury vapor.(153) Marinova et al. (1973) studied 111 women who were occupationally exposed to mercury vapor and thirty women used as controls (not occupationally exposed). The exposed women were working with mercury in dentistry or in mercury rectifier stations. Almost 29% of the mercury-exposed group had hypermenorrhoea, whereas only 0.3% of the controls had the same condition. (*Hypermenorrhoea* is defined by *Dorland's Medical Dictionary* (154) as "excessive uterine bleeding occurring at regular intervals, the period of flow being of usual duration.")

Hypomenorrhea (less than the normal amount of bleeding) occurred in 15.3% of the exposed group and only 0.6% in the controls.(155)

Panova and Dimitrov (1974) investigated menstrual function in seventy-four women between the ages of 20 and 40 who were employed in the manufacture of fluorescent lamps. The exposed group was compared against 100 women of similar ages who were working in a tailoring and clothing business. The incidence of menstrual disturbances was determined by questionnaires. Answers from the exposed group (exposed for more than six months) indicated 36.5% had some type of menstrual problem. The most common problems were little or scanty periods or reduced blood flow, and less commonly, excessive blood flow, or normal blood flow but at irregular intervals, and painful menstruation.(156)

The researchers then carried out microscopic evaluations of vaginal cells taken from sixty of the exposed women during two successive menstrual cycles and in one menstrual cycle for the controls. Relative to the infertility issue, they found the incidence of anovulation (not accompanied with the discharge of an ovum) in the mercury exposed group was 46.7% for the first cycle and 43.3% on the second cycle, while the incidence was only 27% in the control group.(156)

In a 1977 study, Goncharuk investigated menstrual function in 196 women exposed to mercury vapor through the preparation of mercury ore for smelting and in other jobs related to the processing of mercury ore. The exposed women were compared with 204 controls who did not come into contact with mercury in their work. Of the exposed women, 44.7% had menstrual disturbances (67% occurring in women exposed more than three years), compared with only 18.6% of the controls. The most common problems were painful menstruation (dysmenorrhoea) and excessive blood flow with a normal menstrual cycle (hypermenorrhoea).(157)

With regard to the effects of lead on the female reproductive function, a 1986 study done in China by Yang Shixian brings home the point clearly. Although this study was based on industrial exposure, it serves to demonstrate the importance of also considering lead exposure. The study involved 1886 women who were exposed to lead in the work place and 852 controls. The results showed that the incidence of abnormal menstruation, dysmenorrhea, premenstrual tension, and toxemia were significantly higher in the subjects than in the control group. The menstrual disturbances occurred more frequently among young workers and among those with fewer working years.(158)

SPONTANEOUS ABORTION/MISCARRIAGE

The United States Environmental Protection Agency states that "women chronically exposed to mercury vapor experienced increased frequencies of menstrual disturbances and spontaneous abortions; also, a high mortality rate was observed among infants born to women who displayed symptoms of mercury poisoning."(18) This chilling pronouncement is supported by documented studies.

In 1950, Derobert and Tara reported the case of a woman chronically poisoned by mercury vapor who experienced two pregnancies that ended unfavorably. She gave birth to a healthy child after recovery from the overt mercury poisoning.(159)

In 1967, an epidemiological survey was conducted in Lithuania on women working in dental offices where mercury vapor concentrations were lower than 0.08 milligrams per cubic meter. The women experienced an increased incidence of spontaneous abortion and breast pathology that was related to the length of time on the job.(160)

Baranski and Szymczyk (1973) exposed female rats to mercury vapor and found that the rats had longer estrus cycles.

The offspring of these rats died within six days after birth.(146)

Mishonova and associates, in 1980, studied the course of pregnancy and delivery in 349 women exposed via inhalation to low concentrations of mercury vapor in the work place, compared to a control group of 215 nonexposed women. They concluded that the rates of pregnancy and labor complications were higher in the exposed women and depended on the length and concentration of the mercury vapor exposure. The placentas of the exposed women showed signs of functional and structural inadequacy and of compensatory adaptation. In addition, immune disturbances in the mother-fetus system were found at the cellular level.(161)

The incidence of spontaneous abortions in four groups of female workers was studied in Denmark in 1984.(162) Heidam, the author, concluded that the dental assistant group, who were exposed to mercury and nitrous oxide, did not show an increased rate of spontaneous abortions compared to the reference group, which had a rate of 10.0%. Private clinic dental assistants had a rate of 11.2%, and schoolservice dental assistants had a rate of 9.7%. However, the author also examined the rate of spontaneous abortions in female factory workers, painters, and gardening workers and compared them to a different reference group, which exhibited a rate of 7.1%. It would seem that the two groups of dental assistants would have exhibited a significantly higher rate of spontaneous abortions compared to the reference group used for the other three subject groups. The author gave no explanation for the use of two separate reference groups with such divergent rates of spontaneous abortions.(162) Unfortunately, no consideration was given to the numbers and surfaces of mercury amalgam dental fillings implanted in the study subjects. It may have possibly explained why there was so little difference between the dental assistants and their reference group.

In 1981, the International Conference on Mercury Hazards in Dental Practice was held in Glasgow, Scotland. One of the papers presented was entitled "Pregnancy In Female Dentists -- A Mercury Hazard?" by H. Gordon.(163) The reported findings were:

1. Female dentists had a higher rate of spontaneous abortions than a control group of female medical personnel. This increase was especially evident in first pregnancies. The abortion rate in the female dentists was also higher than large population studies reported from Aberdeen, New York, and two large series of private patients in the United States.

2. The perinatal mortality rate for the dentists was 19.5 per 1000, which was significantly higher than the rate for Social Class I in Great Britain, which was 7.5 per 1,000. The rate for Social Class III was 19.6 per 1,000.

The author stated that "it does therefore seem that female dentists who work have a higher than expected incidence of spontaneous abortion and premature labour and perhaps a high perinatal mortality," then blithely concluded that "there is no absolute evidence that mercury is a major factor in the poor reproductive performance of female dentists." Strange logic!!!

Further evidence of the manipulative reasoning of defenders of dental mercury may be found in the November 1985 issue of the *Journal of the American Dental Association* (JADA), Volume 111. A questionnaire survey was mailed to 29,514 male dentists and 30,272 female dental assistants with the expressed goal of examining the "relationship of mercury exposure and pregnancy outcome among dental professionals and their spouses."(164) More than 70%

of the dentists (21,634) and dental assistants (21,202) completed and returned the questionnaire, which was designed to determine the incidence of spontaneous abortions and congenital abnormalities. The authors concluded that "there were no increased rates of spontaneous abortions or congenital abnormalities in the children of men and women who were exposed to low versus high levels of mercury in a dental environment."

An analysis of this study and its methodology casts doubt on the validity of that conclusion. The study subjects were originally divided into three mercury exposure groups, one of which was a no exposure group, but was subsequently revised into two groups. Wives of dentists and dental assistants who placed 0-40 amalgam fillings per week were placed in the "low direct and indirect exposure groups"; those who placed more than forty amalgam fillings per week were placed in the "high direct and indirect exposure groups." The authors stated that "as few dental professionals (less than 10%) reported no exposure to mercury, the zero and low mercury exposure groups were combined for statistical comparison."

The data provided by the authors shows that 17,171 of the 21,634 responding wives of dentists were included in the analysis, but only 7,384 of the 21,202 responding assistants were included. No explanation for this disparity was given. Moreover, 10% of the respondents would total more than 2,000 of each group reporting no exposure to mercury, certainly a sufficient control population. Even so, general population rates for these conditions are readily available. Further, the division of the two exposure groups is extremely broad. In essence, the "low" and "high" exposure groups in this study may well have averaged placing thirty-nine and forty-one amalgam fillings per week, hardly a scientifically valid comparison. One can only wonder why the authors did not compare subjects to controls or general population rates. If anything, all that the study demonstrated was that exposure to smaller levels of mercury vapor (thirty-nine fillings per week) is no less harmful than exposure to higher levels of mercury vapor (forty or more fillings per week).

INFERTILITY AND ENDOMETRIOSIS

Endometriosis is being treated separately because it affects so many women. Data indicates it is a major cause of infertility and pregnancy loss after implantation. We are also proposing that mercury and lead may be hidden or unrecognized factors in the development of the disease.

Endometriosis is a disease in which the tissue that forms the lining of the uterus (endometrium) spreads to organs outside the womb or diffuses and infiltrates into the myometrium. The cause of endometriosis is unknown.(165) It is apparent that nobody really knows the true magnitude of the problem. One report states that endometriosis may affect 1% of women in the United States, and that it is believed to cause 30-40% of female infertility.(166) Other reports indicate there may be as many as twelve million American women who are suffering from endometriosis with many of them not being aware that they have it. For this reason, endometriosis has been named "the hidden disease." Although very common in women between the ages of 30 and 40, endometriosis affects women of all ages.

During every menstrual cycle, the lining of the uterus undergoes physiologic changes that result in an increase in tissue and blood vessels in preparation to receive and nurture a fertilized egg. If fertilization does not occur, then the blood supply to the endometrium is reduced and the tissue detaches and is expelled as the menstrual blood. These physiologic changes that occur are thought to be controlled hormonally by the ebb and flow of estrogen and progesterone through a feedback loop to the hypothalamus and pituitary.(167)

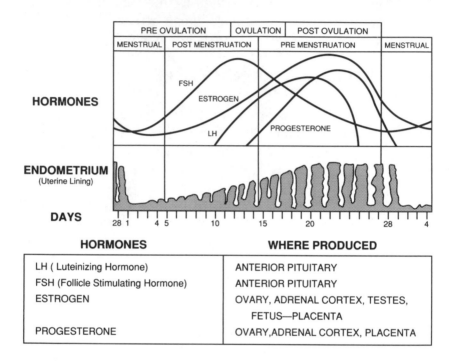

HORMONES	WHERE PRODUCED
LH (Luteinizing Hormone)	ANTERIOR PITUITARY
FSH (Follicle Stimulating Hormone)	ANTERIOR PITUITARY
ESTROGEN	OVARY, ADRENAL CORTEX, TESTES, FETUS—PLACENTA
PROGESTERONE	OVARY,ADRENAL CORTEX, PLACENTA

Figure 8-2: The effect of glandular function and hormones on the endometrial lining of the uterus.

There are several schools of thought related to the etiology of endometriosis. One theory relates the increased incidence of the disease to the changes in our society associated with the women's movement. More women are opting for careers in business and deferring the decision to have a child until much later in life. As a result, some physicians now refer to endometriosis as "the career woman's disease" because of the greatly increased incidence of the disease found in career women. The tremendously increased stress of competing in the work or marketplace causes stress-related changes in normal balances of hormones, vitamins, and minerals.

Dr. Niels Lauersen describes one effect of stress: "It seems that the figures on endometriosis are being pushed upward by the fact that today there are fewer pregnancies, and fewer women on the pill, and lifestyles are often more stressful." Dr. Lauersen feels that once women are under stress, their bodies secrete more steroid hormones from the adrenal glands. These steroid hormones decrease the amount of immune antibodies that a woman produces. Dr. Lauersen concluded: "Since immune antibodies are needed in full force to reject any foreign tissue, as well as to kill infection and viruses, a stressed woman with reduced antibodies will obviously have a hard time protecting herself against endometriosis."(168)

Although the above theory holds that increased stress is the cause for an increased incidence of endometriosis, it appears that the underlying physiological cause may indeed be a diminished immune function. In this regard, there have been several recent scientific reports also suggesting that endometriosis is linked to abnormal immune function.(467,470)

The nagging question that needs to be answered is why do some women get endometriosis and others don't? The ability of a cell or tissue to grow and proliferate in an abnormal location is considered a phenomenon related to some defect or impairment of the immune system. In a normally functioning immune system, it has to be assumed that the foreign tissue--in this case, the presence of endometrium tissue outside the uterus--would be recognized as foreign and rejected. However, in the case of endometriosis, it could also be assumed there is some deficiency in the immune system that does not recognize the displaced endometrium cells as foreign, or the immune system has been weakened to the point that it is unable to effectively control the displaced cells and therefore allows them to proliferate.

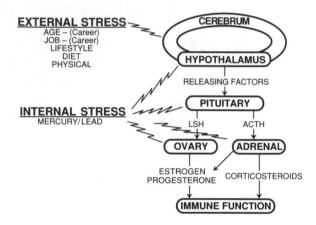

Figure 8-3: Female endocrine stress factors. External stress that affects the hypothalaumus. Internal stress can be applied by mercury and lead through its presence within the producing gland. The end result of chronic stress can be suppression of immune function.

Such a hypothesis was advanced by Dmowski et al. in 1981. In their study, utilizing rhesus monkeys with spontaneous endometriosis, they were able to demonstrate that the animals with the disease responded with a lesser lymphocytic reaction to injected endometrial antigens as compared to control animals. Assuming their hypothesis is correct, then implantation of the endometrial fragments in an abnormal location should occur only in women with a specific type of cell-mediated immunodeficiency. They conclude their study with the following statement: "If endometriosis, as we postulate, is associated with a deficiency in cellular immunity, women afflicted with this disease may have an incidence or a natural course of allergic, autoimmune, or neoplastic diseases different from that of the general population."(169)

We consider the work of Dmowski et al. to be very significant in relation to the basic hypothesis of this book and specifically to the scientific data documenting a suppression of immune function by both mercury and lead as described in Chapter 7.

One of the immune aspects of infertility that has been documented since the turn of the century is the fact that sperm antigens could induce an antibody response resulting in infertility or subfertility. An antigen is defined as any substance capable of inducing the formation of antibodies. An antibody is defined as an immunoglobulin molecule that is produced by the body in response to specific antigens. It has a specific amino acid structure that causes it to interact only with the antigen that induced its synthesis. The immune system of the body is extremely complex but an oversimplified view of it would be that any time there is a foreign substance present, the body initiates a whole cascade of actions designed to immobilize and reject the intruder.

In a recent review of the subject, Sogar (1987) brings out the following points:

1. Male reproductive tissues have long been recognized as antigenic. This includes both the spermatozoa and the seminal plasma.

2. There is a "blood-testis barrier" that should prevent the man from becoming autosensitized to his own sperm. Any breech of the blood-testis barrier can lead to sensitization.

3. Three mechanisms whereby autoimmunity to spermatozoa may interfere with fertility are possible: (1) interference with the production of normal numbers of spermatozoa, (2) reduction in migratory potential of spermatozoa, and (3) impairment of the interaction of spermatozoa with the ovum.(170)

The female genital tract can also have an immune response to the sperm, which is, in effect, an antigenic or foreign substance to the woman. The human cervix is also capable of a local immune response. In other words, women can have antisperm antibodies. Infertile women appear to have higher levels of antisperm antibodies, which could be a cause of their infertility. However, it appears that the issue is much more complex than the presence of antisperm antibodies within the genital tract. Two recent studies bring out the fact that the persistent leakage of sperm components into the general immune system will cause the formation of circulating antigen-antibody complexes. Further, that with an antigen excess, all the antibody will be present in the form of circulating immune complexes.(171,172) Just to make things more perplexing, Witkins et al. (1984) bring out the conflicting facts that although immune complexes are present in 38% of infertile women and in only 3% of fertile women, both groups had approximately the same levels of sperm antibodies. They go on to say, however, that circulating immune complexes without sperm-related components could also contribute to decreased fertility.(173) Circulating immune complexes of mercury and/or lead would fit the latter comment.

As brought out previously in this chapter, the male ejaculate and seminal fluid contains many heavy metals. Could the presence of some of these metals in the fluid and sperm be the factor triggering an immune response in the woman? Is it one particular metallic ion or is it a specific combination of ions that causes the rejection of the sperm in infertile women? These are interesting questions, especially when viewed in context with the information brought out in Chapter 7 regarding the number of individuals in the United States who may be hypersensitive to mercury. The percentage of those affected could range as high as 22.5%, encompassing as many as 30 million individuals. Based on the research that we present later in this chapter, many women could have existent metallic ion antibodies to mercury and/or lead or immune complexes circulating in their blood prior to their first experience with male sperm.

The failure of your own immune system to differentiate between a foreign substance and your body's own tissue is a phenomenon called *autoimmunity*. An autoimmune response occurs when your body's immune system produces antibodies or immune lymphoid cells against the body's own tissues. This can result in hypersensitivity reactions, or if severe, in autoimmune disease. There are several diseases that are now viewed as being related to the autoimmune response phenomenon and two of these--systemic lupus erythematosus, or SLE a generalized connective tissue disorder, and rheumatoid arthritis--are thought to relate to circulating immune complexes.(103)

Therefore, it appears that there are two separate aspects of autoimmunity that exist. The first is that your immune system may not actually recognize or identify a foreign substance, or you have an acquired immune deficiency and your immune system is weakened and therefore does not respond immunologically. The second aspect is just the opposite; that is, your immune system recognizes your own tissue as a foreign substance and responds immunologically, attempting to destroy or reject it in much the same way that transplanted organs are rejected.

In a July 1987 study entitled "Is Endometriosis an Autoimmune Disease?" Gleicher and his associates evaluated fifty-nine endometriosis patients for the presence of autoantibodies. The authors felt the results of their study suggested that endometriosis is associated with abnormal polyclonal B cell activation, a classic characteristic of autoimmune disease.(174)

From the data presented here, it is apparent that immune dysfunction must seriously be considered as an etiological factor in endometriosis. It is also evident that the ability of environmental mercury, lead, and mercury vapor from mercury amalgam dental fillings to alter or suppress immune function should also be considered in a causal relationship when evaluating immune dysfunction of endometriosis patients.

The remaining piece of the immune dysfunction and endometriosis puzzle, which we will now try to put together, relates to how mercury and lead may be involved in the sequence of events leading to endometriosis.

To start with, stress affects the adrenal glands which ultimately can cause an immune dysfunction. During stress, the adrenal glands increase in size as a normal reaction in order to produce more steroids (hormones). Both physical and physiological stress will stimulate the adrenal glands. The outer shell of the adrenal gland is called the cortex and the inner core of the gland is called the medulla. The cortex produces three types of steroids called glucocorticoids. Cortisone is a corticoid essential to life, and functions to maintain stress reactions. Mineral corticoids, such as aldosterone, regulate the balance of blood electrolytes and also cause the kidneys to retain sodium and excrete potassium and hydrogen. They are also involved in gluconeogenesis, which is the process whereby your body converts glycogen to glucose (blood sugar). Small amounts of corticoid sex hormones, both male and female, are also produced by the adrenal cortex.(167)

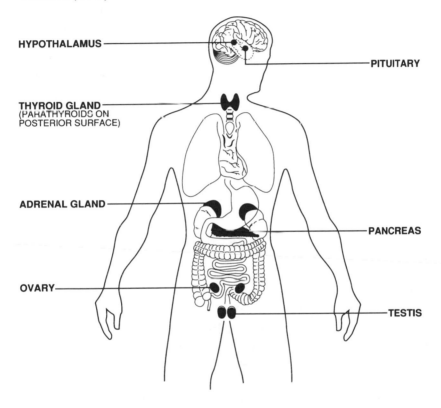

HYPOTHALAMUS

PITUITARY

THYROID GLAND
(PARATHYROIDS ON
POSTERIOR SURFACE)

ADRENAL GLAND

PANCREAS

OVARY

TESTIS

Figure 8-4: Endocrine glands and their locations.

Two primary nutrients for the adrenal glands are pantothenic acid and ascorbic acid (vitamin C). A deficiency of pantothenic acid can lead to adrenal exhaustion and ultimately to destruction of the adrenal glands. A deficiency of pantothenic acid also causes a progressive fall in the level of adrenal hormones produced.(175) One of the largest tissue stores of vitamin C is in the adrenals; it is exceeded only by the level of vitamin C in the pituitary. Physical and mental stress increases the excretion of adrenocorticotropin hormone (ACTH) from the pituitary, which is the hormone that tells the adrenals to increase their activity. The increased adrenal activity in turn depletes both vitamin C and pantothenic acid from the gland. Humans cannot produce vitamin C and attempt to replenish the ascorbic acid needs of the adrenals by taking it from other storage locations in the body. If your overall ascorbate status is low, there may be an insufficient amount available to satisfy the needs of the adrenals. Under these conditions, normal adrenal hormone response may become inadequate.(176,177) This could then also lead to an inadequate immune function. Mercury depletes the adrenals of both pantothenic and ascorbic acid (see Chapter 11). We also know that mercury accumulates in the pituitary, but at this point, there is only very limited data describing its effect on ACTH production. Stress and the presence of mercury would have a very negative effect on the adrenal production of critical steroids. Therefore, if you are under chronic stress, as women are who are infertile or who are competing actively in the business world, and also have a mouthful of mercury amalgam dental fillings chronically releasing mercury vapor, your adrenal glands could be in double jeopardy of developing some dysfunction.

The ability of the adrenal gland to produce steroids is called steroidogenesis and is dependent upon reactions mediated by the enzyme cytochrome P-450. Cytochrome P-450 reacts with cholesterol to produce pregnenolone, which is then converted to progesterone. (The adrenal glands use cholesterol as the base material to manufacture steroids.) Cytochrome P-450 can then convert progesterone to deoxycorticosterone which is then converted to corticosterone or aldosterone by other enzymes in the adrenals. It is generally thought that these adrenal reactions are controlled by the pituitary through the release of ACTH. However, recent research has shown that these adrenal functions can also be affected by metal ions.

In a study with rats, Veltman and Maines (1986) demonstrated that mercury altered heme (heme is the iron pigment portion of the hemoglobin molecule) and cytochrome P-450 metabolism in the adrenal glands. The presence of mercury in the gland altered the ability of the adrenals to produce steroid hormones, which in turn resulted in marked changes of adrenocortical hormones in the plasma. It appeared that mercury had a direct action effect on the adrenal gland itself, as well as markedly reducing the concentration of intact cytochrome P-450. It was also shown that mercury reduced the activity of another critical enzyme identified as 21a-hydroxylase. In humans, a deficiency of 21a-hydroxylase activity is reflected by increased circulating concentrations of both adrenal androgens (male hormones) and progesterone. Veltman and Maines conclude their article as follows: "The present findings strongly suggest that Hg^{2+} could adversely affect the function and the homeostatic control of the adrenal cortex which, in turn could elicit severe physiological consequences. The diminished level of plasma corticosterone along with the increase in the concentrations of progesterone and dehydroepiandrosterone in the plasma of the Hg^{2+}-treated rats clearly indicates that the normal pattern of steroid biosynthesis had become disrupted."(178)

There is another factor that must be considered at this point--alcoholism. It has been estimated that about 50% of all American women experience premenstrual tension syndrome (PMS or PMTS), which occurs during the luteal phase of the menstrual cycle (when the corpus luteum in the ovary is active and has discharged the ovum). Within the group of women in the United States of reproductive age, it has been estimated that two million of them may be alcoholic.

Of this number, 67% relate their drinking to the anxiety and depression experienced during the menstrual cycle.(179)

Although we suspect that there may be direct correlations between PMS and mercury, our concern in discussing alcohol at this point deals with its effect on the distribution of mercury in the body. In a recent study with rats and monkeys, Khayat and Dencker (1984) demonstrated that inhaled mercury vapor (the same as released by mercury amalgam dental fillings) accumulated in the adrenal glands and the corpora lutea of the ovaries. The adrenal cortex portion of the adrenal gland was responsible for most of the oxidation of the mercury vapor into mercuric ions. However, in the monkey, large concentrations were also found in the adrenal medulla. In the ovary, high concentrations were seen in the corpora lutea but not in the follicles. As opposed to other organs measured for mercury content, when alcohol was administered to the animals there was an increased concentration of mercury in the liver and adrenals. The authors felt that the presence of mercury in the endocrine organs may put the active cells (those that produce hormones) at high risk.(65)

It is apparent that the above data applies to a great percentage of American women of reproductive age who (1) have a mouthful of mercury amalgam dental fillings chronically releasing mercury vapor that is being inhaled and may be accumulating in their pituitary, adrenal glands, and ovaries; (2) are not eating a diet rich in vitamin C or pantothenic acid; (3) engage in structured exercise programs (physical stress); (4) drink alcohol in more than social quantities; (5) have deferred the decision to bear children until some future date; (6) are competing in the business world and work place (mental stress); and (7) have increased tension and anxiety related to PMS during their menstrual periods. All of these factors have the potential of affecting proper functioning of the adrenal glands that may lead to hormonal imbalances and immune dysfunction. Is the woman that fits the above description at greater risk of having endometriosis? It is certainly a question that must be viewed seriously, and epidemiological studies to investigate the potential should receive the highest priority for funding.

There is another aspect of immunity and endometriosis that we feel bears directly on the information already provided, and that is the interaction between the reproductive and immune systems. Both clinical and experimental evidence support the theory that gonadal steroid hormones--estrogen, androgen, and progesterone--regulate immune function. In an excellent review of the subject, Grossman (1985) brings out the following points: (1) Immunoglobulin production is greater in females than in males; (2) in mice, estrogens enhance the antibody response. Estrogens also seem to regulate the synthesis of uterine IgA and IgG in rats; (3) research has suggested that estradiol can inhibit suppressor T-cell activity, which leads to an increase in B-cell antibody production; (4) lupus erythematosus is more prevalent in females than in males, and that androgens depress and estrogens accelerate the disease process; (5) women have a greater incidence of rheumatoid arthritis and in many women using oral contraceptives, joint inflammation is reduced; (6) the thymus gland has steroid receptors for estrogen, androgen, and progesterone and two studies have shown estrogen and androgen receptors in T cells; (7) progesterone prolongs survival of allografts and can act as an immunosuppressive agent on lymphocytes stimulated by an allogenic antigen (cell types that are antigenically distinct); (8) in the absence of suppressor T cell and the presence of helper T cell, B cells produce autoantibody to oocytes" (eggs); and (9) the ratio of estrogen to androgen may determine whether the circulating hormones will stimulate or inhibit the immune response.(180)

Since any metabolic disturbance that affects the production of sex hormones has the capability of causing these and other pathological and physiological changes it is important at this point to evaluate how mercury and/or lead may affect these processes.

The major regulator of adrenalcortical growth and secretion activity is the pituitary hormone ACTH. ACTH attaches to receptors on the surface of the adrenal cortical cell and activates an enzymatic action that ultimately produces cyclic adenosine monophosphate (cAMP). cAMP, in turn, serves as a cofactor in activating key enzymes in the adrenal cortex. The adrenal cortex is able to synthesize cholesterol and to also take it up from circulation. All steroid hormones produced by the adrenal glands are derived from cholesterol through a series of enzymatic actions, which are all stimulated initially by ACTH. Steroid biosynthesis involves the conversion of cholesterol to pregnenolone, which is then enzymatically transformed into the major biologically active corticosteroids.(167)

There are two aspects of the above biochemical activities that research has shown can be affected by mercury and/or lead. The first relates to the production of ACTH by the pituitary. cAMP is produced from adenosine triphosphate (ATP) by the action of adenyl cyclase. In a 1980 report, Ewers and Erbe demonstrated that adenylate cyclase activity in the brain was inhibited by micromolar concentrations of lead, mercury, and cadmium. Another finding of their study was that brain activity of phosphodiesterase was also reduced 10-20%. Interestingly, the function of the enzyme phosphodiesterase is to inactivate cAMP.(181,182)

One of the key biochemical steps in the conversion of adrenal pregnenolone to cortisol and aldosterone involves an enzyme identified as 21-hydroxylase. As reported previously, Veltman and Maines demonstrated that mercury caused a defect in adrenal steroid biosynthesis by inhibiting the activity of 21a-hydroxylase. The consequences of this inhibition included lowered plasma levels of corticosterone and elevated concentrations of progesterone and dehydroepiandrosterone (DHEA). DHEA is an adrenal male hormone.(178) Because patients with 21-hydroxylase deficiencies are incapable of synthesizing cortisol with normal efficiency, there is a compensatory increase in ACTH leading to adrenal hyperplasia and excessive excretion of 17a-hydroxyprogesterone, which without the enzyme 21-hydroxylase cannot ultimately be converted to cortisol. It is interesting to note that in the case of congenital adrenal hyperplasia,infertility was the rule until glucocorticoid substitution therapy was instituted to suppress excessive adrenal androgen production.(167) Other scientific data has demonstrated that mercury can cause adrenal hyperplasia. The suppression or inhibition of the 21-hydroxylase system may be the mechanism behind the mercury-induced adrenal hyperplasia, the cause of which has not previously been identified. We should also point out that adrenal hyperplasia can stress the adrenal glands by their accelerated activity to produce steroids to the point that production begins to diminish and the glands will atrophy. The result is a subnormal production of corticosteroids. Thus it appears that both lead and mercury can precipitate pathophysiological changes along the hypothalamus-pituitary- adrenal and gonadal axis that may seriously affect reproductive function, organs, and tissues.

There is another effect of adrenal steroids on the body that is of great importance--the effect of corticosteroids on the immune function, which may also be involved in the mechanisms of endometriosis. Leukocyte production, distribution, and function are markedly altered by glucocorticosteroid administration. The most easily measured effects of steroids on leukocytes are changes in blood cell counts. In Addison's disease (hypofunction of the adrenal glands), for example, neutrophilia occurs 4-6 hours after administration of a single dose of hydrocortisone, prednisone, or dexamethasone.(167) Neutrophilia is an increase in the number of neutrophils in the blood. Neutrophils are also called - polymorphonuclear leukocytes (PMNs) .The initial immune response of PMNs to a foreign substance in the blood is a metabolic reaction called the "respiratory burst." Without this initial reaction, the PMNs cannot carry out their immune system function of destroying the foreign substance.(185) Mercury has been shown to inhibit the respiratory burst of PMNs.(183,184) It would appear, therefore, that mercury could not only cause a suppression of adrenalcorticosteroids that would normally have stimulated an increase of PMNs, but at the same time could also affect the ability of existing PMNs to perform their immune function by inhibiting their respiratory burst.

Systemic lupus erythematosus occurs more commonly in women of childbearing age than in others. This association has been reproduced in the mouse model for lupus nephritis. (These are mice that will develop destructive inflammation of the kidneys (nephritis) when exposed to autoantibodies.) Estrogens increased the production of anti-DNA antibodies and the progression of nephritis, whereas androgens had the opposite effect. Furthermore, in sensitive species such as the mouse, rat, and rabbits, humoral antibody response can be inhibited by steroid administration. However, once either the T or B cells have been activated by an antigen, they become steroid-resistant. (167) As mentioned earlier, mercury can cause anti-DNA antibodies.

Finally, what is the effect of increased production of progesterone in regard to endometriosis? The onset of normal menstruation is triggered by an abrupt decline in progesterone. If the duration of the luteal phase is lengthened by the presence of abnormal concentrations of progesterone, decidual changes in the endometrial stroma similar to those seen in early pregnancy can be induced.(186) During the second half of the follicular phase of the menstrual cycle, the increased plasma estrogen concentration causes a thirty-fold increase in endocervical mucus. Progesterone reverses the estrogen effect and the mucus decreases in amount and consistency.(186) Does the increased production of progesterone affect the cervical mucus to the point where the cervical opening does not let all the menstrual blood escape vaginally, thereby causing a portion of the blood-filled uterine lining to be pushed backward through the Fallopian tubes and subsequently spraying out of the tubes into the abdomen? Is this possibly one of the mechanisms whereby endometrial tissue is transplanted to areas outside of the uterus? Does the routine higher concentration of progesterone then cause the body to react as in a pseudopregnancy, causing metabolic changes in the displaced endometrial tissue similar to preparation for implantation of the egg?

In regard to this last question, there is an important immune function phenomenon that should also be considered. We would like to quote the following statement by Murad and Haynes: "While progesterone is very important for the maintenance of pregnancy, in part because it suppresses uterine contractility, other effects may be equally important. For example, progesterone may contribute to a state of transplantation immunity and prevent immunological rejection of the fetus (Siiteri et al., 1977)."(187) The question then is; Would increased concentrations of progesterone cause the immune system to react as in normal pregnancy where increased levels of progesterone are produced to maintain implantation in the uterus, thus permitting the displaced endometrial tissue to proliferate?

The last aspect we wish to cover is the effect of mercury on the release of follicle stimulating hormone (FSH) and luteinizing hormone (LH). The menstrual and reproductive cycles are controlled by a very complex feedback mechanism between the ovaries, hypothalamus, and the pituitary. In the case of FSH, there is a negative feedback relationship with estradiol at all times. However, with LH there is both a negative and positive feedback relationship; that is, when estrogen levels are low, the release of LH is increased, and when estrogen levels are high, LH is decreased. This ebb and flow controls the hormonal function leading to ovulation and the midcycle changes related to the luteal phase. It is also thought that the midcycle surge of both LH and FSH and the reduction of LH and FSH at the luteal phase relate to a feedback relationship with progesterone. Progesterone is not secreted by the ovary until just before ovulation. This in turn provokes changes in estrogen's effect on both LH and FSH. After ovulation, progesterone secretion undergoes a tremendous increase. The high levels of progesterone and estrogen associated with the luteal phase combine to suppress FSH and LH during the corpus luteum phase.(167,186)

Lamperti and Niewenhuis (1976) demonstrated that mercuric chloride administered to hamsters during one estrous cycle altered the responsiveness of the ovary to physiological levels of FSH. There was also a significantly higher level of FSH in the pituitaries, suggesting that mercury partially inhibits the release of FSH from the pituitary possibly by damaging the membranes of the cells in the anterior pituitary. The levels of LH in the pituitaries did not decrease. This would be expected because failure of FSH to stimulate estrogen secretion from the ovaries would affect the feedback relationship and fail to trigger the release of LH. The authors felt that it appeared from the results of their study that mercury may directly affect the responsiveness of the ovary and pituitary to hormonal stimulation.(188)

There are some additional relationships between mercury and the preceding data that are worthy of special consideration. The onset of clinically observable signs or symptoms of mercury toxicity may take as long as 20-30 years to appear, depending on a person's biochemical individuality. In individuals who inherit a strong genetic predisposition to good health and who practice sound dietary principles, the implantation of mercury amalgam dental fillings during childhood and progressively thereafter may not produce an observable effect for a number of years. However, we feel that the chronic inhalation of mercury vapor from such fillings for twenty years or more could result in accumulation of pathologic quantities of mercury in the brain and other critical organs and tissues. For example, human autopsy studies of accident victims have shown a positive correlation between the numbers of mercury amalgam dental fillings and the concentration of mercury in the brain.(62,63) Other human autopsy studies have shown accumulations of mercury in the kidneys, liver, heart, muscles, lungs, spleen, and pancreas,(189) as well as specific accumulations of mercury in the pituitary.(16,126) Primate studies have shown mercury accumulations in these locations as well as the nasal mucosa and trachea, thyroid, adrenal cortex, spinal ganglia and nerves, testes, ovaries, brown fat, bone marrow, and the eye.(65)

Based on the above, it would appear that the potential for a relationship to exist between the presence of mercury amalgam dental fillings from childhood and the higher incidence of endometriosis in women between the ages of 30 and 40 is very real. Further, it could also be the critical factor associated with the widespread prevalence of endometriosis as well as being the determining factor in why some women get the disease and others don't.

The increasing incidence of endometriosis among women of childbearing age, including those in their teens, could also be related to the presence of mercury amalgam dental fillings and biochemical individuality. In the younger group of women it could well be that their genetic predisposition to good health wasn't very strong at the outset. This inherent weakness could also have been aggravated by a diet centered around "fast foods." Imposition on these women of the additional mercury burden resulting from chronic inhalation of mercury vapor after implantation of mercury amalgam dental fillings during childhood could be sufficient to trigger some metabolic dysfunction that could manifest in much earlier symptomatology such as allergic or sensitive-type reactions, gingivitis, and others. It would therefore seem probable that these women would also experience a greater incidence of premenstrual syndrome and menstrual irregularities that could ultimately be involved in the development of endometriosis.

It should be obvious from the complexity of the physiological and pathophysiological aspects of the data presented that there is no simple answer to the cause of endometriosis. However, we do believe we have presented sufficient data to cause a serious consideration of the metallic ions of both mercury and lead as possible factors in the mechanisms that ultimately lead to endometriosis. The proof or disproof must now rest in the hands of unbiased research scientists who might be intrigued enough by some of the relationships advanced to initiate some detailed investigations.

SUMMARY

Two important aspects of the data presented in this chapter stand out and lend themselves to epidemiological study: (1) There are millions of infertile couples in the United States and it appears that 50% of the problem relates to male reproductive dysfunction; and (2) thirty to forty percent of female infertility is thought to be caused by endometriosis.

Scientific investigation of the biochemical and pathophysiologic effects of mercury and lead on the above two aspects of infertility should be given the greatest priority. It would appear that by using a simple questionnaire, meaningful and clinically useful data could be gathered through a retrospective study of the couples who are infertile. Sample questions could include:

1. Has the participant had any external exposure to mercury and/or lead or other heavy metals?

2. Has the participant had any dental fillings? If yes, how many of them were metal and what kind of metal was implanted?

3. At what age were the first mercury amalgam dental fillings implanted?

4. Did the participant have any dental prostheses?

5. If the participant is female, does she have endometriosis?

6. Do female participants experience any type of menstrual dysfunction and/or PMS?

The results of such a questionnaire would reveal the percentage of infertile males and females that had dental fillings and how many did not have any metals in their mouth. The study would also reveal the number of years metals were present in the oral environment. The researchers could then see if there were any correlations between both partners having amalgam fillings, one partner having amalgam fillings, whether in fact, gender made any difference, and so on. They might also be able to determine possible correlations between metals in the mouth and endometriosis, menstrual dysfunctions, or PMS.

If the findings of such a study showed a definite correlation between the presence of mercury amalgam dental fillings in the oral cavity and infertility, then additional research could be done on these individuals to see if the simple act of replacing their amalgam fillings and detoxifying their bodies of mercury corrected the infertility problems or ameliorated any of the female reproductive organ dysfunctions. If the problems were corrected, subsequent studies could attempt to correlate chronic mercury vapor exposure from mercury amalgam dental fillings with critical biochemical elements of the reproductive system, such as zinc and selenium, and the presence of lead. It might even be possible that a therapeutic course of those vitamins and minerals depleted by mercury and lead would correct the infertility problem without the immediate necessity of having their amalgam fillings replaced. However, if the health impact of mercury amalgam fillings is confirmed, then science should advocate a period of at least six months after mercury amalgam replacement before again undertaking planned parenthood efforts.

9

CAN MERCURY AND LEAD
CAUSE BIRTH DEFECTS?

In the course of a normal day, we are all exposed in some degree to mercury, either in the food we eat or the air we breathe. However, those individuals who have mercury amalgam dental fillings receive additional exposure from the inhalation of mercury vapor released from their dental fillings. Does this extra body burden of a toxic substance place those people at greater risk? What about the woman who is pregnant or contemplating pregnancy? Should she be more concerned if she has a mouthful of "silver fillings"?

The first indications that mercury might be toxic to the fetus occurred during the time mercury was utilized as the treatment for syphilis. It was observed that women undergoing mercury treatment for syphilis frequently aborted, although there was no clear scientific proof that this was directly related to the mercury treatment and not to the disease itself.

Kussmaul (1861) attempted to clarify the distinction between syphilis and mercury poisoning. In 1861, there were no blood tests for syphilis. All that was known was that it was contagious and mercury poisoning was not. In order to describe effects caused only by mercury (inhaled mercury vapor, not effects caused by various mercury compounds), Kussmaul elected to study employees of mirror factories. Mercury is used in the silvering process on glass to produce the reflective surface of the mirror. Kussmaul cites reports from the chief physician for occupational diseases concerning employees at the mirror factories in Furth, Germany who stated, "Even if today no statistical proof can be presented, it appears quite clear that pregnant mirror-makers often have miscarriages or give birth to dead children and that the surviving ones often are scrofulous (primary tuberculosis of the cervical lymph nodes or suppurating abscesses), have rachitis (rickets or inflammatory disease of the vertebral column), and suffer from skin diseases and exhausting fevers." (190)

Subsequent events tend to confirm a relationship between mercury and aborted pregnancies/stillbirths as mercury was detected in stillborn infants of mothers who were being treated with mercury compounds.(191,192)

CATASTROPHIC MERCURY POISONING

During the period 1953 to 1971, a total of 121 people living in villages around Minamata Bay in Japan were poisoned. Investigators determined that the poisonings were due to the consumption of fish having high concentrations of methylmercury. Researchers also found that 22 infants had been poisoned prenatally.(193) Other researchers found that during that same period a total of twenty-five infants were born with brain damage. From 1944 to 1959 approximately 6% of the children born around Minamata Bay developed cerebral palsy. Other neurologic symptoms included chorea (continuous, rapid, involuntary jerky movements), ataxia (irregular and uncoordinated muscle movement), tremors, seizures, and mental retardation. All of these children had been exposed in utero to methylmercury from maternal consumption of fish. (194,195)

A far more devastating and tragic epidemic of methylmercury poisoning, resulting in hundreds of deaths, occurred in

Iraq during 1971-1972. Methylmercury fungicides had been used to treat wheat and barley seed grains. Instead of being planted, the grain was used to make bread. A total of 6,530 cases of poisoning were admitted to hospitals throughout Iraq. Of this number, 459 recorded hospital deaths were directly attributable to methylmercury poisoning. Thirty-one pregnant women were admitted. Paired blood samples taken from both the mother and child, born after hospital admission, revealed that most of the infants had mercury blood concentrations substantially higher than the mothers. Several of these infants had signs of severe brain damage. Researchers concluded that methylmercury readily passed through the placenta and crossed from mother to fetus and that the concentration of mercury in the blood of the newborn was equal to, if not higher than, that in the mother.(67)

The catastrophe gave scientists a rare opportunity to study the effects of prenatal exposure to methylmercury. Thirty-two infants (fifteen male and seventeen female), all full-term pregnancies, prenatally exposed to methylmercury, and their mothers were examined over a five-year period. Eighteen of the infants were younger than two months of age at the time of first clinical observation. Thirteen infants were initially exposed during the first trimester, seven during the second, and twelve during the third. Twenty-nine of the infants were nursed and received additional doses of mercury from the breast milk.

For evaluation purposes, the fourteen infants displaying early signs of abnormality were placed in one group and the other eighteen not displaying any clinical manifestations of abnormality were placed in a separate group. Of the fourteen in the first group: ten had cerebral palsy-type symptoms, were irritable and showed an exaggerated reaction to sudden noise; six of the ten infants were blind, two had minimal sight, and two had apparently good sight; five of the fourteen had abnormally small head circumference; the mentality of all fourteen children in the first group was severely affected and their language development was poor or nonexistent.

Of the eighteen infants in the second group, half of them had neurological signs and delays in psychomotor development that only became obvious as time passed (2-5 years of age). These later developments were not severe enough to cause mental and physical incapacitation.

Nine of the thirty-two children in the study died within three years. Two died within one month of birth and the other seven died at home at the ages of 2-2 1/2 years. This mortality rate of 28% compared to a 6% mortality in the children used as a control group who had not had any prenatal exposure to mercury.(67)

One other very important result of this research was the determination that mercury was being excreted in the breast milk and passed to the infants in very appreciable quantities, resulting in higher blood mercury levels during the period of breast feeding. In another group of infants born prior to the epidemic, it was determined that at least eight had been exposed only through breast feeding. These infants had blood mercury levels paralleling the minimum toxic dose established by a Swedish expert committee. It should be pointed out that none of the eight infants exposed solely through breast milk exhibited any signs or symptoms of poisoning.(193)

Several important factors were determined by these studies. It was scientifically established that maternal exposure prior to conception, as well as after conception, could cause passage of methylmercury through the placenta to the embryo or fetus. After birth, further contamination occurred during the entire period of breast feeding. Infants born to mothers who had been exposed, in most instances, had higher blood mercury levels than their mothers. Children born to mothers who had been exposed to mercury prior to or during gestation had an abnormally high number of birth defects. Some of the women who had been poisoned aborted their pregnancies, and in five deliveries there was prolonged labor which had not been noted in their earlier pregnancies. Tragically, - fourteen of the thirty-one pregnant Iraqi women who were hospitalized died from unexplained causes.(67)

In this country, there was an incident of mercury poisoning that resulted from eating contaminated pork (the animals had subsisted on contaminated feed that had been sprayed with a mercury fungicide). A 40-year-old woman ate this contaminated pork for three months during her third to sixth month of pregnancy. The woman experienced and displayed minimal symptoms of mercury toxicity. An apparently normal child was delivered at term. However, at three months of age, the infant's electroencephalogram showed abnormal activity. When the infant was six months old, he developed myotonic (increased muscular irritability and muscle spasms) jerks with a very abnormal electroencephalogram. It was assumed because the child was never breast-fed that his symptoms were the result of in utero exposure to maternal mercury.(196,197) This investigation demonstrated that the effects of prenatal exposure to mercury may not be apparent until well after birth.

The preceding events clearly indicate that there is a need for women contemplating pregnancy to be concerned about mercury. Although the information presented dealt only with catastrophic events primarily related to organic mercurials, we feel that the balance of information provided in this chapter will convey a similar importance and concern about exposure to mercury vapor as well as some of the other heavy metals.

As discussed in preceding chapters, mercury and lead have the ability to penetrate the placenta and be taken up by the fetus. We have also shown how these toxic metals accumulate in the male and female reproductive organs, and possess the potential to affect the quality of the male sperm and the female ovum. The scientific information that follows will show the potential of mercury and lead to cause birth defects, and why the additional body burden of mercury from mercury amalgam fillings may increase the possibility of physical defects or mental deficits.

It is no longer possible to ignore the additive or synergistic effects of lead when addressing the toxicity potentials of mercury. Both of these heavy metals are everywhere in our environment and there is no escaping the fact that both will be present in the human body. Both of these metals share some other unique distinctions:

--neither has any demonstrated biological need in humans

--blood levels of lead and mercury only relate to current or acute exposures and do not indicate tissue or body burden

--science has been unable to identify a threshold level below which some type of metabolic or health effect will not occur

--both have an affinity for central nervous system (CNS) tissue, especially in the embryo or fetus.

PHYSIOLOGICAL CHANGES DURING PREGNANCY

When a woman becomes pregnant, several major physiological changes occur.(102,198) We feel these important changes may have been overlooked by many scientists evaluating the possible effects of toxic metals during pregnancy. For example, there is an increased tidal volume (the amount of air taken into the lungs and expelled during one respiratory cycle) and a reduced amount of air remaining in the lungs. There is also an increase in the respiratory rate and an increase in oxygen consumption. Therefore, there will be increased absorption of substances such as mercury and lead in aerosol or vapor form. To our knowledge, no one has yet evaluated this phenomenon in regard to mercury vapor released from mercury amalgam dental fillings.

The output of the heart increases by 30-50% during pregnancy. Increases in both the heart rate and volume of blood pumped account for this change. These changes begin about the sixth week of pregnancy. During labor, heart output increases another 30%. This increase in blood circulation could result in increased tissue burdens of mercury and lead. Because mercury vapor is both lipid soluble and has no electrical charge, this could result in increased levels in the maternal brain, uterus, and placenta, and increased accumulation in the fetal brain and gonads, as well as possible contamination of germ cells.

Along with the increase in heart output, there is an increase in plasma volume of approximately 50%. At the same time, there is a decrease in plasma-binding proteins. As mercury and lead both bind to plasma proteins, this could further reduce available plasma protein. There is also a 70% elevation of the extracellular fluid space, which causes the swelling, or edema, associated with normal pregnancy.

There are also changes that occur in the gastrointestinal tract, liver, and bile. Interestingly, these changes may also relate to mercury and lead homeostasis during pregnancy. Constipation may occur, and there is also an increased incidence of gallbladder disease during pregnancy. One of the possible factors in the increased incidence of gallbladder disease is an impairment of the sodium and potassium ATPase enzymes. It is well documented in the scientific literature that mercury inhibits the ATPase enzymes. Another aspect of the gastrointestinal-liver-bile physiology is that both mercury and lead are excreted through this pathway. Consequently, customary changes that may occur during pregnancy could be further aggravated by the presence of mercury and lead. More importantly, these same changes could result in reduced excretion of these toxic metals in the feces, resulting in an increased recirculation of lead and mercury from the colon through the portal vein back to the liver.

During pregnancy the function of most endocrine glands is altered with noticeable changes occurring in the thyroid and adrenal glands. There are also changes in glucose metabolism, with an increased need for insulin. The placenta may be involved in the insulin requirements because it manufactures insulinase (an enzyme that destroys or inactivates insulin) during pregnancy. Placental insulinase may function to protect or control the fetal insulin levels. In this regard it should be noted that insulin has three disulfide cross-linkages which also makes it a potential target for binding by both mercury and lead. We consider these endocrine changes to be of extreme significance because of the scientifically documented biochemical effects that mercury and lead have on thyroid and adrenal glands, hormones, and glucose metabolism. Because of these effects we found it interesting that the *Merck Manual* indicates that women who were diagnosed as prediabetic prior to pregnancy frequently develop more positive diabetic symptoms during pregnancy. There are no published scientific studies evaluating any of the potential effects of mercury and lead mentioned in this paragraph.

Although the research is very scanty, the existing evidence of increased blood mercury levels during pregnancy could in fact be a reflection of the physiologic changes outlined above, causing a redistribution of some of the tissue mercury body burden. More importantly, it could also cause an increase in fetal body burden of both mercury and lead, which could also be involved in some of the other fetal changes that occur for which there is no clear scientific explanation.

SPONTANEOUS ABORTION

Spontaneous abortion could be classified as an infertility problem because it is considered a cause of reproductive failure. However, it can also be considered a birth defect in that some abnormality probably caused the rejection/miscarriage. There are various estimates indicating the frequency of spontaneous abortion. We have seen statements indicating spontaneous abortions of all recognized pregnancies to be 15% to 25%.(198) We have also seen information stating there is a 78% spontaneous abortion rate. The 78% figure would include all the unreported spontaneous abortions (usually less than 20 weeks) and all the other spontaneous abortions that occur prior to having the pregnancy recognized.(198,199)

According to a 1980 National Center for Health Statistics Report, of approximately three million infants born alive each year, 13.1 per thousand die within the first year.(200) A U.S. Environmental Protection Agency report indicates approximately 900,000 newborns may be at potential risk of lead intoxication via their mothers.(201) In their 1980 facts report, The National Foundation/ March of Dimes indicated that 2-3 percent of infants born alive have major congenital defects that are detected within the first year of life. The figures do not take into consideration the defects that only become apparent at some later stage in life. Chung and Myrianthopopoulos (1975) estimate that when these types of birth defects are included, approximately 16% of all live births would have incurred some type of birth defect.(202)

REPRODUCTIVE EFFECTS

As of 1985, there was only one published scientific experiment (an animal study) investigating the effects of mercury vapor on the adult reproductive system (146), and no published studies on prenatal or early postnatal effects. Since 1985 there has only been one additional study. This appeared in March 1987 as an abstract of a study on prenatal effects, done by the American Dental Association Health Foundation, Research Institute.(203) The authors investigated the effects of elemental mercury vapor on prenatal development in pregnant rats. Subjecting the animals to both chronic exposure and acute exposure, they reported that exposure at 0.1 milligram mercury per cubic meter of air revealed no gross congenital malformations or resorptions when compared to the controls. The abstract concluded with the following statement: "These findings indicate that acute exposure of pregnant rats to 0.5 milligrams of mercury vapor per cubic meter produced fetotoxicity and that 1.0 milligram per cubic meter of mercury vapor additionally resulted in maternal toxicity." We were unable to obtain the actual study data supporting this abstract even though we requested this data from the author. Consequently, there are many factors concerning the validity of the study which cannot be answered. For example, why weren't developmental, metabolic, and central nervous system effects evaluated, since the purpose of the study was to investigate the effects of mercury vapor on prenatal development? Further, there is no data on how long the offspring survived after birth.

The results reflected in the above abstract notwithstanding, the ADA has not taken a public position on whether women should or should not have mercury amalgam fillings placed or replaced during their pregnancy. This is in spite of the fact that some of the world experts have now taken positions that mercury amalgam dental fillings should not be placed in children or pregnant women. The World Health Organization has also taken a position that women should not be subjected to mercury exposure during their pregnancy.(70)

The conclusions of some of the world experts on toxicology of metals, in a recent report on the subject, contained the following statement which captures the essence of the overall problem: "Surprisingly, mercury vapor and inorganic mercury, the two forms of mercury to which people are occupationally exposed, have received very little attention despite the fact that animal work suggests that effects might be expected at least in certain times in the life cycle....However, for vapor, metallic, and inorganic mercury, data from animal studies indicate that we should focus on human exposure in the developmental period."(204)

There have been some epidemiological studies attempting to correlate reproductive effects of mercury vapor on groups of women who are exposed on the basis of their work. However, here again, most of the studies used questionnaires which participants were asked to fill out to the best of their knowledge and recollection. Therefore, some of the results and conclusions drawn from the data were based on subjective data. Regardless of the findings of these studies, none of them attempted to separate amalgam versus nonamalgam participants.

Perhaps the greatest problem confronting anyone investigating the health effects of mercury is the design or protocol of so many of the published studies. The traditional protocol used is to inject either mercuric chloride or methylmercury into the test animals and then determine the effect of the dosage administered. How do you extrapolate such research results to the real-life situation confronted by an individual with amalgam fillings who may be routinely subjected to the chronic inhalation of significant amounts of metallic mercury vapor for a great many years? How do you equate the effects of a single acute dose in an animal experiment to the chronic accumulation of mercury in the brain and other critical organs over the entire lifetime of the amalgam fillings?

For example, Khayat and Dencker (1983), in experiments with mice (utilizing radioactive mercury), have clearly demonstrated that the distribution pattern of inhaled mercury vapor was much different than that seen after the injection of mercuric chloride. They also demonstrated that the blood concentration was considerably lower after elemental mercury vapor inhalation than after mercuric chloride injection. Their autoradiography studies revealed additional sites of mercury accumulation, not shown on previous studies, that included the thyroid, adrenal cortex, spinal ganglia and nerves, interstitial tissues of the testes and epididymis, and corpora lutea of the ovaries.(66)

Another aspect revealed by various animal studies is that the embryo of each species has a critical period of developmental sensitivity during which there is chemical susceptibility, particularly during the days of rapid organogenesis. The organogenesis period is characterized by the division, migration, and association of cells into primitive organ rudiments. During this time for example, relatively low levels of methylmercury can produce a high fetal mortality.(205) The phase of organogenesis for the human embryo is from about days 18 to 20 until about days 55 to 60.(206)

Nishimura et al. (1974) tried to determine a normal level of mercury in human embryos and fetuses in Japan. Total mercury was measured. Mercury was detected in all of the sixty-seven embryos from five to seven and one-half weeks old and in all the fetal organs of twenty-eight fetuses between four and ten months old. No significant differences were found between mercury levels in the brain and any of the trimester stages. However, there was a significant decrease in the average mercury level of third-trimester livers. The authors thought this might be due to the onset of detoxication by the fetal liver.(207)

In regard to the preceding two studies, we think it important to point out the work of Clarkson et al. (58) who stated in their 1972 report: "The blood-brain barrier is known to discriminate against ionic mercury but to allow transit of the dissolved vapor [Berlin et al., 1966; Magos, 1968]. Our results indicate that the placenta has similar properties. Thus mercury vapor now shares with the short-chain alkylmercurials the ability to pass across two important diffusion barriers in the body." What these researchers have determined is that elemental mercury vapor, from mercury amalgam fillings, could pass into the maternal brain as well as having the ability to pass through the placenta and enter the fetal brain just as easily as methylmercury. The reader should also bear in mind that both forms of mercury have an affinity for nerve tissue.

Another finding of Clarkson and his associates was that after injection of elemental metallic mercury, the fetal content was over *ten* times greater and after inhaling mercury vapor, approximately *forty* times greater than after an equivalent dose of inorganic mercury (mercuric chloride).

Results of various animal studies demonstrate that exposure to methylmercury can produce congenital as well as embryolethal effects in the uterus. Intrauterine death is usually manifested by fetal resorption or stillbirth, whereas congenital effects cover a wide spectrum of defects. The cause of brain damage in children is largely unknown. As any review of the court records will confirm, more and more women and society as a group, seem to be placing sole blame for delivery of a less than perfect child on their obstetrician and gynecologist. A recent study in Israel sheds some revealing light on this subject. Jaffe et al. (1985) sought information on the possible occurrence of cerebral insult during two critical stages--gestation, a period during which fetal insults are often not detected, and the perinatal period, when the condition of the fetus and neonate may be monitored by clinicians.

Dr. Jaffe and his colleagues did a comparison evaluation of forty-six brain-damaged children with fifty-three healthy children used as controls. They evaluated unusual dermatoglyphic patterns (patterns of ridges of the skin of the fingers, palms, toes, and soles) and abnormal dental enamel markers, based on the hypothesis that if the brain-damaged children had a higher incidence of these markers, it would indicate that some insult causing the abnormalities would have occurred prior to delivery. The evidence revealed by this study supports the contention that most brain damage in children originates during gestation, not from delivery itself. What was extremely interesting was that the dental findings were the predominant marker, suggesting that the insult was sustained after the fourth month of pregnancy.(208)

In evaluating for gestational or perinatal insult, does the chronic inhalation of mercury vapor from dental amalgam fillings during pregnancy constitute one of the possible insults involved in brain damage? Or is it possible that electrogalvanic potentials being generated by dissimilar metals in the oral cavity are also involved in some obscure way? Recent publications concerning the electrical/magnetic phenomenon, in relation to living matter, clearly indicate that there is an electrical energy balance as well as a chemical balance involved in cellular homeostasis. Consequently, one must wonder whether the galvanic currents emanating from the dental fillings are capable of disrupting the electrical balance or energy flow through the placenta to the embryo, thereby affecting the energy homeostasis of the growing organism. Is it also possible that this disruption could then cause congenital abnormalities? (209,210)

There is not much question that environmental agents can produce preconception mutations in the maternal or paternal germ cells, resulting in adverse reproductive outcomes. Janerich and Polednak, in a recent review paper on birth defects, stated the magnitude and breath of the problem in a single paragraph:

"The exploration of the environmental causes of birth defects must be extended beyond simple teratogenesis. Risk from long-term occupational or environmental exposures to the mother or father requires greater detailed consideration than is generally now being given, and future studies will need a greater degree of precision in reporting and recording of exposure data than contemporary studies are using." Agents that have a long metabolic clearance time are a particular problem. Were these agents used during pregnancy or were they used within the ordinary clearance time prior to pregnancy? The authors felt that this information is essential before an investigator can make certain statements about the safety or risk associated with exposure to these agents. Janerich and Polednak also felt that "An environmental exposure that has the ability to affect permanently the female or male germ cells or the female reproductive organs (cervix, endometrium, etc.) requires a precise and comprehensive history."(211)

In regard to the preceding statements, how long mercury remains in the body after exposure assumes added importance. Mercury has a long metabolic clearance time, at least 100 days for the slow component, and up to twenty-seven years in the brain. There is evidence that as differentiation of the various embryonic systems progresses, the vulnerability to anatomical defects decreases. However, do not be misled by that statement. Science has also shown that the development of the central nervous system continues during the last third of intrauterine life. Consequently, the central nervous system may be vulnerable for much longer than other organs or systems in the developing fetus. The presence of foreign chemicals or substances during the late intrauterine period may therefore interfere with brain development. This might then cause subtle abnormalities that only reveal themselves as behavioral alterations or functional disturbances.(212)

In experimental animals, methylmercury's impact on the developing organism has resulted in a variety of congenital malformations such as cleft palate (205,213-215), limb defects (205), brain and facial malformations (213,216), changes in form or structure of the fetal liver (217), and changes in form or structure of fetal kidneys.(218,219)

The phenomenon of cleft palate is perhaps one of the most common congenital malformations reported from animal exposures to methylmercury. Su and Okita (214), in their study utilizing six consecutive injections of methylmercury on days 7-12 of gestation, produced a 97% incidence of cleft palate in 129 mouse fetuses. Why cleft palate is so prevalent or what metabolic mechanisms are involved have not been discerned or elucidated as yet. However, Olson and Massaro (215) have suggested that because mercury can inhibit protein synthesis, this could then disrupt the regulatory processes controlling closure of the palate. Here again, exactly when the exposure occurs in the reproductive cycle is critical to the degree of toxicity or teratogenic (physical defect) effect induced.

For example, Harris et al. (205) found that a single intraperitoneal injection of methylmercury on the eighth day of gestation resulted in a 42% incidence of fetal death and a 36% incidence of grossly malformed offspring. However, when the same dose was given on the fourth day of gestation, the results were drastically different--only 5% incidence of fetal death and only an 8% incidence of malformations. Finally, when the same dose was administered on day ten of gestation, there was a 30% incidence of fetal death but no incidence of gross malformations.

Rizzo and Furst (1972) set out to determine if mercuric oxide, which does not produce immediate toxic effects, would be teratogenic if given orally to pregnant rats. Three experimental groups (A,B,C) of rats were established and each group received their mercuric oxide at a different day after conception. Group A was treated five days after conception, Group B twelve days, and Group C on day nineteen post-conception. The offspring of Group A had 29.7% deformities, Group B decreased to 6.8%, and Group C decreased further to 3.4%. The mothers did not demonstrate any toxic effects. The authors concluded: "This pilot study, which should be repeated, does suggest a potential human hazard. In this test, a relatively inert mercuric compound was found to have teratogenic properties. There may exist in the environment more hazardous compounds, and investigations should be made concerning the effects of mercury from both natural and man-made sources." (220)

Although we might be prejudiced, we don't believe there is any such classification as a "relatively inert mercuric compound." For example, a recent case report from Belgium involved a 4-month-old infant who died from the repeated application to the skin of yellow mercuric oxide ointment. The infant was being treated for infected eczema. Toxic levels of mercury were measured in blood, urine, cerebrospinal fluid, and tissues.(23)

It is apparent from the Rizzo and Furst study that the timing of the exposure has a bearing on the teratogenic effect. This is not peculiar to mercury alone; the same has been shown to be true when assessing the teratogenicity of lead. When rats were given a single injection of lead nitrate, teratogenic effects could be observed only when the injection was given on the ninth day of pregnancy. In this same context, the embryo- and fetotoxic effects were most pronounced when the lead injection was given between the tenth and fifteenth day of the pregnancy. If the injection was given after day sixteen, the fetotoxic effects were minimal.(221)

The same criticality of exposure seems to be true whether it involves a xenobiotic or a virus. In a small study, 80% of the embryos of mothers who had rubella in the first trimester were malformed.(222) This same scenario could be ascertained for the Thalidomide disaster of 1961.

What about something as innocuous as mercurochrome, which contains mercury? Yeh et al. (1978) describe a case history of a newborn infant with an omphalocele (part of the intestine protrudes through a large defect in the abdominal wall at the umbilicus, covered with only a thin transparent membrane). The omphalocele was dressed with 2% mercurochrome for four days and discontinued for four days. On the eighth day, 0.5% mercurochrome dressing was applied and continued until the death of the infant on the eleventh day. Autopsy results suggested that the infant had died of heavy metal poisoning. Yeh and colleagues cite a German study of thirteen infants with omphaloceles who were also treated with 2% mercurochrome and subsequently died. The report concluded with the following statement: "Infected omphalocele remains a critical problem in neonatal surgery and local application of metallic antiseptics should be avoided."(223)

Mercurochrome is still a widely used antiseptic, both in the home and in the medical profession. Most people who use it have no idea that it contains mercury. Consequently, there is a serious question regarding just what contribution of mercury this common antiseptic makes to total mercury body burden. Its use is so widespread that in a nationwide allergy sampling in the United States, 8% of the people tested positive to mercurochrome.(97) In Japan, some researchers have concluded that the widespread sensitivity reaction to mercury is directly related to the routine use of mercurochrome.(224)

Determining the actual effect of chronic exposure to mercury vapor from amalgam fillings during conception and gestation is a very difficult task. The phenomena of metal-to-metal interactions and metal-to-element interactions within the maternal and fetal systems is extremely complex, and to our knowledge has not been addressed by the scientific community. However, research is beginning to appear showing that when two metals--for example, lead and mercury--are present at the same time, they both will be competing for cellular receptor sites, which in turn can disrupt normal metabolic function or have the effect of increasing the potential toxicity of one of the metals.

SUBTLE BIRTH DEFECTS

Another aspect of complexity is related to the subtlety of some birth defects. The severe forms of congenital heart disease are readily diagnosed at birth. However, the milder cases may not be diagnosed for varied periods, sometimes even years. By the time such cases are diagnosed the cause may be attributed to events or environmental exposures that in reality were not the true etiological factors.

In regard to the above thesis, a 1986 study by Howard and Mottet (225) demonstrates the point very clearly. Sprague-Dawley female rats were given 12.5 ppm of methylmercury in their drinking water starting on the second day of pregnancy. There was no evidence of maternal toxicity nor were any gross malformations observed in the offspring, although whole-body weights were 18.6% less than those of the controls. Litter size was normal. However, 32.8% of the offspring died within 48 hours of birth and the specific cause of death was not clear.

Perhaps the most subtle finding of these researchers related to their investigation of the effect on the brain, specifically the cerebellum (the area concerned with coordination of movements). They found a 23.6% reduction in cerebellar weight which was considered statistically significant when compared to the whole-body weight reduction. Other researchers had determined that continuous low-dose methylmercury exposure, similar to what might occur in environmental contamination, resulted in high mercury tissue burdens. Chen et al. (1979), who also used rats in their study, found that organ weights were significantly subnormal. The results of the study confirmed that the cells in the kidneys and liver were of normal size but were fewer in total number.(226) In both of the studies referenced, peak burdens of mercury were observed at the time of birth, immediately prior to the major phase of cell proliferation in the cerebellum. What Howard and Mottet had concluded from their findings was that the mercury exposure had resulted in significant reductions in the total cell population of the cerebellum.

The results of the Howard and Mottet study also suggested that impaired cell proliferation, resulting from chronic low-dose exposure, is central to the mechanism of mercury toxicity. Further, other researchers, according to the authors, had determined that chronic low-level methylmercury exposures similar to that used in their study had been associated with learning deficits in infant animals.

Much the same can be said for lead. Lead crosses the placenta, readily producing an increase in blood lead levels in the fetus, with fetal blood lead levels matching those found in the mother's blood.(227) Lin-Fu (1973), in discussing the subtle effects of lead during the postnatal period, brought forth the following information: the first ten postnatal days of neural development in the rat approximates the first two and a half years of human life, and that it requires only one-quarter the amount of lead to cause the same decrease of learning abilities in one-to-ten-day-old rats as in rats that are eleven days or more in age.(228)

The major point of all this is the subtleness of the birth defects. The only way these types of birth defects were determined was by performing autopsy studies on the prenatally exposed infant animals, certainly not a procedure that can be employed for clinical diagnosis with humans. However, it is significant to note that in the Minamata Bay epidemic in Japan, the results of autopsy studies done on two children who had died showed depletion of cerebellar granular cells and damage to the cerebral cortex of a nonspecific nature, similar to the lesions seen in the adult form of fatal Minamata Disease. Dying infants had high levels of mercury in their brains, livers, and kidneys approximating the levels found in adults dying of mercury poisoning.(229) It would appear that the animal studies showing depletion of cerebellum cells as a result of mercury exposure represent a confirmation of what was discovered by the autopsy studies done almost 20 years earlier on Minamata Bay victims. It is interesting to note that the ADA researchers involved in the previously mentioned study (203) failed to consider all of these well-documented effects. Their study investigated only grossly observable birth defects.

Although these studies dealt only with the effects of chronic methylmercury exposure, the same could be true for chronic exposure to elemental mercury vapor from mercury amalgam dental fillings. Clarkson et al. (204) stated: "After inhalation of radioactive vapor, the differences in fetal uptake were greater. The fetal content was approximately 40 times greater than after an equivalent dose of mercuric chloride, the maternal blood to fetal ratios differed by a factor in excess of 1,000, and the placental/fetal ratios were 122 after inhalation as compared to unity after ionic mercury." ("Unity" means one, and in this case would mean "the same.")

There is no way that anyone can state categorically that low-dose chronic exposure to elemental mercury vapor, such as that released from mercury amalgam dental fillings with its continual accumulation in the fetal brain, is not the primary etiological cause of learning deficits, or other types of birth defects of unknown etiology, in some children. Further, the pro-amalgam advocates, in making their statements about no possible effects from low-dose mercury vapor from mercury amalgam dental fillings, have totally neglected to also consider the potential for increased central nervous system damage when both lead and mercury are present in the brain simultaneously.

IODINE, MERCURY, AND THE THYROID

There is another facet of the potential toxicities of mercury and lead that has been largely overlooked and it is related to thyroid dysfunction and iodine deficiency. In a 1983 study,

Hetzel and Potter stated, "Iodine deficiency has only recently been proven to be a cause of retarded human brain development." (230) We found this statement both startling and provocative. Startling because we had not previously considered iodine deficiency to be related to this type of birth defect. Provocative because we could immediately visualize, from a biochemical standpoint, the potential of mercury to affect iodine metabolism and availability.

Normally, iodine deficiency is associated with some type of enlargement of the thyroid gland which is medically termed as *goiter*. Goiter was endemic in many parts of the world, including areas of the United States. However, the widespread use of iodized salt and the addition of iodine to bread and water has been an effective means of correcting endemic iodine deficiency.

Cretinism is defined by *Dorland's Medical Dictionary* as "a chronic condition due to congenital lack of thyroid secretion, marked by arrested physical and mental development, dystrophy of the bones and soft parts, and lowered basal metabolism." It was during the mid-nineteenth century that cretinism was identified with hypothyroidism. This was a broad category which has been refined during the last twenty years into two classifications-- hypothyroid cretinism, a condition responsive to thyroid hormones; and neurological cretinism, a condition that usually does not respond to thyroid hormones. The signs or symptoms of neurological cretinism usually encompass mental deficiency, deafness, deaf-mutism, and squint and spastic diplegia (muscular weakness, walking difficulties, and usually convulsions). Symptoms related to hypothyroidism are characterized primarily by skeletal problems and mental retardation.

The results of recent epidemiological studies (231-233) have revealed relationships between maternal iodine and thyroid hormone status and fetal brain development. Motor coordination defects in otherwise apparently normal children have been related to iodine deficiency during pregnancy. In others, there was a relationship between maternal serum thyroxine and significant reductions of certain motor skills in the offspring. As a result of their findings, Pharoah et al. (1981) suggested that the maternal thyroxine status could exert metabolic effects on the fetus without the necessity for thyroxine to cross the placental membrane.(233)

Animal studies related to maternal iodine deficiency have also demonstrated observable effects at birth. In rats there were significant reductions in body weights, brain cholesterol content, and reductions in whole-brain weights.(234) In sheep there were reductions in body weights, brain weights, brain DNA, and protein content. Fetal brain development (cerebellum) was retarded with an increased density of large neuron cells (Purkinje's cells). There was also evidence of retarded myelination in the cerebral hemispheres and brainstem related to lowered brain cholesterol content.(234,235)

In both human and animal studies during the prenatal and early perinatal periods, hypothyroidism is accompanied by a variety of alterations to the central nervous system. If hypothyroidism is not corrected during pregnancy, mental retardation may result from the slow growth and maturation of the central nervous system. Scientists have not clearly defined during what period of gestation the fetal brain is most vulnerable to defective development of the thyroid. However, the critical effects of thyroid hormone on brain development in humans are believed to occur during the last trimester of pregnancy and the first postnatal year. Consequently, fetal iodine deficiency could have a significant effect on fetal brain development in humans.(230)

There are several aspects of iodine deficiency and hypothyroidism-related effects on fetal and perinatal brain development that can be aggravated or otherwise affected by the presence of mercury. Earlier we discussed the research demonstrating the ability of mercury to reduce cerebellar brain weight through significant reductions in total cell population of the cerebellum. Evidence was also presented showing reductions of total body weight at birth related to maternal exposure to mercury. Lead and mercury have also been shown to have a direct effect on neuronal development leading to learning deficits. These are the same type of birth defects produced by maternal iodine deficiency and hypothyroidism. As you will see from the information that follows, mercury can have a negative effect on both iodine and thyroid status. Therefore, it is not illogical to conclude that the pregnant woman with a mouthful of mercury amalgam fillings has a much greater chance of experiencing some degree of hypothyroidism and/or iodine deficiency during her pregnancy than her counterpart without mercury amalgam fillings.

Recent scientific studies have shown that in humans, both the pituitary and the thyroid display an affinity for accumulating mercury.(63,126,236,237) There have also been animal studies showing that the enzymatic effects of mercury intoxication could be overcome by the administration of the thyroid hormone thyroxine.(238,239) With regard to mercury accumulation in the pituitary, it is important to point out that through a feedback loop, the pituitary releases thyrotropin-releasing hormone, which in effect tells the thyroid how much thyroxine hormone to release into the blood. The effect of mercury on this function of the pituitary has not been defined.

Trahktenberg (1969) reported that mercury first stimulates the thyroid and then suppresses thyroid function.(2) This was also confirmed with animal experiments by Goldman and Blackburn in 1979. More importantly, this latter study demonstrated that chronic intake of mercury for more than ninety days resulted in signs of mercury poisoning, together with decreased uptake of iodine and depression of thyroid hormonal secretion. The animals that survived the mercury intoxication were then placed on diets devoid of mercury to see if there was a recovery of thyroid function. Their results revealed that there was no amelioration and that the toxic effect of chronic mercury intake on the thyroid was permanent and irreversible.(240) There have also been a number of reports demonstrating stimulatory and depressive effects of lead on thyroid function.(237,240)

Kawada et al. (1981) conducted comparative studies on acute and subacute effects of organic and inorganic mercurials on thyroidal functions in rats and mice. They concluded that acute administrations seemed to exert more drastic effects on thyroidal functions than the prolonged treatment. They thought that inorganic mercury created more hazards on the thyroid than organic mercury in lower concentrations. However, organic mercury caused severe damage to both the endocrine and neural systems at the higher concentrations.(241) Another effect of iodine in the diet was determined by Kostial and Kargacin in 1982. Their study demonstrated that increasing the iodine contents of the rats' diets caused an increase in the whole-body retention of radioactive mercury after oral, but not after intraperitoneal, administration. The authors felt that iodine increases the gastrointestinal absorption of inorganic mercury and could therefore be a factor to consider in conditions where simultaneous exposure to both elements occurred.(242)

Friden and Naile (1954) found that the administration of thyroxine reversed the phenylmercuric chloride inhibition of the enzyme ascorbic acid oxidase. Further, thyroxine and related compounds react with phenylmercuric chloride at relatively low concentrations. These reactions cause a lessening of the thyroxine effect on the oxidation of ascorbic acid (vitamin C). (239) In this regard, Sillen (1949) proved the existence of a complex of mercury and iodine when both were present in the media used in their in vitro experiments.(243)

Biochemical aspects and relationships of mercury and lead are covered in detail in Chapter 11. However, we would just like to touch briefly on some details here involving other nutrients, mercury/lead, and the thyroid. It is apparent from the scientific information presented in Chapter 11 that there is a relationship to thyroid function and the nutritional status of folate, vitamin B_{12}, and methionine. There is also a current study demonstrating a strong association of lowered zinc intake and lowered basal metabolic rate, and lowered thyroid hormones and lowered protein utilization. (244) With regard to protein intake, a critical factor during pregnancy, a 1977 animal study demonstrated that the thyroid function of prenatally protein-deprived rats was significantly affected.(245) Mercury can affect the nutritional status of folate, vitamin B_{12}, methionine, and zinc, as well as protein nutriture.

If we put all the information related to the thyroid together, it appears very plausible to conclude that the chronic inhalation of mercury vapor from mercury amalgam dental fillings, together with mercury and dietary lead intakes, may constitute one of the most serious threats to fetal brain development. It is also not unreasonable to assume that the woman contemplating conception who has a number of mercury amalgam implants in her teeth and who may also have some degree of thyroid dysfunction, could be at much greater risk of giving birth to a child who may have many of the characteristics described in the preceding paragraphs.

NEUROLOGICAL DEFECTS

Murakami et al. (1956) did a study in which they investigated the effects of phenylmercury contraceptives on mouse embryos. The study was done at a time when phenylmercuric acetate was considered to be one of the most effective spermatocidal agents and was being prescribed as a contraceptive. The researchers wanted to investigate whether the contraceptive might in itself be teratogenic to embryos if it was used continuously after conception. The experiment demonstrated that approximately 15% of the embryos had abnormalities. The authors also concluded that the phenylmercuric acetate might affect embryos not only directly, but also indirectly, and that the predominant abnormalities involved the central nervous system.(194)

In another study, Snell et al. (1977) investigated the exposure of pregnant rats to low doses of methylmercury during gestation. Postnatal rats exposed to methylmercury in utero exhibited higher liver glycogen concentrations and decreased body weights compared to the rats used as controls. The authors felt the results of their study pointed to a derangement of perinatal carbohydrate metabolism in the offspring, which also caused a severe and protracted hypoglycemic response in the newborns. Perhaps even more importantly, the researchers felt that the postnatal hypoglycemic episode in exposed rats may contribute to the pathogenesis of the neurological disturbances revealed by these animals in later life.(246) Is there a parallel here with human offspring born with a derangement of their carbohydrate metabolism and severe blood sugar problems? Until physicians accept the fact that mercury vapor and mercury dissolution from amalgam dental fillings have the potential of causing chronic mercury toxicity, it will never be considered in any diagnosis of health problems in newborn infants or, for that matter, during the first several months or years of life.

The outbreak of Minamata Disease in Japan provides added emphasis to the necessity of universal acceptance of mercury as an etiological factor in many diseases or health conditions. For example, from about 1955 to 1960, 6% of children born in the villages near Minamata Bay developed cerebral palsy, convulsions, and/or mental retardation; their symptoms developed by six months after birth. All of the victims of Minamata Disease had been poisoned by eating fish contaminated with methylmercury. However, many of the mothers whose children developed these health problems did not display any symptoms of mercury toxicity. This demonstrated a fetal toxicity far outweighing maternal toxicity. Twenty years later some of the stricken children had improvements in their motor and cerebellar function, but many remained profoundly retarded.(229,247,248)

In regard to the neurotoxic effects, Diewert and Juriloff (249), who were investigating the cleft palate phenomenon associated with mercury exposure said, "Prenatal exposure to methylmercury is known to have neurological effects and affect postnatal behavior of treated mice with no detectable gross congenital malformations.(250) Since the fetal brain achieves a level of methylmercury that is twice that of the maternal brain level (251), altered neural development may affect fetal body development. When corrections are made for different blood levels, the concentrations in the fetal brain are 4 to 5 times that in the maternal brain and 2 to 2.6 times as great in the fetal liver than in the maternal liver."

It is now some thirty years after the Minamata Bay disaster, and within the United States, there has been a proliferation of cerebral palsy throughout the country. We have not come across even an inkling that science, the medical profession, or the Cerebral Palsy Foundation have attempted to evaluate a single child afflicted with this terrible disease to determine if in utero mercury exposure was a possible etiological factor. Unlike the Minamata Bay disaster, there is no common identifiable environmental exposure threat such as the eating of fish contaminated with high levels of methylmercury. Consequently, there is no obvious reason to suspect that mercury may be the indirect cause. This will continue to be the case until someone accepts the premise that elemental mercury vapor and mercury dissolution from mercury amalgam dental fillings may be the missing common environmental factor. Once that mental leap is made, then research to prove or disprove this simple hypothesis could be designed and funded, either independently or by the National Institutes of Health.

The newborn infant who is being nursed may be subjected to hidden burdens of toxins contained in the mother's milk. Both lead and mercury are present in mother's milk and can constitute a viable source of both of these toxins. There is a great deal of disparity between the various studies indicating the exact amount of mercury being transferred via the milk. The data related to lead indicates that the amount transferred can be substantial. Kostial and Momcilovic (1974) demonstrated that 10.1% to 14.2% of radioactive lead injected into female rats was transferred to the suckling pups via lactation, while transplacental transfer amounted to only 3%.(252)

Mansour et al. (1973) demonstrated that both organic and inorganic mercury are transferred through the milk at about the same extent. The authors felt that because of this, milk could play an important role in the accumulation of mercury in nursing infants. Although rats were used in their experiment, their conclusions contained the following statement: "If the same is true for humans, it would seem prudent for mothers with known history of exposure to mercury not to nurse their babies."(253)

Yang et al. (1973), utilizing rats as test animals, also investigated the transfer of mercury via milk. Only 1% of the dose required to produce neurological symptoms in adult rats was used. Five days after administering the mercury to the mother rats, their brains contained 0.218% of the administered dose. The concentration of mercury appeared to be highest in the pituitary.In the nursing pups, the quantity of labeled mercury deposited in the brain increased from day 1 to day 5 of suckling. At the end of five days the pup brain contained a higher concentration than the mother's brain.(254)

It seems apparent that in the newborn, whose immune function may have been compromised in utero because of exposure to these elements, the additional body burden derived from nursing has the potential of (1) further depressing the immune function and (2) aggravating other health problems that might be present at birth.The subtle latent effects on the central nervous system that may be aggravated by the additional burdens to toxic metals derived from nursing warrant special attention.

As described in Chapter 11, the importance of an adequate selenium status in offsetting toxic effects of mercury may be of extreme importance to the nursing mother and her infant. Data by Smith et al. (1981) showed that 60% of human milk-fed and 95% of formula-fed infants had selenium intakes below the 10-40 micrograms a day proposed by the National Research Council for infants 0-6 months of age.(255) Consequently, children born to woman with mercury amalgam fillings will be at greater risk from both inadequate selenium nurture during gestation and inadequate selenium intake during nursing.

ALCOHOL AND MERCURY

It is fairly well established in the scientific literature that alcohol is a potent teratogenic substance and in fact, may be one of the prime causes of mental retardation in the western world.(256) That statement was both startling and intriguing to us because of the scientific data related to latent mental defects caused by mercury. There was another parallel that immediately came to mind--that of the liver, where alcohol causes damage and where mercury also accumulates. Please understand that we are not saying, or implying, that it is mercury and not alcohol that is causing the problems related to consumption of alcohol. Nor do we want the reader to construe any of the following information to mean that consumption of alcohol during pregnancy is acceptable. As we have done in Chapter 11 and elsewhere in this book, we merely wish to point out some of the relationships between the toxicity of certain substances and nutritional status.

A recent study by Halmesmaki et al. (1986) evaluated the effect of drinking alcohol during pregnancy on maternal and fetal selenium nutriture. Some interesting data emerged. In abstinent pregnant women, serum selenium decreased with advancing gestational age. In pregnant women who drank heavily, serum selenium increased. Of the 17 women in the study who drank heavily during pregnancy, nine of them (53%) gave birth to infants with fetal alcohol syndrome. The study also found that selenium levels in umbilical serum of drinking women were lower than umbilical levels of abstinent women.(257)

The authors were not able to determine the significance of their findings or the relationship to the infants born with fetal alcohol syndrome. No consideration was given as to whether the women in the study had mercury amalgam fillings. However, it is not unreasonable to assume that most of them did. Therefore, if the results of the study are viewed in the context of the study population being exposed continually to a source of mercury vapor from their mercury amalgam fillings during their entire pregnancy, the findings are more understandable. Alcohol changes the distribution and retention of inhaled mercury vapor.(66,258) In a 1984 study, Khayat and Dencker demonstrated a high capacity for oxidizing mercury vapor to the ionic form in the respiratory epithelium (nasal mucosa, trachea and bronchial tree), cortex of the kidney, lung, myocardium, and spleen. They also found high concentrations in the liver, pancreas, eye (retina and pigment epithelium), adrenals, thyroid and salivary glands. Additionally, high levels were seen in the corpora lutea of the ovary, in the grey matter of the brain, and in skeletal muscles.(65)

When the same experiments were done after pretreatment of the animals with ethyl alcohol, the effects were characterized by a decreased accumulation in most organs and in the whole body. However, the liver and adrenal increased in mercury concentration. The same effect was seen in the testis. The effect in the brain was different, as ethyl alcohol decreased the activity, especially in the grey matter.(65)

Alcohol is known to deplete the following nutrients: folic acid, thiamin, riboflavin, niacin, ascorbic acid, vitamin B_6, vitamin B_{12}, magnesium, zinc, and protein.(259) Mercury has the ability to affect the homeostasis of each one of the nutrients listed, either through depletion or reduction of metabolic capacity (see Chapter 11).

Mercury binds to selenium, making it unavailable for normal metabolic function. One of the important functions of selenium is to cause a chemical reaction that results in the formation of the enzyme glutathione peroxidase. Glutathione peroxidase, in turn, functions to eliminate free radicals such as hydrogen peroxide and lipid peroxide. These free radical byproducts, if not controlled, are capable of causing a variety of cellular damage. Hydrogen peroxide is one of the byproducts that is produced from normal oxidation processes and lipid peroxides are an abundant byproduct during the body's metabolism of ethanol (alcohol). (260) Consequently, the increased redistribution of mercury caused by ingestion of alcohol, together with the probable tissue redistribution of mercury caused by alcohol/liquids diluting the blood, could cause more metabolically inert selenium to be present in the serum. This could account for the increased serum selenium levels Halmesmaki et al. found in the pregnant women who were drinking.

The true significance of the above relationships is reflected in the scientific literature dealing with the ability of nutritional deficiencies during pregnancy to cause birth defects. Pantothenic acid deficiency causes edema and cleft palate. Folic acid deficiency causes cleft lip, cleft palate, oblique facial clefts, and atrophy of nostrils. Vitamin C deficiency causes diminished bone formation, hemorrhages in the bone marrow, and formation of medullary substances. Vitamin E deficiency causes hydrocephalus, scoliosis, agnathous, cleft mandible, receding maxilla and mandibles, cleft lip, cleft palate, and harelip.(260) These genetic defects are related primarily to defects of the mouth and head, and are given only to illustrate the magnitude of the problem. More importantly, mercury affects the maternal status of each of the nutrients indicated. When the effects of lead and alcohol are added to those of mercury, the potential effects on the embryo and fetus could be devastating.

We feel very strongly that the U.S. government has an obligation to the American people to seriously consider the information presented. Certainly it is not unreasonable to suggest that out of the billions of dollars allocated for medical and dental research, an adequate amount could be set aside expressly for specific research on this subject. Whether the research is done by the National Institutes of Health or at various universities or colleges, the hypothesis that birth defects may be associated with an increased burden of mercury derived from dental fillings must not be ignored any longer. Setting aside any considerations related to the emotional, and psychological consequences of caring for and raising children born with physical or mental defects, or the diminished quality of life of such children, the bottom line warrants that research go forward. Looking at the problem in a pure dollars and cents fashion, the proving of the theory has the potential of ultimately saving hundreds of billions of dollars in health care costs, which should make it a project worthy of consideration even by those politicians not obsessed with the bottom line.

10

CANCER

There is scientific evidence showing that the fetus is very vulnerable to various types of chemical insult and a variety of substances can pass through the placenta to the fetus. Some of these may be carcinogenic in themselves, while others may cause a series of events to occur that may ultimately result in the development of cancer at some future time.

Many scientific studies have been done on cancer that describe metabolic processes related to the production or causation of tumors that involved thiols/sulfur/sulfhydryls and the transsulfuration pathways. A thiol is any organic compound containing a univalent radical called a sulfhydryl and identified by the symbol -SH (sulfur-hydrogen). This means that a thiol can attract one atom of mercury in the ionized form and have it combine with itself. It also means, that because it is a radical, that it can enter into or go out of this combination without any change. Mercury and lead both have a great affinity for sulfur and sulfhydryls and are capable of affecting the transsulfuration pathways in the body. Accordingly, we felt it important to bring together research having a direct bearing or showing the potential of these two toxic metals to be involved in biochemical or immunological events that could lead to the development of cancer.

Substances that can produce cancer are called carcinogens. Transplacental carcinogenesis is the medical term used to describe the passage of carcinogens through the placenta to the fetus and producing a carcinoma (cancerous tumor). Some statistics and data related to this phenomenon are:

1. The period from completion of 28 weeks of gestation and ending approximately 1 to 4 weeks after birth is called the perinatal period. Researchers have concluded that during the perinatal period of life the fetus has a high susceptibility to chemically induced carcinogenesis.(198)

2. It is also suspected that some types of cancers are of perinatal origin because they appear so soon after birth. Further, there is some suggestion that embryotoxic insult may predispose the offspring to secondary tumor induction later in life.(261)

3. In their 1980 report on cancer statistics, the American Cancer Society indicated that in 1976 cancer was the chief cause of death in children under the age of 15 in the United States. Lymphoma and leukemia were the major killers, accounting for over 50% of the deaths. Cancers of the brain and central nervous system, soft tissues, kidney, and bone accounted for the remaining deaths.(262)

MERCURY AND OTHER METALS IN CANCER

While mercury in itself is not considered a carcinogen, it does participate in a cascade of biochemical events that could ultimately produce cancer. The possible involvement of metals in the development of cancer is not a new idea. For example, a 1973 report concluded that metals may induce or activate an oncogenic virus (a virus that is capable of inducing a tumor) causing it to produce a tumor. The report went on to say that "the affinity of a metal for a specific tissue may largely determine its activity on a virus in that tissue. An oncogenic virus and cell may be in a 'homeostatic state,' and a chemical insult may suppress interferon, antibody, specific enzyme, hormone, or a combination of these defense factors to permit the virus to produce its carcinogenic effects; also the chemical may increase the activity of any one or more of these defensive factors and result in reduced activity of the virus."(263)

Cancer researchers appear to state, without any reservations, that healthy persons routinely defend/contain or destroy cancerous cells that form in our body throughout our lifetime. Therefore, foreign substances, such as mercury and lead, that affect this normal protective biochemical function might, by a continuous chronic onslaught on the immune defenses for years, make the body vulnerable to cancer and other major diseases. The two studies that follow seem to reflect that basic premise.

A 1981 study by Mangal and Sharma investigated the concentration of some trace elements in human whole blood of leukemia victims. Concentrations of eight trace elements (iron, zinc, cobalt, chromium, selenium, rubidium, scandium, and mercury) were determined in normal and leukemic human whole blood. There was a significant decrease in the concentrations of cobalt, chromium, rubidium, and iron in leukemic blood. There was also a slight decrease in the concentrations of zinc and scandium. However, the concentrations of selenium and mercury were increased in leukemia.(264) When the concentrations of these trace elements in leukemic blood were compared with the leukocyte cell counts in each subject, it was found that the concentrations of iron, zinc, cobalt, chromium, mercury, and selenium decreased, and those of rubidium increased uniformly with increases in the leukocyte cell counts. The increase in the level of rubidium and the decrease in the level of mercury as a function of leukocyte cell counts was in contradiction to the changes in the concentrations of these elements in leukemia, when compared to those in normal blood samples. The authors expressed the view that the results of their study suggested some special role of rubidium and mercury (both nonessential elements) in the initiation and progress of leukemia.(264)

What we found so interesting about the above study in relation to our theory of mercury being involved in the cancerogenesis process, is that rubidium and selenium both bind to mercury, thus reducing their biological availability. It is also well established in the scientific literature that distribution of mercury within the blood varies between different components of the blood. Consequently, we interpret the results of Mangal and Sharma's experiments to reflect similar results. The blood concentrations of selenium and mercury increased in leukemic patients which reflects the binding of selenium to mercury. Although the authors did not check for glutathione peroxidase (GSH-Px) levels, it would appear logical to assume that the reduced availability of selenium would also cause a reduced level of glutathione peroxidase. Conversely, there was approximately a 35% reduction in blood rubidium levels in leukemic patients. Where did the rubidium go? It appears from the study that it was taken up by the leukocytes as a defensive mechanism against leukocyte mercury which, because of rubidium's ability to avidly bind to mercury, also appears feasible. As you will see in the following study, science is finding that rubidium may in fact play an important role in the overall metabolic processes related to cancer.

In a 1984 study by Rizk and Sky-Peck, the researchers compared the concentrations of trace elements in normal and neoplastic human breast tissue. In neoplastic breast tumors the researchers found significantly large increases in calcium, vanadium, copper, zinc, selenium, and rubidium and a lesser increase in nickel. When these results were compared with normal breast tissue from the same individual, zinc and rubidium were found to be consistently higher in the tumor, whereas calcium, copper, and vanadium levels varied from normal to high. In no instance were the tissue changes in calcium, copper, zinc, or rubidium reflected in the blood levels, which were within normal limits. However, excretion of rubidium in the urine was consistently elevated. Tissue levels of mercury and lead were about the same in normal and neoplastic breast tissue.(265) Although the authors did not comment on the presence of mercury and lead in normal and cancerous tissue, we found their presence to be very provocative.

One of the experimental cancer therapies being tested involves inducing a high pH (alkaline) level in the tumorous tissue. A 1984 study by Brewer demonstrated that potassium, rubidium, and especially cesium are efficiently taken up by cancer cells (all three are alkali metals). Further, this uptake was enhanced by vitamin A, vitamin C, zinc, and selenium. The quantity of cesium taken up was sufficient to raise the cell pH to 8 (mild alkalinity). At this pH, cell mitosis ceases and the life of the cell is shortened. Tests on mice that were fed cesium and rubidium showed marked reduction in tumor masses within two weeks. In addition, the mice showed none of the side effects of cancer. Tests have been carried out on over thirty humans. In each case, the tumor masses disappeared. Studies of the food intake in areas where the incidence of cancer is very low showed that it met the requirements for the high pH therapy.(266)

Cesium and rubidium are potassium analogues. This means that cesium and rubidium are both similar to potassium in structure but differ chemically in some component of the structure. However, because of the difference, they may have a similar or opposite action metabolically. In this particular instance, it appears that cesium and rubidium can or may replace the potassium metabolite. Furthermore, there is a mercurial-invoked accumulation of potassium within cells which is thought to collapse the mitochondrial membrane potential, ultimately resulting in inhibited phosphorylation of adenosine diphosphate (ADP) and decreased adenosine triphosphate (ATP) production.(267)

This is a very vital process in the body. ADP, ATP and inorganic phosphate are stored in every cell in the body and serve as an energy-transmitting system. During the process of producing energy, ATP is broken down to ADP and phosphate. The cycle starts all over again as ADP is phosphorylated (one molecule of phosphate is added), thus regenerating ATP. Therefore, any process that inhibits any part of this energy cycle can result in serious metabolic problems.

There are certain biochemical aspects involved in the above studies that are extremely intriguing. In the first study, breast tumors had increased levels of calcium, vanadium, copper, zinc, selenium, and rubidium. In the second study, administration of cesium and rubidium caused resorption of tumors. The uptake of these elements by the tumor was increased by vitamin A, vitamin C, zinc, and selenium. Another factor required for cellular uptake of rubidium is the presence of ATP. (268) Each of these factors has some negative metabolic or biochemical relationship to mercury. Mercury can inhibit or modify how the body uses ATP, zinc, selenium, rubidium, vitamins A and C, and calcium. We haven't researched copper and vanadium, but are aware of some data indicating lead and mercury can affect their status as well.

The tumors assayed in both studies reflected higher levels of some of the nutrients involved, with the exception of ATP.

Additionally, levels of mercury and lead appeared to be the same in normal and tumorous tissue, a fact which neither set of investigators commented upon. One aspect of the way a normal healthy tissue rejects cancer could be by inducing very high uptakes of critical defensive nutrients and enzymes, such as the alkali metals indicated above and glutathione peroxidase (GSH-Px) to control free radicals. Their influx is enhanced by the other nutrients mentioned. However, although the tissue assays in the tumors showed higher levels than nontumorous tissue, let's hypothesize about some of the factors that might be involved.

Cancer cells have altered sodium and calcium transport and reduced oxygen transport through the cell membrane. The oxygen deficiency within the cell reduces or eliminates the ability of the cell to oxidize glucose to carbon dioxide, which in turn results in glucose being converted to lactic acid, lowering cellular pH into the acid range. These combined effects radically change cell metabolism and ultimately DNA replication.

Mercury can alter sodium and calcium transport and also reduces the amount of oxygen transported. Mercury competes with calcium for cellular binding sites and through this mechanism can decrease cellular calcium or increase extracellular calcium. Mercury binds avidly to rubidium and selenium. Decreases in available selenium can also reduce available GSH-Px which in turn causes a proliferation of free radical cellular damage. Mercury, at extremely low levels, can inhibit the respiratory burst of killer cell leukocytes, reducing their effectiveness in controlling cancer cell proliferation.

It is possible for rubidium to replace potassium, thereby reducing the amount of glucose carried into the cancer cell. This results in a reduction in the amount of lactic acid produced, which would also tend to raise the pH, ultimately leading to reversal of cancer cell metabolic processes.

Our hypothesis is based on the effects of mercury and lead modifying cellular availability of key nutrients utilized by healthy tissue in fighting off the development and implantation of a cancerous cell. Normal defensive mechanisms would cause a spontaneous rise to significantly higher levels than those demonstrated after induction of the tumor. This theory would seem to be supported by the results of Brewer's study. If that hypothesis is correct, then the presence of lead and mercury, which inhibit or reduce the bioavailabiliy of these same key factors and ATP, could significantly diminish their availability. Consequently, although the tissue attempting to suppress the cancer is preferentially accumulating these nutrients, the available stores are inadequate to reach the level required for suppression. At the same time, mercury and lead have also reduced available intracellular oxygen leading to an increase in production of lactic acid and a reduction in pH, both conditions conducive to proliferation of cancer cells.

One of the problems in advancing a hypothesis such as the one above and proving its validity is the very nature of the pathogenesis of cancer. Cancer cells have a usual growth pattern of doubling approximately every 100 days. Therefore, as in the case of breast cancer, if you have had cancer for three and a half months, you would have two cancer cells in your breast. The growth is microscopic and a pathologist would be unable to find it. At the end of six years, a breast tumor would contain one million cells, and it would be no larger than the period at the end of this sentence.(269) Because of the microscopic growth, it is difficult to visualize how a laboratory analysis could be structured to prove the hypothesis. However, it does appear that there are some epidemiological studies that could be done. For example, in the case of breast cancer, which strikes about 120,000 women each year, you could determine (1) how many women with breast cancer have mercury amalgam dental fillings, how many fillings they have, and how long they have had these fillings; (2) how many women with mercury amalgam dental fillings also have gold or nonprecious metals (such as chrome, nickel, beryllium, or aluminum) present in their mouths; (3) how many women have low blood selenium and glutathione peroxidase levels; (4) how many women have low blood zinc, calcium, rubidium, vitamin A, and vitamin C levels; (5) how many women are excreting higher than normal levels of any of the nutrients or their metabolites in their urine; (6) what their blood erythrocyte and hair mercury levels are; and (7) the spectrum of heavy metal as well as essential mineral content present, with specific emphasis on mercury and lead, by using magnetic resonance imaging analysis techniques.

The data derived from women who had developed breast cancer would then be compared against a control group of women who did not have breast cancer and who had no metals present in their mouth and no excessive amount of lead in their bodies. It would also be possible to do comparative analyses of breast tissue of women with no breast cancer who have died accidental deaths against tissue samples from women who have had breast cancer.

The role of metals in carcinogenesis was evaluated by Jennette in 1981. In his discussion he states: "The divalent ions of beryllium, manganese, cobalt, nickel, cadmium, mercury, and lead are stable forms of these elements which may mimic essential divalent ions such as magnesium, calcium, iron, copper, or zinc. These ions may complex small molecules, enzymes, and nucleic acids in such a way that the normal activity of these species is altered. Free radicals may be produced in the presence of these metal ions which damage critical cellular molecules." (270)

In our research on this subject, we found only one article _[Druckery et al. (1957], in which the experiment concluded that there was a direct relationship between the administration of mercury and the development of cancer. In Sweden, Dr. Mats Hanson had also been looking for relationships between mercury and cancer. Dr. Hanson found three German articles (one of which was Druckery et al.) which he translated and forwarded to us. We considered these articles to be of great significance, even though two of them did not fulfill strict scientific construction. Therefore, we would like to stipulate at the outset that the articles by Ledergerber (1949) and Schwarzkopf (1959) fall more in the category of anecdotal, or case history evaluations, rather than expressions of hard scientific data derived from experiments. Nevertheless, we view them as presenting real-life experiences that are significant and certainly food for thought.

In 1949, E. Ledergerber published an article entitled "On deaths and diseases leading to death among workers producing detonators." What is so fascinating about this article is that the author investigated causes of death from 1918 to 1942 in workmen exposed to mercury in the work place, and attempted to establish an occupational connection between mercury and the actual cause of death.(271) It should be noted that although the detonators contained mercury-fulminate, an organic mercury compound, the workers were exposed mainly to inorganic mercury during the manufacturing process. The causes of deaths recorded were influenza, kidney inflammation, lung tuberculosis, suicide (resulting from kidney disease), abdominal tumor, brain inflammation from sinusitis, explosion, lymphogranuloma, acute myeloblastic leukemia, and colitis. Ledergerber concluded that an occupational connection was not considered likely in the case of influenza, tuberculosis, suicide, and abdominal tumor. Moreover, the deaths due to kidney disease were not thought to be connected with the work and were therefore not investigated.(271)

Ledergerber's paper presents data on two of ten deaths among workers employed at the time of death, as well as information on workers who had retired. The two specific case histories were given because of the data related to blood diseases and their subsequent cancer.

In case 1, there was a malignant disease of the lymphatic system, and in case 2, there was a systemic disease of the bone marrow. In the first case, symptoms of a mercury intoxication are relatively sparse: enlarged throat glands, irritation, tachycardia, loss of potency and sweating.

In case 2, however, there were numerous symptoms which indicated mercury poisoning: tiredness, nose bleeding, headache, loss of weight, thirst, disturbed sleep, uremia, and coughing with bloody discharges. The proof that these symptoms were caused by a chronic mercury poisoning is that the patient, after appearance of the first symptoms (skin eruptions), was transferred to another section of the factory with the consequence that the symptoms were reduced and only appeared again when he returned to the detonator section.

Ledergerber stated that it could not be proven that the cause of these two diseases was mercury poisoning. However, the fact that within one year, two relatively rare diseases appeared during a period of time where the possibility of mercury poisonings prevailed because of intense production, makes it impossible to dismiss the notion of a connection between mercury and an occupational disease.

To obtain more knowledge concerning the effects of mercury on the hematopoietic system, Ledergerber conducted a serial study of all employees in the mercury-fulminate division. He was amazed by the wide variations that occurred without any evident cause in the same individual worker within a short time. He found that the number of erythrocytes, for example, could increase or decrease within a few days by 2 million and the leukocytes could vary between 2-5,000 more or less.

The described cell changes in the blood could be absolute or relative. When the number of leukocytes rose, the lymphocytes could, for example, fall sharply. For other workers it was the reverse; a falling leukocyte number was accompanied by a relatively large elevation of lymphocytes. Still others showed parallel changes. To illustrate how rapidly changes could occur, the blood values for two workers are shown here:

Case 1	May 22, 1944	May 30, 1944
Hemoglobin	92%	97%
Leukocytes	12300	4600
Neutrophils	78.5%	60.5%
Eosinophils	0.5%	2.5%
Basophils	0.5%	0.5%
Lymphocytes	13.5%	27.5%
Monocytes	7%	9%
Sedimentation Rate	10/32 mm	8/19 mm

Case 2	Mar 26, 1943	Apr 27, 1943	May 18, 1943
Hemoglobin	113%	99%	85%
Erythrocytes	5,600,000	4,900,000	4,300,000
Leukocytes	4500	12000	7400
Eosinophils	3%	3%	1%
Neutrophils	53%	37.5%	27.5%
Lymphocytes	31%	55.5%	63.5%
Monocytes	13%	4%	5%

Ledergerber commented on the complexity of the conditions encountered and speculated that apparently there must have been some damage to the bone marrow caused by irritation or some type of inhibition. As a consequence there is an unusual and very variable export of cells from the bone marrow into the blood. Ledergerber thought that these many-sided deviations of blood values demonstrated the profound damage that could be caused by mercury fulminate. Ledergerber cited other literature that had demonstrated that the use of mercury medicines had caused severe agranulocytosis (a decrease in the number of granule containing leukocytes that can manifest as lesions of the throat and other mucous membranes), partly with toxic and partly with allergic conditions.

Among the thirteen workers who died after retirement, heart disease predominated. Among sixteen pensioners still living in 1943 (mean age 68.7 years), eleven had heart disease. The blood pressure was normal in only four cases, with an average of 140/85 mm/Hg. The other twelve cases showed elevated values, with an average of 170/110 mm/Hg.

The workers who had retired between 1939 and 1943 reported that they had felt successively better after the pensioning. The nervousness of those who had been pensioned earlier had been reduced somewhat; those who were pensioned later had not noticed any reduction of these troubles. Impaired hearing improved slowly. Four of the sixteen had unimpaired hearing, while the other twelve were more or less hard of hearing. Rheumatic troubles, especially in the shoulders, were common, and it was more common on the right then on the left side. All complained of being very thirsty. Remarkably, all pensioners had a fairly developed goiter. However, most of them reported that the goiter had diminished after pensioning. Women who worked in the factory almost universally had goiter. Among active men, the hypothyroid changes were less common in relation to the mercury poisonings.(271)

****

Schwarzkopf's article, entitled "Dental Materials and Cancer," appeared in 1959. A dentist colleague had raised the point that with the increase in dentistry there also appeared to be an increase in the incidence of cancer. In thinking about what his colleague had said, Schwarzkopf rationalized that prior to the advent of filling materials, teeth were simply pulled. Oddly enough, there wasn't any cancer then, either.(272) Accordingly, he set out to investigate oral conditions of some cancer patients. Of four cancer patients evaluated, the following was found:

Case 1: A large number of silver amalgam fillings and a steel crown.

Case 2: Two silver amalgams, one upper plastic denture with a steel suction piece.

Case 3: A complete upper denture of India rubber (contains mercury) with a steel suction piece since 1935, and a complete lower denture of plastic placed in 1942.

Case 4: Seven silver amalgams and one copper amalgam filling.

Schwarzkopf decided to treat these patients by removing the metals from their mouths. In Case 3 he also replaced the India rubber denture with one of plastic. Following are his results.

Case 1: Male 62; diagnosed in 1951 as having a recurrence of stomach cancer that had been operated on in 1927. In 1951 it was considered inoperable. Beginning in February 1952, the silver amalgam fillings were removed and replaced with Drala-stone-cement fillings. The tooth with the steel crown had a granuloma at the root apex and was pulled, after which the granuloma cleared up. Between February and April of 1952 the patient improved and clinical symptoms disappeared, including the stomach tumor which was no longer visible from the outside. The patient continued smoking ten cigarettes a day. When last seen by Dr. Schwarzkopf in 1959, the patient's cancer was still in remission.

Case 2: A 66-year-old female who had received radium therapy in 1949 for carcinoma of the uterus, which her physician considered inoperable. Beginning in February of 1952, the tooth with two amalgam fillings was extracted, and the steel suction part of the upper denture was removed. Between February and September of 1952, the patient showed steady improvement and loss of all clinical symptoms. When last seen in 1959, her cancer was still in remission.

Case 3: A 63-year-old female with carcinoma of the uterus; existent since 1947 and who, by 1951, was unable to walk. On March 8, 1952, the India rubber denture with steel suction plate was replaced with one made of plastic without steel. The patient improved through July 1952 and was able to walk. She experienced a relapse in August 1952, and was given ten x-ray treatments. Her condition worsened and she died in 1953.

Case 4: Female, 38, with carcinoma of the uterus who had received radium treatment in May 1948 and x-ray treatment six weeks later. Since then she had been bedridden with violent pains in lower back and legs. In February of 1952, the seven silver amalgam and one copper amalgam fillings were removed. From then until June 1952 there was amelioration of much of the symptomatology. However, in June her condition worsened and she died that July.

In his article, Schwarzkopf analyzes his findings and relates many anecdotal cases of other health conditions that showed dramatic improvement after removal of metals from the mouth. He goes on to say that certainly not every person who has silver amalgam fillings or India rubber dentures (mercuric sulfide is used to color the rubber) will have cancer. Most humans are very resistant against these compounds and have them in their mouths for years without any ill effects. If, however, usual methods fail to heal the described disease, one should think of a poisoning from the materials deposited in the mouth.

This next paragraph from the same article reflects how journals can seriously limit the flow of controversial information within a profession simply by rejecting the article.

I have written this paper in 1952 without having been able to publish it in a professional journal despite several attempts! In the meantime I have

often had the possibility to stop metal and mercury poisonings, almost always with good results
on various diseases. In some cases I had not
success until several years later when I found
out that there were still amalgam fillings under a
bridge or a crown.(272)

****

The article by Druckerey et al. (1957), entitled "Cancerogenic effects of metallic mercury after intraperitoneal
injection in rats," describes how liquid elemental mercury
was injected into the abdominal cavity of rats. The researchers
found that the normal 800 day life span of the rats was reduced
to 580 days in the experiment animals, whereas the controls
(no mercury exposure) lived 780 days.(273)

There were thirty-nine animals that received the mercury
injection. Of that number twenty-seven died by the 22nd
month, when the first tumor appeared in one of the twelve
remaining rats. Abdominal tumors appeared in four other
rats as well. There was no relation to sex of the animal. After
the animals died, the tumors were dissected and mercury
droplets were found in their inner parts. Most of the mercury
droplets could be seen with the naked eye.

All of the tumors had developed, without exception, in the
regions where there had been immediate contact with the
metal. The authors relate the work of other researchers who
had demonstrated that different metals and metal salts were
capable of causing cancer. Perhaps the most significant statement pertained to research by Zollinger that showed repeated
injections of a 2% lead-phosphate suspension produced kidney carcinoma and -adenoma. This particular experiment
demonstrated that the tumors did not appear at the site of application but far from the application site, indicating a clear
effect caused by absorption.(273)

We think the significance of the preceding articles have
been totally overlooked by scientific and medical researchers
throughout the world. Cancer researchers have spent an
average of one billion dollars a year since 1972 on everything from the ridiculous to the sublime, in the quest to find
a cause and/or cure for this dreaded killer disease. In that
context, it is almost beyond belief that the basic theory of
cancer induction by mercury embodied in all three articles
has been ignored.

HYPOTHESIS:

MERCURY AND/OR FOREIGN SUBSTANCES
INHALED, INGESTED, OR PLACED IN THE
ORAL CAVITY CAN CAUSE CRITICAL EVENTS
TO TRANSPIRE IN THE HUMAN BODY, LEAD-
ING TO THE DEVELOPMENT OF CANCER
YEARS LATER. REMOVAL OF THESE SUB-
STANCES FROM THE MOUTH MAY BE PALLIA-
TIVE OR CURATIVE.

TRANSSULFURATION PATHWAY

The great binding affinity that mercury and lead have for the
sulfur atom forms the basis of our hypothesis. Think of the
tremendously complicated metabolic mechanisms of the
human defense system, which includes the immune system,
as a house of cards. Throughout the fragile structure of the
house are cards labeled "sulfur atom." As in any building,
there are certain critical weight-bearing structures that hold
the building up by carrying the weight of the structure built
above them. Think of the sulfur atoms as the weight-bearing members of your defense/immune system. Now think of
what termites in a wooden house can do. Completely hidden

from sight, they can destroy a critical support structure. We feel that mercury and lead function in a similar manner in your body's defense/immune system, or house of cards. It may take years of attacking and reducing the number of sulfur atoms holding up the house, but eventually enough sulfur atoms are missing so that the system comes tumbling down!

With that in mind, let's look at some of the sulfur-related aspects considered critical to life sustaining biochemical functions. An oversimplification of the transsulfuration pathways could be depicted as a biochemical road map. For example:

TRANSSULFURATION PATHWAYS

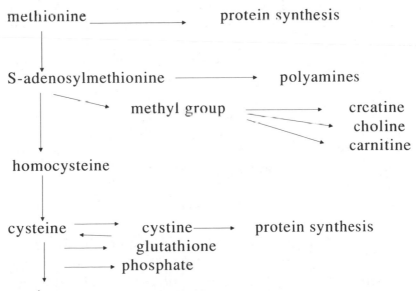

From this basic transsulfuration pathway, there are a myriad of other biochemical functions that take place, including those described in Chapter 11 involving folic acid and vitamin B_{12}. One of the critical aspects of metabolism relates to the transfer or the reduction of the methyl group. The primary methyl donor in the body is S-adenosyl-methionine. If you look at our "road map," you will see that it is metabolized from methionine. It is here that methionine functions as a primary carrier and donor of the methyl group through S-adenosylmethionine. The first two letters of *methionine* stand for "methyl." Many critical metabolic functions are contingent upon an adequate supply of the methyl substance first derived from methionine. The importance of this function is discussed later in this chapter.

The liver is one of the most important organs in the body when it comes to detoxifying or getting rid of foreign substances or toxins. Glutathione, which appears to be the most abundant sulfhydryl in the body, functions to chelate and detoxify heavy metals; mercury and lead both have been shown to combine or complex with glutathione. Once complexed together, the bile becomes a major route used by the body to excrete the complex, thereby reducing the amount of glutathione available.

Another piece of the pie relating to glutathione is that xenobiotics (drugs) can also cause a reduction in its availability. Although the exact mechanism is not known, it is thought to be by complexing and excretion, the same as for mercury and lead. If you look at the transsulfuration pathway above, you will see that cysteine is a precursor (has to be present) in the formation (synthesis) of glutathione. Consequently, if an adequate supply of cysteine is not readily available, the rate of production of glutathione will be reduced. Therefore, you could say that cysteine is the limiting factor in the biosynthesis of glutathione.

The primary source of the sulfur portion of cysteine appears to be methionine. Cysteine cannot be taken up by hepatocytes (liver cells) easily, whereas methionine is taken up more readily, and is then metabolized into S-adenosyl-methionine, homocysteine, cystathionine, and cysteine. Therefore, if the availability of methionine is reduced, not only will the capability of the liver to detoxify be impaired, but there will also be less glutathione available to complex with foreign substances.

In 1984, Ghoshal and Farber conducted research on the effects of a dietary deficiency of methionine and choline in relation to subsequent development of liver cancer. As early as 1946, research by Copeland and Salmon (274) had demonstrated the occurrence of neoplasms (uncontrolled or abnormal growth of a new tissue) in the liver, lungs, and other tissues of rats fed a prolonged choline deficient diet. This was subsequently confirmed by several other researchers under various experimental protocols. In their experiment, Ghoshal and Farber fed a choline-methionine-deficient diet to Fischer male rats for 13-24 months. There was a 100% incidence of precancerous liver cell nodules and a 51% incidence of hepatocellular carcinoma (developed liver cancer). The addition of 0.8% choline chloride completely prevented the development of both the nodules and the cancer.(275)

Latta and Donaldson (1986), using chicks, investigated whether dietary methionine and choline could affect the toxicity of lead. In one experiment, a methionine-deficient diet was fed to the chicks; in the second experiment, a choline-deficient diet was fed to the chicks. The experimental variable was the addition of choline to a methionine-deficient diet or the addition of methionine to a choline-deficient diet. Concurrently with either diet, the chicks were given either zero or 1,000 parts per million of lead in their diets as the other variable.

In both experiments, lead depressed growth while methionine stimulated growth. Growth depression by lead was less with the methionine-adequate diet. There were no differences in growth with the choline-marginal diet or the choline-excess diet. Lead-induced depression of growth was exacerbated by added choline when methionine-inadequate diets were fed. The authors concluded that their results suggested that lead lowers the chicks' choline requirement and that the methyl portion of methionine does not participate directly in lead detoxification. The amelioration of lead toxicity by methionine appears to be related to increased excretion of lead.(276)

One very interesting aspect of this study was the finding that adding dietary choline, when methionine was deficient, further aggravated the depression of growth. The authors did not know the reason for this reaction but because of one other report in the literature indicating choline could inhibit the conversion of methionine to cysteine, thought this might have also occurred in their experiment and felt that the presence of toxicants in the diet may alter requirements for some nutrients.

These two studies clearly demonstrated that the deficiency of methionine could, in itself, cause liver cancer without the presence of a carcinogen, and also that the deficiency of methionine could permit a heavy metal to cause toxic effects.Throughout this entire chapter we ask you to keep firmly fixed in your mind that the presence of mercury or lead in the body can cause disruptions in every biochemical process that we will discuss. With that in mind, let's look at some of the research that has been done investigating the role of methionine in cancer.

Previous research on methionine and cancer had concluded that cancer cells required methionine in order to grow and proliferate. Based on that research, one of the cancer treatment protocols utilized has been to administer a class of drugs that inhibited the availability of methionine and to also feed cancer patients methionine-deficient diets. However, current research investigating this phenomenon has arrived at different conclusions. Following are abstracts of two 1985 articles on this subject.

Methionine metabolism and transmethylation are frequently altered in cancer cells. The alteration is often expressed as an inability of the cancer cells to grow when methionine is replaced by homocysteine in the culture medium, a condition that allows the growth of normal cells. This metabolic defect is termed methionine dependence. Methionine dependence may reflect an overall imbalance in transmethylation which results in the overmethylation of some substances and undermethylation of others within cancer cells. Many carcinogens affect various stages of methionine/ transmethylation metabolism. The ultimate effect of the alteration of methionine/transmethylation metabolism may be the disruption of the regulations of genes involved in the oncogenic process. The known protective effect of methionine against cancer may be due to prevention of altered methionine/transmethylation metabolism or compensation of the altered metabolism.(277)

A 1985 paper by van der Westhuyzen summarizes recent developments linking methionine metabolism and S-adenosyl-methionine to DNA methylation and gene expression in relation to cancer.

Methionine, obtained in the diet and synthesized by several reactions in the body, is the sole precursor of S-adenosylmethionine, the primary methyl donor in the body. Disruptions in methionine metabolism and methylation reactions may be involved in cancer processes. S-adenosylmethionine is involved in, inter alia, the methylation of a small percentage of cytosine bases of DNA. Recent evidence suggests that enzymatic DNA methylation is an important component of gene control and may serve as a silencing mechanism for gene methylation, and thus may allow oncogene activation. Demethylation may be a necessary, but not always sufficient, condition for enhanced transcription. DNA hypomethylation has been observed in many cancer cells and tumors. The hypothesis that oncogenic transformation may be prevented or even reversed by a diet containing excess methionine and/or choline needs to be further investigated.(278)

We believe both of these articles are bringing out the fact that cancer or tumor-cell dependence on methionine for growth is an artificial condition, brought about by some earlier failure in the transsulfuration and transmethylation pathways. As a consequence, normal metabolic processes that would prevent the cancer or tumor cells from growing are not in place. In other words, normal homeostasis mechanisms have been disrupted. The same thing can be stated another way, as was so aptly done by Hoffman and Erbe in a 1976 article: "Methionine-dependence can not be considered as the inability of a cell to grow on methionine endogenously synthesized from a precursor, but depends on the precursor used, and possibly, on a toxic effect of the precursor in the absence of methionine."(279)

Mercury and lead also can cause disruptions of the metabolic reactions in both the transsulfuration and transmethylation pathways. Remember, both metals have the ability to complex with sulfur atoms and sulfhydryls. Furthermore, when you consider the wide-ranging metabolic effects of both of these toxic metals, the hypothesis that they can both be involved in the etiology of cancer becomes more probable.

For example, research has clearly shown that zinc availability can be reduced by mercury. In a 1985 article, Wallwork and Duerre demonstrated that the uptake of methionine by the rat liver was significantly less when the rats had been fed a zinc-deficient diet. They also found that the synthesis of methionine, S-adenosylhomocysteine, and S-adenosylmethionine was not impaired in the livers of zinc-deficient rats. However, the methyl group of S-adenosyl-methionine turned over more slowly (a slowing of metabolic reactions). This was reflected in the depressed rates of methylation of various macromolecules, particularly DNA and histones (simple proteins). The synthesis of nuclear proteins (histones and nonhistone chromosomal proteins) was depressed in the livers from zinc-deficient rats. This was consistent with the finding that DNA biosynthesis and cellular proliferation are markedly depressed in zinc-deficient animals.(280)

Most people have read newspaper accounts of the cancer-causing effects of asbestos and diethylstilbestrol (DES). The unique feature of both of these substances is that they cause a particular type of cancer. It was this characteristic that permitted some scientific confirmation of their latent malignancy. In other words, because they caused a particular type of cancer to occur, it was possible to look back at when the patient may have been exposed to the substance causing this particular form of cancer. For example, the scientific world was confronted with the fact that DES was a transplacental carcinogen. Suddenly, scientists and physicians of the industrialized nations of the world were confronted with the spector that a drug, aggressively prescribed to pregnant women to prevent morning sickness and miscarriages, was capable of causing cancerous-type cell changes in the fetus that could ultimately cause cancer, months, years, or decades later.

There are several aspects of the DES debacle that we consider quite remarkable and for which medicine and science have no logical explanation. For example, not all children of women receiving DES during their pregnancies were stricken with cancer. Those that did get cancer were between the ages of fourteen and twenty-two (the largest occurrence at age 19). It appears that the cancer death rate among DES mothers was twice that of non-DES mothers, and the primary malignancies were mainly breast cancer. DES daughters had an increased incidence of menstrual problems. About 25% of DES sons had various genital abnormalities--low sperm counts, with 40% having abnormally shaped sperm--DES sons had an increased rate of testicular cancer.(281-283)

What we find so important about the entire DES disaster is that it clearly demonstrates that transplacental latent malignancies and other more subtle dysfunctions capable of causing sterility, infertility, and birth defects years later, can be caused by maternal exposure to a foreign substance during pregnancy.

Medicine and science have been unable to provide an acceptable rationale for the hit-or-miss manner in which DES took its toll. However, we feel strongly that the DES tragedy supports the hypothesis advanced by both Chapter 11 and this chapter. For example, there are burning questions that arise in our minds: How many mothers receiving DES treatment had a mouthful of mercury amalgam dental fillings or partial dentures or caps containing nickel, chrome, or beryllium? What were the maternal and fetal cord blood levels of mercury and lead? Did the DES mothers undergo dental restorative work during their pregnancies, where mercury amalgam fillings were placed or replaced? Did the DES sons and daughters have mercury amalgam dental fillings in their teeth? Perhaps more importantly, at what age did the children have their first mercury amalgam fillings placed, and how many were placed prior to puberty?

The rationale behind these questions is quite simple, especially if one views them in the context of how scientists conduct laboratory and animal experiments to determine how one substance might change the toxicity of another substance. For example, when scientists want to test whether vitamin E or selenium can reduce the toxicity of mercury or other poisons, the protocol usually involves administering the poison to an animal and then seeing if administration of vitamin E or selenium will reduce the lethal effects of the poison. Variations of the protocol involve first feeding the animal a diet rich in vitamin E or selenium and then administering the poison, or, giving the vitamin E or selenium at the same time the poison is administered. The results of such studies are usually given in terms of how effective the vitamin E or selenium was in reducing or preventing the lethal effects of the poison.

The same type of experiments are done when science is attempting to determine if a substance is effective against the prevention of cancer. There are special strains of animals that are prone to develop certain types of cancers. If a scientist wants to determine if a vitamin or a drug has anticarcinogenic properties, they set up an experiment where the animal gets a known carcinogen, and then see if the vitamin or drug is able to prevent the animal from getting cancer. The same technique can be used to determine the combined effects of substances, such as co-administration of a known carcinogen with mercury and/or lead.

The purpose of discussing this information is that the scientific literature reflects literally hundreds of experiments that have demonstrated that deficiencies of key nutrients will permit increased incidences of everything from viral infections to cancers. More importantly, the scientific literature also has demonstrated that the effects of poisons, such as mercury and lead, can also be reduced or eliminated when certain nutrients are provided in adequate quantities.

Moreover, it is an established fact that most drugs have side effects that affect some normal metabolic process in the body, some of which can be life threatening, and a great many of which cause nutritional deficiencies. For example, Dr. Daphne A. Roe, in her classic book entitled "Drug-Induced Nutritional Deficiencies," states: "Drugs in five major groups have been shown either to function as vitamin B_6 antagonists, or to increase the turnover of vitamin B6 in the body...Drugs in ten major groups have been shown to affect the absorption of folate; to act as folate antagonists; or to increase the turnover or loss of folate from the body...Drugs in four groups have been shown to affect the absorption of vitamin B_{12}." Dr. Roe goes on to point out the fact that the depletion of one vitamin can affect the requirement for another vitamin.(259) Coincidentally, isn't it interesting that mercury can cause similar deficiencies or metabolic changes in the way the body handles these same three vitamins (see Chapter 11)? What happens to the nutritional status of a woman taking the pill and who is also chronically inhaling mercury from her mercury amalgam dental fillings? Is she more vulnerable to the potential cancerous effects of exogenous estrogen?

In relation to the DES tragedy and the implication that estrogens were the controlling factor, one of the drugs that affected vitamin B_6 and folate status was oral contraceptives. Further, Dr. Roe went on to cite research indicating the pill could also cause decreases of ascorbic acid, vitamin B_2 (which caused a fall in erythrocyte glutathione reductase activity), vitamin E, and zinc. So, here we have evidence showing that an estrogen-containing pill can cause a variety of nutritional deficits.(259) Here again, and as shown in Chapter 11, mercury can affect nutriture status of these same nutrients.

When the chronic lifetime inhalation and absorption of mercury from amalgam fillings is coupled with chronic lead exposure; the routine intake of both prescription and non-prescription drugs; and poor dietary regimes and/or high-fish diets rich in methylmercury, the effect on an individual's nutriture, and ultimately on the body's immune system and other defense mechanisms, could be devastating. To place the defense mechanisms of the body in better perspective to this statement, let's look at some of the research.

Wulf et al. (1986) evaluated the mutagenicity of the chromosomes of the peripheral lymphocytes of 147 Greenlandic Eskimos living in both Greenland and Denmark, by means of a sister chromatid exchange (SCE) test. They found that SCE correlated linearly with mercury concentration. "This may imply that mercury is mutagenic/carcinogenic in concentrations far below the level of methylmercury intoxication (Bernstein 1975; Kitamura et al., 1976). Mercury exposure is related to the amount of marine food (seal, whole fish, etc.) consumed...."(284)

Heimburger et al. (1987) evaluated whether changes in folate and vitamin B_{12} nutriture modify the severity of cytological lesions in sputum samples of smokers. The tests were conducted on smokers with bronchial squamous metaplasia (scaly abnormal cells within the windpipe). Their conclusion: "Our findings provide preliminary evidence that atypical bronchial squamous metaplasia, an intermediate step in the progression from normal bronchial epithelium to cancer, may be improved by supplementation with folate and vitamin B_{12}."(285) A question could logically be asked here: Did the test subjects have mercury amalgam dental fillings, and did that mercury exposure initiate the nutritional deficiencies/decrease in immunocompetence that permitted the squamous metaplasia to develop in the first place?

Sara Benum (1987) brings out some interesting data concerning viruses and the immune function. She quotes several authorities who indicate that a person who has had hepatitis B has 100 times the normal risk of later developing liver cancer; Epstein-Barr virus has been linked to at least two types of cancer; at least 80% of all cervical cancers are linked to the human papillomavirus (HPV); human T-cell lymphotropic virus type 1 (HLTV-1) is a retrovirus which causes a type of adult leukemia. She quotes Dr. Thomas Merigan of the Stanford School of Medicine: "There is a very intimate relationship between viruses and immunity. If our immunity is a little deficient for one reason or another, then we are more likely to have progressive disease."(286) Does the person with mercury amalgam dental fillings have a lower immunocompetence status than the person without poisons implanted in their mouth? Does this make them more vulnerable and allow these viral infections to overwhelm their defense mechanisms?

Shannon and Demos (1977) investigated the influence of estrogen treatment of cystathionine enzymes in relation to vitamin B6 status. Although their research showed estradiol reduced cystathionase, they felt the implications of their findings to women taking estrogen-containing oral contraceptives were a matter of conjecture. However, they concluded their article with the following statement: "We feel that more definitive investigations are needed in regard to effects of estrogens on methionine metabolism, particularly in relation to women taking estrogen-containing oral contraceptives."(287) We know that mercury can also affect methionine nutriture!

There are several studies that show lead and mercury are capable of mutagenic effects, such as inhibiting the mitotic spindle (which causes C-mitosis). Chromosomes in human lymphocytes have also shown evidence of damage from exposures to either lead or mercury. Although some of the researchers have presented conflicting data, there are many factors which could have influenced the outcome of some of the reports not showing chromosomal damage such as, nutritional status of the blood donor, degree of exposure prior to the blood sample being taken, and so forth. Kazantsis (1981) provides an excellent overview of the mutagenicity and carcinogenicity of lead and mercury.(288)

As we have stated earlier, the carcinogenic data on mercury is extremely limited. However, with regards to lead there is much more evidence of a direct causal relationship. Animal studies have shown adenoma and carcinoma of the kidney; interstitial cell tumors of the testis; and adenomas of the pituitary and prostate glands. In experimental studies on humans with long industrial exposures in the work place, the data is less conclusive and only shows a marginal increase in cancer deaths attributed to lead exposure.(288)

Unfortunately, most scientific studies, by their very nature, only evaluate the toxicity of an individual substance. Consequently, little is known about the interaction of lead with mercury compounds in animals or humans. Some studies however, are beginning to appear. A study with rats in 1979 demonstrated that when both lead and mercury were administered, the kidneys accumulated more mercury.(289) A 1985 study with mice demonstrated that when lead and mercury were co-administered, there was an increase of mercury in the spleen. Damage to circulating erythrocytes also occurred more rapidly than the individual elements alone caused.(290) The effects of both studies, if the same reactions transpire in humans, could be a significant factor in immune incompetence.

There are literally hundreds of articles on nutrition and the immune system. We think the summary in a recent 1985 article on the subject by Dr. L.C. Corman sums it up beautifully: "The importance of nutrition in every aspect of human physiology slowly is being appreciated clinically. However, it is clear that immune function is highly dependent on the nutritional status of the individual. That status, in turn, is dependent on the nutritional intake and the metabolic machinery of the individual."(291)

One of the current prevalent cancerogenesis theories being investigated by scientists around the world deals with free radical pathology. There is research demonstrating that mercury can cause free radicals as well as other pathological and metabolic conditions that have the potential of being cancer causing. However, our intent in including a chapter on cancer was not so much to treat the subject of cancer itself as it was to point out the potentials of mercury, lead, and other metals to be involved in the etiology of cancer. The potential of mercury and lead as transplacental carcinogens and the phenomenon of latent development of cancer in offspring subjected to chemical insult during gestation was and is our primary concern. Although we may personally feel that mercury and lead are significantly involved in the etiology of adult cancers, our immediate concern is to alert women of childbearing age and their mates to the devastating potentials of mercury vapor from mercury amalgam dental fillings. If the information presented in this chapter is instrumental in just one child being born without a latent predisposition to cancer because of reduced maternal and paternal body burdens of mercury, it will have served its purpose.

11

BIOCHEMICAL PATHWAYS

MERCURY TOXICITY HYPOTHESIS

In developing this chapter, we may also have developed the biochemical basis for mercury toxicity. Although over 7000 articles have been published on mercury, there is much that scientists do not know regarding exactly how mercury exerts its toxic effect. In a review paper, Chang (1977) concluded with a proposed working hypothesis on the pathogenetic mechanism of mercury as a neurotoxin: "The pathogenetic effects of mercury may be divided into two main categories; (i) disruption of the cellular metabolism which will eventually lead to cell death, and (ii) a direct degradation of the cellular constituents."(292)

What we are hypothesizing is that mercury exerts its toxic effects through disruption of critical biochemical pathways related to various vitamins and minerals required to maintain homeostasis. If one looks at the myriad of symptomatology that can be caused by mercury, the question of how this single element can cause all of these problems has to assume great significance.

When we started to review the literature related to this chapter --especially that pertaining to folic acid, vitamin B_{12}, and thiamine--it became increasingly evident that deficiencies of these vitamins produced a galaxy of symptoms that closely paralleled those caused by mercury. To determine if we were right in this assumption, the following chart of symptoms was developed. Symptoms of mercury toxicity are shown on the left and symptoms of deficiencies of folic acid, vitamin B_{12}, and vitamin B_1 (thiamine) in the three columns to the right.

MERCURY	FOLIC ACID	VITAMIN B12	**VITAMIN B1**
Anemia	Anemia	Anemia	
Irritability	Irritability	Agitation	
Muscle weakness			Irritability
Weight loss	Weight loss		Muscle weakness
Apathy	Apathy		Weight loss
Anorexia	Anorexia	Appetite loss	Anorexia
Emphysema	Dyspnea		Dyspnea
Irregular respiration	Dyspnea		Dyspnea
Ulceration of tongue	Sore tongue		
	Glossitis		Glossitis
Headache	Headache		Headache
Irregular heartbeat	Palpitations		Palpitations
Forgetfulness	Forgetfulness		
Loss of memory			Bad memory
Outbursts of anger	Hostility		
Hallucinations	Paranoid behavior	Hallucinations	
GI Disturbances	GI Disturbances	GI Disturbances	Gastric upset
Diarrhea	Diarrhea	Diarrhea	
Constipation		Constipation	
Fatigue	Weakness	Fatigue	Asthenia
Dizziness		Dizziness	Dizziness
Numbness		Numbness	Numbness
Tingling		Tingling	Tingling
Incoordination		Ataxia	Ataxia
Dimmed vision		Dimmed vision	
Paralysis		Degeneration of spinal cord	Paralysis
Depression		Moodiness	Depression
Confusion		Confusion	Confusion
Emotional instability		Delusions	Personality change
Paresthesias of hands and feet		Paresthesias of hands and feet	Paresthesia
		Increased RBC hemolysis	
Alterations of blood pressure		Postural hypotension	ECG changes
Joint pain			Neuritic pain
Insomnia			Insomnia
Drowsiness			Asthenia
Low body temperature			Low body temperature
Chest pain or pressure			
			Hyperesthesia

We didn't chart symptoms for the other vitamins and minerals affected by the presence of mercury in the biological systems as all we wished to do was see if a positive correlation appeared to exist. We think that it is obvious from the chart that there is both individuality and overlap in the deficiency symptoms spectrum that correlate extremely well with the acknowledged symptoms of mercury toxicity. In our discussion of each one of the nutrients outlined in this chapter, we have provided the plausible biochemical pathways showing where and how mercury can inhibit, deplete body stores, or render normal metabolic functions of these various nutrients inoperative. If we are correct in our hypothesis, then there is also a parallel in the course of time required for mercury vapor to exert its toxic effects and for overt clinical symptoms to develop related to nutrient deficiencies. Both can take upwards of twenty years to develop, unless there are critical inherited deficiencies at the outset, which would also encompass our natural biochemical individuality.

Herbert and his colleagues (293) defined nutritional deficiency as meaning that there was an inadequate usage of a nutrient in one or more intracellular systems to sustain normal biochemical functions. Such inadequate usage falls into six basic categories:

1. Inadequate ingestion

2. Inadequate absorption

3. Inadequate utilization

4. Increased requirement

5. Increased excretion

6. Increased destruction

Any one or combination of these three inadequacies and three excesses may result in nutritional deficiency. In each of the categories defined, there is a metabolic or biochemical pathway influenced by mercury and other sulfur-sensitive heavy metals that could ultimately affect nutritional status.

There is also another aspect of life, relating directly to the overall purpose of this book, to which the hypothesis may be equally applicable. Although the following statement is contained in chapter 1, we consider it important enough to reiterate here.

There are believed to be well over 2000 kinds of human genetic defects or diseases, and the number continues to increase rapidly. More than 120,000 infants with genetic diseases are born each year in the United States.(13,page 542)

In effect, we are saying that the chronic inhalation of mercury vapor derived from dental amalgam fillings may be the unrecognized and uninvestigated possible cause of serious health problems in millions of people. It is our fervent hope that research investigating the metabolic and physiological effects of chronic inhalation of low doses of elemental mercury vapor will eventually be funded.

THE ATTRACTION BETWEEN SULFUR AND MERCURY

We have established in earlier chapters that mercury, in its various forms, has a great affinity for certain minerals, and protein and nonprotein molecules in the body. For example, science has demonstrated that mercurials have a great attraction to the sulfhydryls, or thiols.(294) What this means, all other aspects being equal, is that the mercury atom or molecule will tend to bind with any molecule present that has sulfur or a sulfur-hydrogen combination in its structure.(295) This process of combining with a metal to form a complex in which the metallic ion is sequestered and firmly bound is called chelate or chelation.

The primary sulfur-containing protein amino acids in the body are cystine, cysteine, methionine, and taurine. There is also a sulfur-containing tripeptide (having three amino acids) called glutathione that is composed of glutamic acid, cysteine, and glycine. Sulfur exists in a reduced form (-SH) in cysteine and in an oxidized form (-S-S-) as the double molecule, cystine. Whenever mercury binds to one of these sulfur-containing molecules, it reduces their availability for normal metabolic functions. Sulfur is present in all proteins, which makes it universally available throughout the body for binding with mercury.

Some of the important biochemical sulfur-containing compounds of the body besides glutathione are insulin (a protein hormone that regulates carbohydrate, lipid, and amino acid metabolism), prolactin (one of the hormones of the pituitary gland that stimulates and sustains lactation), growth hormone, and vasopressin (a hormone secreted by the pituitary gland involved in the control of blood pressure, muscles of the intestinal tract, and some muscular control of the uterus). These are not exactly unimportant functions within the body, and science has not yet investigated the effect of mercury upon them.(296,297)

Mercury has a particularly high affinity for thiol groups and progressively less for other groups in the following sequence: Sulfur, amides, amines, carbon, and phosphate.(298) Because of this capability mercury has the potential of binding to proteins throughout the body. Mercury compounds are formed by the binding of mercury to the biological binders albumin or cysteine.(299)

The principal biological reaction of mercury is with thiols to form mercury mercaptides.(295) The sulfur groups are often referred to as mercaptans because of their marked affinity for mercury. Mercaptan is defined as any compound containing reduced sulfur bound to carbon. When a metal, such as mercury, replaces the hydrogen ion of the reduced sulfur, the resulting compound is called a mercaptide.(154) It has been demonstrated that mercury can form at least three compounds with cysteine in which all or a part of the mercury is bound firmly as a mercaptide. (300)

A number of researchers have suggested that mercury may cause damage, especially to the placenta, by inactivation of sulfhydryl groups in cellular enzymes.(155,301-303) According to Winship, "Mercury interacts with sulfhydryl groups and disulfide bonds, as a result of which specific membrane transport is blocked and selective permeability of the membrane is altered. Mercury also combines readily with phosphate and heterocyclic base groups of DNA. It also combines with other ligands: amide, amine, carboxyl and phosphoryl groups."(301)

CYSTEINE AND CYSTINE

According to Sturman, "Cysteine [pronounced "sis-tee'in"] is a unique amino acid, largely by virtue of its sulfhydryl group. It is an important constituent of proteins in which it is largely responsible for their molecular configuration, either by forming disulfide bonds with other cysteine molecules incorporated into the same protein or by forming disulfide bonds with free cysteine. It can link together a number of separate proteins or polypeptides by forming disulfide bonds between cysteine residues in different molecules. Cyst(e)ine is an important precursor of the tripeptide glutathione and theoretically, also of taurine, which may have an important role in development."(304)

Cysteine is made from two other amino acids, methionine and serine. Methionine furnishes the sulfur atom and serine furnishes the carbon skeleton in the synthesis of cysteine.(296) Cysteine is produced by enzymatic or acid hydrolysis of proteins. Cysteine can be oxidized to cystine [pronounced "sis-tin"], which is rather insoluble in water.(154) It is this characteristic of cysteine that can cause problems. Sometimes it can be found in the urine and in the bladder in a crystal form where it will frequently form cystine calculus (stones) in the kidneys or bladder. Cystine is the main sulfur-containing compound of the protein molecule. Upon reduction, cystine produces two molecules of cysteine. Heavy metals catalyze the oxidation of cysteine to cystine and also react with cysteine to form mercaptides.(305)

Cysteine is very soluble in water and therefore can be easily eliminated via the urine. However, cysteine can be oxidized to cystine, which can then present the potential of stone problems. Research has demonstrated that if an adequate supply of vitamin C is available, it will help keep cysteine in its reduced and soluble form, thereby preventing the formation of stones. To accomplish this, the ratio of vitamin C to cysteine should be three to one.(306)

In a series of experiments with mice it was found that when an excess of cysteine was given at the same time mercury was given that it reduced the mercury content in the liver three hours after being administered. Six hours after treatment with the cysteine, levels in the kidney were lowered. However, the administration of excess cysteine had no effect on brain mercury levels or blood mercury levels.(307)

Cystathionase, an enzyme that is necessary to change cystathionine into cysteine and which is present in humans postnatally, is not present in human fetal liver or brain. It has also been reported that cystathionase activity was absent from the liver of many preterm infants who died shortly after birth, and was low in normal-term infants who died shortly after birth. Cysteine is not considered an essential amino acid in adults. However, the results of this study indicated cysteine was an essential amino acid for the human fetus, and possibly for prematurely born and even full term infants for a short period after birth.(308) This would make the fetus dependent on the mother's circulation to obtain cysteine. In this regard, cysteine is unique among free amino acids found in the plasma in that its concentration in maternal plasma is greater than or equal to that in fetal plasma. This study also suggested that cystathionine which is present in human brain in large concentrations, may not be needed until some time after birth.(308)

METHIONINE

Methionine is one of the essential amino acids required by humans, whereas cysteine is considered to be nonessential. The daily methionine requirement of young adult men was estimated to be 800-1100 mg. Eighty to 90% of this requirement could be replaced by cystine. The ability for one sulfur to replace another is called transsulfuration and represents an important route for the formation of either cysteine or cystine.(304)

A recent paper by Ogawa et al. (1985) provides some insight as to the possible importance of methionine in regard to the transsulfuration pathway. Free amino acids, including sulfur amino acids such as taurine and methionine, were determined in the plasma of twelve controls (normal blood pressure) and twelve patients with essential hypertension. The plasma levels of taurine, serine, methionine, and threonine were significantly lower in the patients with essential hypertension (high blood pressure). The levels of these four amino acids, as well as total sulfur amino acids, correlated inversely with systolic blood pressure. The authors concluded that in as much as taurine, methionine, and serine are involved in the metabolism of sulfur amino acids, the decrease in plasma sulfur amino acids may be a factor contributing to hypertension.(309) We wonder how many individuals with high blood pressure have mercury amalgam dental fillings and low plasma sulfur amino acids?

Mercury has been shown to affect methionine use. In experiments with rats, Trahktenberg (1969), utilizing radioactive methionine, clearly demonstrated that low concentrations of mercury inhibited methionine uptake by a factor of 2. That is, when compared with the control animals, the percentage of uptake of radioactive methionine in the mercury exposed animals was less than half of what it was in the unexposed controls.(2)

TAURINE

Taurine is a sulfur-containing amino acid that the body makes from cysteine. Methionine is a precursor for cysteine and taurine biosynthesis.(310) Fats in your diet are broken down (emulsified) in the small intestine so that they can be absorbed through the intestinal wall. This is accomplished by acids contained in the bile excreted by your gall bladder. There are two primary bile acids needed to break down fats and one of them, taurocholic acid, cannot be produced without taurine. Other studies have determined that taurine is highly concentrated in the brain where it is believed by some investigators to function as a neurotransmitter and/or as a modulator of neurotransmission preventing spontaneous excess electrical activity, such as that occurring during epileptic episodes.(311) Scientists have also determined that taurine plays a major role in the transport regulation of blood electrolytes such as calcium and potassium and because of this, may play an important role in the heart and cardiovascular system.(312)

Although the exact role that taurine may play in maternal reproductive functions has not been defined, it is known that excretion of taurine in pregnant women falls dramatically starting at week 9 of pregnancy. It is thought that this is the mechanism whereby maternal reserves of taurine are increased for use during the latter phases of pregnancy. It is also known that concentrations of taurine are higher in the fetal liver and brain and some researchers believe that it plays a role in brain development and also functions as a growth modulator.(313-316)

We were unable to find any research investigating or demonstrating the possible effect of mercury and lead on the metabolism of taurine. However, and as stated previously in this chapter, both mercury and lead have a great affinity for the sulfur atom. More importantly, we have shown that mercury can seriously interfere in the transsulfuration pathway at many different locations. It is therefore not unreasonable to assume that the effects of mercury and possibly lead, could ultimately lead to a deficiency or reduction in available taurine. The potential toxicological importance of mercury induced taurine deficiencies will have to be determined by future scientific investigation as the metabolic functions of taurine become more fully documented.

GLUTATHIONE

Glutathione is present in almost all cells in the body in rather high concentrations. Glutathione serves as a storage and transport form of cysteine and also as a respiratory carrier of oxygen, both extremely important functions. Within the cell itself it has some very important metabolic functions such as protecting the cells against damage that can be caused by free radicals and hydrogen peroxide.(317,318) In the liver, glutathione acts as a reservoir of cysteine which is utilized whenever necessary for protein synthesis. Glutathione can also replace cysteine derived from methionine, thus exerting a methionine sparing action.

One of the wonderful processes employed by the body is to recycle certain key nutrients so they can be used over again after they have performed certain functions. Vitamins C and E are two key nutrients that go through this recycling process. Once they have performed their function as an antioxidant, scavenging free radicals, they are reduced to an inactive state and must be regenerated to their original form. This process requires an adequate supply of reduced glutathione.

In addition to ensuring the clinical effectiveness of vitamins C and E, glutathione plays a double role in the effectiveness of selenium. Selenium is an essential component of several enzymes, particularly glutathione peroxidase (GSH-Px). GSH-Px is an antioxidant enzyme that protects unsaturated phospholipids and cholesterol in cell membranes from free-radical attack, and research has demonstrated that oxidized cholesterol can lead to abnormal calcium buildup within cells and connective tissue.(318,319) Therefore, if there is an abundance of mercury available it will tend to bind to both glutathione and selenium, thereby reducing the available supply to accomplish the critical metabolic functions just outlined.

Reduced glutathione (GSH) is present in red blood cells where it is functionally associated with the enzyme glucose-6-phosphate dehydrogenase (G6PD) and the coenzyme reduced nicotinamide-adenine dinucleotide phosphate (NADPH). Both G6PD and NADPH are needed to maintain red blood cell integrity. (318,319) Glutathione also plays a part in how our immune system functions. When the supply of glutathione is low or has been depleted this can inhibit the activation of lymphocytes, and may also have a bearing on the response of cytotoxic T-lymphocytes (also called killer T cells because they are able to destroy the foreign cell or substance.)(320,321) The ability of mercury to affect the available supply of glutathione would also affect the lymphocyte functions just described. Mercury will also inactivate G6PD which could result in altered red blood cell membrane permeability and blocking of active glucose transport into cells.(298) There is also evidence showing that mercury itself will increase red blood cell membrane permeability.(322) The altered membrane permeability resulting from the effects of mercury could in turn disrupt a large number of essential membrane functions ultimately leading to cell death.

In 1985, Ansari et al. set out to determine if there was normal GSH-Px activity in human brain autopsy samples and fresh surgical brain samples, based on the following data: (1) membrane phospholipids of the brain normally have a high concentration of unsaturated fatty acids; (2) the presence of high concentrations of unsaturated fatty acids should make the brain vulnerable to damage from peroxides; (3) lipid peroxides can be produced in the brain from oxidation of unsaturated fatty acids by oxygen radicals; and (4) other authors have demonstrated the presence of GSH-Px activity in non-human brains. Consequently, Ansari and his associates felt it important to determine if the human brain contained GSH-Px, which is the enzyme system that protects against free radicals and peroxides.(323)

They determined that there was in fact GSH-Px activity present in the human brain. The importance of this is that when polyunsaturated fatty acids, which are located primarily in the brain, are oxidized, organic hydroperoxides are formed that can only be reduced by GSH-Px. Ansari and his associates felt that alterations in GSH-Px activity and tissue damage caused by peroxide accumulation might be of significance in regard to the development of senility and some degenerative neurological diseases.(323)

In 1981, Ridlington and Whanger discussed their research findings that showed silver was most effective in the promotion of liver necrosis in selenium and vitamin E-deficient rats and that silver and mercuric chloride significantly depressed GSH-Px activity in the liver, kidneys, testes, and erythrocytes.(324) Bear in mind that mercury amalgam dental fillings contain approximately 30% silver, which can also be released through the corrosion process.

The ability of mercury to affect the availability of vitamin E and selenium, and the ability of mercury and silver to suppress GSH-Px activity places anyone with mercury amalgam fillings at much greater risk than individuals who have no amalgams or, for that matter, other metals in their mouths. The effect of such a GSH-Px deficiency caused by mercury, silver, and/or selenium depletion on a pregnant woman and the embryo or fetus has not, to our knowledge, been investigated. Consequently, it would appear that, because of the other metabolic changes that occur during a "normal" pregnancy, the pregnant woman with a mouthful of amalgam fillings has a health impairment risk factor that is greater than her nonpregnant counterpart.

One of the primary ways the body gets rid of mercury compounds, as well as other heavy metals, is through a pathway that goes from the liver into the bile where it is then transported to the gut and excreted in the feces. Interestingly, research has indicated that inorganic mercury is complexed with glutathione in the bile, suggesting that glutathione status would be a major consideration in the biliary secretion of mercury.(325,326) This same pathway may be affected by a mercury induced reduction of available taurine needed to produce bile acid.

With regard to the above excretory pathway, there is scientific evidence that when the microflora of the intestine has been reduced through stress, poor diet, use of antibiotics and other drugs, fecal content of mercury is greatly reduced. What the researchers found was that instead of being excreted in the feces, the mercury was being recirculated back to the liver.(327) Consequently, the person that is under stress, eating a poor diet, and/or taking antibiotics will tend to maintain a higher body burden of mercury derived from dietary sources. There are millions of prescriptions written for antibiotics each year; it is therefore not unreasonable to believe that those individuals will be at greater risk, especially if they also are eating diets high in fish.

In 1980, investigators had demonstrated that methylmercury binds to glutathione in the red blood cells of humans, rabbits and mice.(328) In a 1986 study researchers demonstrated that when methylmercury was administered to mice it caused a depletion of glutathione in various organs, that was thought to be caused by a direct binding of mercury to glutathione. To determine if glutathione protected against mercury transport or toxicity, a substance known to deplete

glutathione was administered prior to giving the mice methylmercury. What the researchers found was that three hours
after administration of the methylmercury, mercury concentrations in the brain and blood had increased. This was
thought to be due to the decreased glutathione content of
various tissues that had also caused or resulted in a redistribution of mercury from the organs where mercury was normally deposited.(307)

One other facet of the previous study dealt with the distribution of inorganic mercury. One day after administration
of inorganic mercury, it was equally distributed in blood
cells and plasma. Thereafter, there was a gradual increase in
the red blood cell to plasma ratio, with the distribution reaching the same ratio as in the case of methylmercury. The
authors thought that it was possible that inorganic mercury
in vivo is slowly converted to an organic form, even though
the levels of mercury in the blood were rapidly declining.(307)

SELENIUM

Selenium closely resembles sulfur in its physical and chemical properties. The selenium concentration in the blood is
19-25 micrograms per 100 milliliters (U.S. population
studies). It is found in the highest concentrations in the kidney, heart, spleen, and liver, and to some degree in all other
tissues except fat. A provisional Recommended Dietary Al-
lowance of 50 to 200 micrograms per day for adults has been
given.(329)

It is paradoxical that, although selenium can be toxic by
itself, it also prevents the toxicity of several other metals
such as silver, mercury, cadmium, and lead.(330) Chmielnicki et al. (1986), utilizing white female rats, demonstrated
that after a single injection of mercuric chloride, there was

a threefold increase in the daily excretion of endogenous copper and a fourfold increase of zinc excretion in the mercury-exposed group, in comparison with the control groups of rats. When the rats were administered sodium selenite at the same time as the mercury, it prevented the urinary excretion of endogenous copper and partially prevented the excretion of zinc.(331) This means that mercury causes the loss of the needed metals copper and zinc, and that selenium helps to prevent that loss by binding the mercury.

Low selenium intakes have been related epidemiologically to a higher incident of death from cancer of the digestive organs, lung, breast, and lymph when compared to populations living in areas having a high-selenium content in the soil and forage crops. Significantly lower levels of selenium have also been seen in patients with various types of cancer such as lymphocytic leukemia, breast, pulmonary carcinoma, gastrointestinal, colon, genitourinary carcinoma, skin cancer, and Hodgkins's disease. (332,333)

Autopsy studies done by Kosta, Byrne, and Zelenko in 1975 revealed that, contrary to accepted belief that the kidney was the prime accumulator of inorganic mercury, the thyroid and pituitary had retained and accumulated more inorganic mercury than the kidney. These same authors went on to see if there was a correlation between mercury and selenium. Using other postmortem samples of exposed humans and analyzing both elements, they found an approximate 1:1 molar ratio for those organs which accumulate and retain mercury strongly, such as the thyroid, pituitary, and kidney. In brain samples, the same 1:1 molar ratio was observed in various sections of the brain. The co-accumulation of selenium was not the result of comparable exposures to both elements and may represent a natural or autoprotective effect. (236)

The source and accumulation of mercury in the brain is a very complex problem that is under investigation by many scientists. The initial results of a Swedish group investigating the possible contribution of mercury from dental fillings to brain mercury was published in 1986.(63) The group headed by Dr. Lars Friberg revealed a direct correlation between the amount of inorganic mercury in the brain and the number and surfaces of amalgam fillings. The autopsy specimens were from accidental death victims. One of the researchers from the Friberg group, Dr. Magnus Nylander, a dentist himself, published the results of autopsy studies on three dentists that showed high levels of mercury accumulation in the pituitary in comparison to controls.(126) This affinity of mercury for the pituitary gland was first identified by Stock in 1940.(334) Unfortunately, the Friberg group has not as yet investigated any relationship between mercury and selenium in the brain even though Sweden is one of the low selenium areas of the world.

Kling and Soares (1978) postulated that since mercury tends to combine with selenium, part of the damage caused by mercury when administered alone might be associated with decreasing the bioavailability of selenium.(28) This theory was supported by the results obtained by Wada et al. in 1976. They found that mercuric chloride inhibited GSH-Px in mice and that simultaneous administration of the same molar dose of sodium selenite eliminated any reduction in GSH-Px activity.(335) Remember, selenium is required for the formation of GSH-Px.

In an ongoing research project in Sweden, blood selenium and GSH-Px levels are being assayed in people with amalgam fillings. The researchers have found below-normal levels of both selenium and GSH-Px that required five months of therapeutic supplementation of selenium and glutathione to bring blood selenium and GSH-Px levels back to normal.

They were startled when one of their study participants who had achieved normal levels of selenium and GSH-Px suddenly displayed pre-supplementation values. The blood test was run again to determine if it was laboratory error that caused the precipitous drop in selenium and glutathione peroxidase levels. The results were the same. When the individual was interviewed it was revealed that he had just been to the dentist and had an amalgam filling placed in his mouth. Hopefully, this study will be published in the near future. It appears to represent a major breakthrough that will provide scientific evidence of a direct relationship between amalgam fillings and a metabolic dysfunction.(336)

There seems little doubt that selenium is an essential nutrient and that deficiencies or low dietary intakes have a bearing on mortality and morbidity associated with several major diseases. The four studies that follow clearly demonstrate this association.

In a rather unique study published in 1983, Willet et al. had taken blood samples five years before 111 individuals developed cancer. The blood selenium levels of these cancer victims was compared against blood selenium samples taken from 210 cancer-free subjects. Dr. Willet and his associates found that the mean blood selenium level of the cancer victims was significantly lower than the blood selenium levels of the individuals who did not get cancer.(337)

The results of a seven year Finnish study evaluating the relationship of blood selenium levels to heart disease in 8113 men and women was published in 1982. Blood samples were taken and then frozen and stored. During the next seven years, the researchers monitored the 8113 individuals to determine the number of hospital admissions for heart disease and the number of deaths because of heart disease. These statistics were compared to those of a matched control group.

Their findings revealed that a blood selenium level of less than 35 mcg/l was associated with a six- to sevenfold increase in risk of death from heart disease and a twofold increase in the risk of myocardial infarction. (338)

In a very recent study involving twelve AIDS (acquired immunodeficiency syndrome) patients, Dworkin et al. determined that blood selenium levels were significantly reduced. The authors concluded that selenium deficiency is a common component of the malnutrition seen in AIDS patients and that aggressive nutritional support should be considered an integral part of the therapy of AIDS patients.(339)

Guidi et al. (1986) measured the GSH-Px activity in twenty-five healthy individuals and in twenty-five patients affected with well documented coronary artery stenosis (narrowing or stricture of the arteries of the heart). The authors found that the mean blood platelet GSH-Px activity of the coronary patients was significantly reduced. The authors hypothesized that a low enzyme activity may be a risk factor for the development of coronary artery disease.(340)

Mercury's ability to complex with selenium, increase its excretion, and reduce its bioavailability for primary metabolic functions must ultimately have a deleterious impact on homeostasis, as was demonstrated in the studies cited here. The effect of low maternal selenium levels in relation to the reproductive cycle and effect on the embryo and fetus remains to be determined. However, it may be well to keep in mind that the baby depends on the mother's blood for its nutrients and protection!

ZINC

It is apparent that our knowledge of minerals lags far behind that of vitamins. In the case of zinc, this is especially true. It wasn't until 1974 that zinc was determined to be an essential element and included in the Recommended Dietary Allowances (RDA's) established by The National Academy of Sciences.(341) Since 1974, extensive research has associated zinc deficiency in humans with retarded growth, anorexia, hypogonadism, diminished sense of taste and/or smell, inadequate bodily development, dermatitis, dystrophy of the fingernails, and impaired wound healing.(342)

Zinc is an essential component of approximately 100 different enzymes. It is also involved in the synthesis of metallothionein, which research indicates is a complex involved in the storage or detoxification of cadmium, mercury, and copper.(342) It has also been shown that zinc resembles cadmium and mercury in its ability to form complexes with thiols. (343,344) Investigations by Day and his colleagues demonstrated that mercury could displace zinc in accordance with the binding affinities that metallothionein had for various metals. In order of attraction these were mercury, copper, cadmium and zinc.(345) Their study, as well as many other studies, consider zinc-induced synthesis of metallothionein as perhaps the primary factor in reducing the toxicity of many heavy metals.

Zinc also works together in the body with vitamin B6 (which increases zinc absorption significantly) and vitamin E. With regard to vitamin E, a recent study has suggested that lipid and/or vitamin E malabsorption may be a consequence of zinc deficiency. Further, zinc deficiency may intensify vitamin E deficiency and thereby increase the requirement for vitamin E under these conditions.(346)

In the rat, bile is considered to be an important excretory route for zinc. In a 1981 paper, Alexander et al. concluded that their results indicated that the process of excreting zinc through the bile appeared to be glutathione-dependent, with the glutathione molecule acting as a carrier. Consequently, they felt that this might involve competition with other heavy metals such as copper, cadmium, and methylmercury, which also use glutathione as a carrier for biliary excretion and which ultimately could affect zinc balance in the body.(347)

The exact actions by which mercury exerts its toxic effect or causes pathological damage is not well defined. One action actively considered is the ability of mercury to stimulate lipid peroxidation. Yonaha et al. (1982) observed that lipid peroxidation (severe oxidation that results in damage to the fat molecules in cell membranes) occurred in the kidneys of rats given mercuric chloride and that the urinary excretion of enzymes was increased.(348) This was subsequently confirmed by Fukino et al. (1984). Moreover, Fukino and his associates were able to reduce the mercury-induced lipid peroxidation and renal damage by pretreatment with zinc.(349)

Fukino and his associates offered two possible mechanisms by which zinc suppresses mercury toxicity -- (1) zinc induces the synthesis of metallothionein to which mercury binds, and (2) that zinc pretreatment increases intracellular glutathione, which in turn increases GSH-Px and G6PD activities in the rat kidney, thus reducing mercury-induced lipid peroxidation. They also theorized that because zinc pretreatment caused a significant rise of reduced glutathione in the kidney and serum, this might indicate that reduced glutathione synthesized in the liver could be mobilized to protect the kidney against the toxic effects of mercury.

In 1984 Gale, using pregnant hamsters, conducted a study designed to determine if zinc could modify the embryo-lethal effects of inorganic mercury (mercuric acetate).(350) The results of this experiment were consistent with other experiments that had demonstrated the ability of zinc to protect vertebrate embryo from the harmful effects produced by several different agents that cause birth defects. Unfortunately, exactly how mercury causes the great number of embryo abnormalities and how zinc affords protection against this damage remains speculative.

Bjorksten et al. (1980) found that the serum level of zinc in patients with Down's syndrome was markedly reduced.(351) Anneren et al. (1985) found the concentrations of selenium in the erythrocytes (red blood cells) of Down's syndrome patients was higher than in controls. They also found a sex difference (higher values in females) both in GSH-Px activity and in plasma and red blood cell selenium levels. Other research has also shown sex differences for mercury status.(352) Does mercury play some part in the metabolic differences discerned in Down's syndrome children?

There is evidence indicating that in some inflammatory diseases there are alterations in the concentration of essential and nonessential elements in various tissues and body fluids. For example, Aaseth et al. in 1981 observed increased concentrations of copper and decreased concentrations of zinc and selenium in the serum of patients with rheumatoid arthritis.(353) A recent study by Alroth-Westerlund (1985) attempted to determine if there could be clinical significance in interpreting macro and trace element variations under various health conditions. Red blood cells and granulocytes (white blood cells) from venous blood of the patient group had increased concentrations of mercury and strontium which were not present in the control group. The patient group also displayed a decreased zinc concentration in red blood cells and neutrophil white blood cells. There seemed to be a general permeability disturbance in blood cells resulting in elevated calcium and strontium and lowered zinc concentrations. (354)

Carmignani and Boscolo (1984), in a study designed to determine cardiovascular homeostasis in rats chronically exposed to mercuric chloride, found that mercury exposure induced baroreflex (relationship to weight or pressure) hyposensitivity and produced a drastic alteration of the levels of copper and zinc in the brain and kidney. As the rats did experience cardiovascular changes, the authors felt that this might have been due to the altered (increased) concentrations of copper and zinc in the brain induced by the mercury.(355) Here again, the mechanism of increased zinc and copper may be related to the augmented synthesis of metallothionein as a protective device against mercury toxicity.(356,357)

A study by Oleske et al., published in 1983, sheds some other very interesting light on zinc and copper relationships. Fifty-eight patients with secondary immunodeficiency syndrome were tested for plasma copper and zinc levels. They had low-serum zinc and elevated-serum copper levels. When given zinc supplements, the patients with primary or secondary immunodeficiency conditions apparently improved. The authors concluded that zinc and copper balance are significantly altered in many immunodeficiency disorders and may be the cause of immunodeficiency.(358)

A very recent paper by Edman et al., 1986, adds to the knowledge of zinc status on cell-mediated immunologic mechanisms. These cell mediated mechanisms are important in preventing mucocutaneous infections caused by candida albicans. Recurrent vulvovaginal candidiasis in women is a very mentally stressful condition that remains an enigma. In their study, Edman et al. have found that mild zinc deficiency is associated with and may play a role in the susceptibility of women to recurrent vaginal candidiasis.(359) Mercury impairs zinc's biological function, and there are clinical case reports indicating that current candida treatment protocols, in some individuals, were not totally effective until mercury amalgam dental fillings were replaced.(360)

Perhaps the most important aspect of mercury's biochemical effect on zinc will be its inhibitory effect on zinc-responsive enzymes and coenzymes. Hopefully, future research will expand greatly on some of the preliminary work in this area. At present, we do know that mercury will inhibit the following zinc-involved enzymes or coenzymes: alcohol dehydrogenase, delta-aminolevulinic acid dehydrogenase, carbonic anhydrase, alkaline phosphatase, and aldolase.(361) Continued research may help to determine whether or not the chronic inhalation of mercury vapor from amalgam dental fillings increases the overall body burden of mercury enough to represent a significant metabolic factor in development of the imbalances of selenium, zinc, and copper. More importantly, in the context of this book, it may also shed some light on the maternal status of these key minerals in the woman with amalgam fillings.

CALCIUM

In 1986, calcium became the predominant topic in medicine, nutrition, and the pharmaceutical industry. Calcium was the cure-all for most ailments of mankind. Formulations for such over-the-counter drug staples as antacids were modified to include calcium. Even breakfast cereals didn't escape the need to be fortified with calcium. Calcium was the panacea for everything from correcting high blood pressure to preventing osteoporosis.

It is paradoxical that in prior years, calcium was the bad guy in cardiovascular problems. Medical journals extolled the virtues of the new "calcium channel blockers." These were a family of drugs that inhibited calcium uptake by the cardiovascular system. The rationale behind their use involved the biochemical function of calcium in stimulating or causing muscle contraction. Therefore, if the contractile response was blocked, the muscle would, in effect, relax and not remain in a constricted state.

As we have indicated previously, one of the major effects of systemic exposure to mercury is neurological. Muscular function is controlled neurologically by the transmission of nerve impulses, which involves calcium and sodium. There are many scientific reports documenting the effect of mercury on the normal metabolic functions of calcium. We will discuss three of them here.

Miyamoto (1983) investigated the effects of mercury ions on motor nerve terminals and specifically looked at whether ionized mercury entered the nerve terminal through calcium channels only. Miyamoto reported that mercury causes (1) irreversible depolarization, (2) increase in transmitter release, and (3) subsequent irreversible block of transmitter release. He concluded that the neurotoxic action of mercury is at an intracellular site and that entry is gained through both sodium and calcium channels. This suggested that metals may inhibit transmitter release at either the calcium channel or at the release site, but that irreversible toxicity was due to an intracellular action, possibly involving sulfhydryl groups.(362)

At almost the same time in 1983, there was another report that appeared related to calcium and mercury. In this report the researchers, Shier and DuBourdieu, were investigating the reasons behind the stimulation of phospholipid hydrolysis and prostaglandin release by mercuric chloride. What intrigued them was the fact that the action of mercury was similar to that of the calcium ion in regard to the stimulation of phospholipid hydrolysis and prostaglandin release. The authors felt their results were consistent with ionized mercury interacting with calcium ion-dependent enzyme(s). Moreover, their results were consistent with ionized mercury acting by a novel mechanism that mimicked that of the calcium ion. The real significance of that statement relates to the fact that mercury competes for the same cellular binding site as calcium and through this mechanism can induce cell death.(363)

The last paper, by Tomera and Harakal (1986), investigated the hypertensive process related to calcium, mercury, lead, and cadmium. They performed in vitro experiments utilizing normotensive thoracic aorta (Dorland's defines aorta as the main trunk from which the systemic arterial system proceeds) from rabbits. We feel the findings of their study are of great significance to anyone experiencing cardiovascular problems who also has mercury amalgam dental fillings. Mercuric chloride and lead acetate caused contraction of rabbit aortic segments. Cadmium had no direct effect. Moreover, the report provides evidence that mercury ions and lead ions can directly induce active tension on processes which rely on extracellular calcium.(364)

This means that mercury and lead can cause contraction of major systemic blood vessels and that this contractile potential is substantial. When the major blood vessels contract, one of the first effects is hypertension (high blood pressure). However, an angiogram reflects this contraction of the artery as a narrowing or blockage, which is considered to be the major cause of cardiovascular problems. The costs of cardiovascular by-pass surgery in 1984 exceeded three billion dollars. It would be interesting to see how many of the people undergoing by-pass surgery had mercury amalgam dental fillings and what the mercury and lead content of the surgically removed cardiac vessels were. More importantly, perhaps, is what effect these metabolic dysfunctions created by mercury and lead have on the pregnant woman and the embryo or fetus.

MAGNESIUM

Until very recently, this essential element had the distinction of "being forgotten" by science and medicine. Magnesium is so plentiful on Earth that it was just not considered to be a serious candidate for evaluation as a factor in nutritional deficiencies. That situation is now being corrected. Scientific studies are producing new data monthly affirming that magnesium is one of the most critical and necessary metals involved in the maintenance of good health.

There are two indispensable functions for cellular life-- the generation of energy in a usable form and the need to be able to reproduce. "All forms of life on earth have basically the same system for these two purposes. They are summed up in the familiar initials ATP and DNA (deoxyribonucleic acid)."(365) ATP, which is the abbreviation for adenosine triphosphate, is the primary mechanism by which living cells capture, store, and transport energy in a chemical form. ATP is involved in most of the normal body processes: membrane transport; generation and transmission of nerve impulses; contraction of muscles; transfer of methyl groups; utilization of glucose; synthesis of fat, protein, nucleic acid, and coenzymes; and so on.(365,366) The importance in all of this is that magnesium is required for activation of hundreds of enzymes in the body, including all those utilizing ATP.

There are several scientific studies demonstrating that mercury can inhibit or reduce many of the magnesium-catalyzed functions. Jennette (1981) demonstrated that mercury and lead may mimic essential divalent ions such as magnesium, calcium, iron, copper, or zinc, and that these ions may then complex small molecules, enzymes, and nucleic acids in such a way that the normal activity of these species is altered. Jennette also felt that in the presence of these metal ions, free radicals could be produced which damage critical cellular molecules.(270)

Thompson and Nechay (1981) demonstrated that mercury, silver, gold, and uranium could cause a 50% inhibition of canine renal calcium or magnesium-activated adenosinetriphosphatase (ATPase) enzymes. Mercury was the most inhibitory, followed by silver. Their experiment also demonstrated that organic mercury was less potent than inorganic mercuric chloride. They also found that if the magnesium concentration was increased while the ATP concentration remained constant, the inhibition by mercury increased. Changes in the calcium, magnesium, and ATP concentrations did not alter the inhibition produced by mercury, silver, and gold.(367)

Mehra and Kanwar (1986) studied the alterations of selected enzymes in the liver, kidneys, and brain of mice following repeated administration of mercuric chloride for ten, twenty, and thirty days. They found that mercury-induced changes in ATPase were complex, inasmuch as the nature and magnitude of these changes varied with the tissue being evaluated, as well as the duration of the treatment. Whereas the liver ATPase declined after each treatment interval, kidney and brain ATPase increased following administration of mercuric chloride for ten days. However, both the kidneys and brain registered a substantial fall in ATPase activity when administrations were continued for thirty days. The levels of both mercury; glucose-6-phosphatase and succinic dehydrogenase decreased in all the tissues following mercuric chloride administration. Invariably, the magnitude of decrease was the highest after thirty days treatment with mercuric chloride.(368)

It is obvious from the data that mercury can affect not only magnesium-controlled ATP, but also the major magnesium-activated enzymes related to the metabolism of ATP, such as ATPase. This, in turn, has the ability to affect a myriad of critical and required biochemical reactions in the body. Some of these reactions are responsible for the maintenance of neuromuscular transmission, heart muscle and blood vessels, bone structure (with calcium), the central nervous system, proper calcium balance, and proper glucose metabolism.(329,365,366)

VITAMIN C

One usually identifies vitamin C as the antiscorbutic vitamin because its discovery was related to prevention and treatment of scurvy. The antiscorbutic factor of the fruits used to treat and prevent scurvy was isolated from lemon juice by Szent-Gyorgi in 1928; in 1933 the name of this factor (hexuronic acid) was changed to ascorbic acid. The symptoms of clinical scurvy include swollen joints, muscular aches, bone pain, edema, weakness, fatigue, anemia, loose teeth, hyperkeratosis (especially around hair follicles), impaired wound healing, and possibly a breakdown of scar tissue. Behavioral changes may include apathy, depression, and emotional disturbances. There are also a number of characteristics probably related to a weakening of the walls of blood vessels such as swollen and bleeding gums, ocular hemorrhages, bruising, and varicosities of small blood vessels which are seen under the tongue.(369) Although frank clinical scurvy is rarely seen today, there is evidence that chronic subclinical vitamin C deficiency may exist in a large segment of the population. This subclinical deficiency has metabolic and clinical aspects and symptoms different from clinical scurvy, but can lead to impaired health and increased susceptibility to other diseases.(370,371)

The known physiological functions of vitamin C are synthesis of polysaccharides and collagen; formation of cartilage, dentin, bone, and teeth; antioxidant; absorption of iron; cold tolerance; maintenance of the adrenal cortex; metabolism of tryptophan, phenylalanine, and tyrosine; growth; wound healing; and maintenance of capillaries.(329) There is also considerable evidence that vitamin C is directly involved in proline and lysine hydroxylation; carnitine synthesis; dopamine hydroxylation; drug and cholesterol breakdown; sulphation; lymphocyte and neutrophil function; and folate reduction.(369)

Vitamin C apparently has a protective effect against mercury poisoning. In experiments with guinea pigs done in 1951, Vauthey demonstrated that a specific dose of mercury cyanide injected into the guinea pigs killed all of the animals within one hour. However, if the guinea pigs were given high levels of ascorbic acid prior to the administration of the mercury, 40% of the animals survived.(372) This same protective effect was demonstrated against other forms of mercury.(373,374)

For many years, mercury diuretics were used extensively by the medical profession. The toxicity of these mercurial diuretics could be reduced if the patient was given ascorbic acid prior to or simultaneously with the mercurial diuretic.(375) Exactly how the ascorbic acid reduced the toxicity of mercury was not determined. However, there is a possible biochemical pathway that appears plausible. When vitamin C is metabolized, part of it is metabolized to vitamin C-sulphate, with the sulphate being derived from sulphur-

C + cysteine

containing amino acids such as cysteine. Vitamin C competes with certain drugs for sulphate conjugation, which could affect the pharmacological activity and toxicity of drugs. (376)

In 1977, Basu demonstrated that a 3-gram dose of vitamin C per day would reduce the excretion of cysteine in the urine to 50% of the pre-vitamin C values. The researcher postulated that the cysteine was being used to metabolize the vitamin C. Experimental and clinical evidence suggest that the detoxification of cyanide takes place by its conversion to a sulphur-containing metabolite called thiocyanate, and that the reaction may require cysteine.(377) Furthermore, Basu demonstrated that the urine levels of thiocyanate were markedly decreased by administration of high doses of vitamin C and that administering 10 mg/day of cysteine restored the urinary thiocyanate to normal levels. Basu also stated: "When excess vitamin C is ingested and the protein intake is limited, it is possible that cystine would be monopolized for sulphate conjugation by the vitamin, and as a consequence render one of the body's detoxification mechanisms less effective."(377)

Mercury competes actively for the sulphur-containing amino acids cysteine and methionine, as well as the cysteine molecule of the tripeptide glutathione. Consequently, it would seem from the data presented that anyone with amalgam fillings should routinely eat a diet rich in sulphur-containing foods to offset the depletion of cysteine and methionine caused by the inhalation of mercury vapor being continually released from amalgam fillings. The problem of cysteine depletion could be further aggravated by the dietary presence of mercury, lead, arsenic, and cadmium, because they are all thiol sensitive.

Mercury is also known to inhibit collagen synthesis.(378) The synthesis of collagen is impaired in vitamin C deficiency. This appears to be due to lowered ability to hydroxylate lysine and proline. There is considerable evidence that the reducing agent in the hydroxylation of both lysine and proline is the reduced form of vitamin C. Consequently, in vitamin C deficiency, it is believed that the amount of effective collagen fibre present in connective tissue is reduced.(369) In severely scorbutic patients, swelling, hemorrhages, and secondary bacterial infections of the gingival margins are common. It is not the actual deficiency of vitamin C that causes the inflammation, but rather the lack of adequate vitamin C impairing the normal defensive responses of the mucous membranes. Thus, the massive gingival enlargement so characteristic of scurvy results from the combined effects of lack of vitamin C and nonspecific inflammation.(379)

It is fascinating to note that the adrenal glands are one of the target glands of mercury deposition. They also contain the body's second highest tissue levels of vitamin C. The physical response to stress is an increased secretion of the hormones of the adrenal glands. It is also interesting to note that physical and mental stress increases adrenal activity which, in turn, depletes ascorbic acid from the gland. In mammals which produce their own ascorbic acid, this depletion is rapidly replenished. However, humans, who don't produce ascorbic acid, attempt to replenish the adrenal stores of vitamin C by taking it from other stores in the body. If tissue values of ascorbic acid are low, there may be an insufficient amount available to replenish or satisfy the requirements of the adrenals. Under these conditions, normal adrenal hormone response may become inadequate.(176)

Trahktenberg (1969) reported that prolonged exposures to low mercury concentrations depress the adrenal ascorbic acid content. Perhaps more importantly, the effects of chronic exposure to low concentrations of mercury were insignificant during the first 4-9 weeks of exposure. However, the reduction of adrenal ascorbic acid content became statistically significant with increased length of exposure thereafter when compared to the start of the experiment. (2)

The person with amalgam dental fillings who is being exposed to chronic intakes of mercury vapor would also be subjecting the adrenals to depletion by chemical stress. This relationship of mercury and vitamin C is not a new discovery. To quote from a paper by Blackstone et al.: "Shun mercury as poison' was Kramer's advice to scorbutic patients according to George Budd, a London physician, in 1840. Budd himself claimed that in cases of scurvy ...'mercury in every form should be religiously avoided [as] we have met with instances in which the scorbutic symptoms seemed to have been much aggravated by mercury taken before the scurvy made its appearance." According to Blackstone, "The observations of Budd indicated that low tissue levels of ascorbic acid increased a person's susceptibility to mercury poisoning (or, conceivably, that an increased intake of mercury exacerbated the scorbutic condition)."(310)

In the paper cited above, Blackstone and his associates determined that mercury did induce adrenal hypertrophy (overgrowth) and that this could be prevented by large doses of ascorbic acid. Biochemically, they felt that thiol groups have a direct role in the preservation of tissue ascorbic acid and its reduced form, and that any decrease in the biological reducing capacity of tissue thiols would presumably result in lower levels of tissue ascorbic acid.

There is another aspect of vitamin C and mercury that is extremely important. One function of the liver tissue is to reduce dehydroascorbic acid to ascorbic acid. This ability guarantees the preservation of the body's vitamin C reserves, so necessary to normal function. Trahktenberg (1969) demonstrated that in animals exposed to low concentrations of mercury, the ability of the liver to reduce dehydroascorbic acid to ascorbic acid was decreased significantly in comparison to controls.(2)

VITAMIN E

Vitamin E is a fat-soluble vitamin, as are vitamins A, D, and K. Fat-soluble or water-soluble relates to the original discovery findings on vitamins. The first vitamin categorized in this manner was called fat-soluble vitamin A because it was found that is was soluble in fat and fat solvents (alcohol and ether). Subsequent discoveries found that certain vitamins were only soluble in water.

Fat-soluble vitamins differ from the water-soluble group in other ways. They can be stored in the body whereas water-solubles cannot. Fat-soluble vitamins are excreted chiefly by the fecal pathway versus the urinary pathway for the water-soluble vitamins. The most important difference lies in the fact that they are absorbed along with dietary fats, and conditions of extremely low fat intake or impaired uptake of fats will also interfere with their absorption. Antibiotics and certain other drugs, as well as certain disease states such as malabsorption syndromes, decrease the absorption of fat-soluble vitamins from the intestinal tract.

The chemical name for vitamin E is tocopherol, which is derived from the Greek tokos (childbirth) and pherin (to bear). The ending "ol" is the chemical suffix to denote an alcohol. The name tocopherol was bestowed on this vitamin in 1938. It relates directly to the original work by Evans and Bishop in 1922 who found that rats, given a purified diet containing all the then-known nutrients, could not reproduce. When fresh green leaves or dried alfalfa was added, the rats could again reproduce. The unknown factor was called substance X, and in 1924, Sure named it vitamin E (or the antisterility vitamin). (329,380-382).

The exact physiological function of vitamin E in man is still not completely understood, although recently some of its functions have been identified. It appears that one of the primary biological functions of vitamin E relates to its role as an antioxidant. Vitamin E's antioxidant ability is enhanced by selenium. This synergistic effect preserves membranes from destruction by oxidation products and especially retards breakdown (hemolysis) of red blood cells.(329)

The literature shows that vitamin E can reduce the toxic effects of mercury. In laboratory tests, vitamin E was able to reduce the chromosomal breakage caused by mercury. Researchers also demonstrated the protective potential of vitamin E against genotoxicity (reproductive toxicity) of methylmercury.(383) Fukino et al. (1984) demonstrated lipid peroxidation and a decrease in vitamin E content in rat kidneys twelve hours after mercury administration.(384) Vitamin E also has been shown to have sulfhydryl-protective activity.(385) Vitamin E was able to protect mouse spleen cells from lipid peroxidation and thereby enhance their primary antibody response and other metabolic responses.(386)

In a recent paper, Marsh et al. (1986) demonstrated that a deficiency of selenium and vitamin E can affect the maturation of the bursa, thymus, and in some instances, the spleen, in chickens. The authors concluded that their data suggested that the primary lymphoid organs are major targets of selenium and vitamin E dietary deficiencies and provide a possible mechanism by which immune function may be impaired.(387)

In another study dealing with cell-mediated immunity, Meekes et al. (1985) performed experiments with mice to determine the effect of vitamin E and/or selenium deficiency on cell-mediated cytotoxicity. Natural killer cell-mediated cytotoxicity (NKCC) was depressed in eight weeks on diets deficient in vitamin E and/or selenium. T-lymphocyte-mediated cytotoxicity (TCMC) was found to be depressed by combined selenium-vitamin E deficiency after seven weeks on diets.(388)

In experiments with rats, Addya and his associates (1984) demonstrated that chronic treatment with mercuric chloride caused a decrease in available glutathione and the enzyme glutathione reductase. When the animals were supplemented with vitamin E normal glutathione levels were restored.(389) Glutathione peroxidase and reductase enzymes and reduced glutathione are involved in antioxidant functions related to free radicals or peroxides, as are other cofactors such as the trace elements manganese, copper, zinc, and selenium. Vitamin E, however, is not a cofactor; it is an independent antioxidant that has its main effect in the lipid phase of the cell, protecting the membrane from auto-oxidative damage.(390,391)

As indicated earlier, vitamin E is involved in reducing the toxic effects of mercury which, in turn, reduces the amount of vitamin E available for normal metabolic functions. It also appears that vitamin E protects the enzymes G6P, G6PD, GSH-Px and glutathione reductase from auto-oxidative damage and at the same time protects the biological supply of glutathione. The presence of mercury in combination with a vitamin E deficiency has the potential of producing toxic reactions in the body.

In the disease cystic fibrosis, one of the distinguishing features is fat malabsorption. Cystic fibrotic patients almost always have a deficiency of vitamin E. Farrell et al. (1977) showed a significant reduction in red blood cell half-life in cystic fibrosis patients not receiving vitamin E supplementation. In six patients who were then treated with vitamin E, the red blood cell survival time approached normal.(392)

Patients with G6PD deficiency have less capacity to generate reduced glutathione, and their red blood cells have a greatly reduced half-life.(393) Corash et al. (1980) treated twenty-three patients with G6PD deficiency for ninety days with 800 IU per day of oral vitamin E. They found increased red blood cell survival time as well as increasing hemoglobin concentration. The authors summarized: "This study demonstrates that supplementation with vitamin E, at a dose without known toxicity, was associated with a reduction in the mild chronic hemolysis (separation of the hemoglobin from the red blood cells and its appearance in the plasma) in our G6PD-deficient patients....Our investigation suggests that it will be important to explore the possibility that long-term vitamin E administration might reduce or ameliorate the severity of acute hemolytic crises, or that vitamin E supplementation might decrease the level of neonatal hyperbilirubinemia due to G6PD deficiency."(394)

Based on these two studies it would not be unreasonable to investigate the possible relationship of cystic fibrosis to mercury as it has been clearly demonstrated that mercury inhibits G6PD activity and also reduces available vitamin E. It would also make an interesting study to determine maternal blood levels of G6PD and vitamin E in pregnant women with a mouthful of amalgams that are chronically inhaling mercury vapor all during their pregnancy.

PANTOTHENIC ACID

Pantothenic acid participates in a variety of pathways involved in normal metabolic functions. The physiological active form of pantothenic acid is coenzyme A, which is required for many different enzymatic actions. It is at the center of energy metabolism and fat, acetylcholine, and antibody synthesis.(13,22,329,395)

Coenzyme A, which is synthesized from pantothenic acid, is abbreviated as CoA or CoA-SH, and functions as a transient carrier and a cofactor for a variety of enzyme-catalyzed reactions involving the transfer of acetyl (two carbon) groups. The CoA-SH designation reflects the fact that the coenzyme A molecule has a reactive thiol (-SH) group, to which acyl groups become covalently linked to form thioesters during acyl-group transfer reactions.(13) All known acyl derivatives of CoA and related pantetheine derivatives are thiol esters.(13,395,396) Because of these derivatives CoA is involved in the metabolism of carbohydrates, lipids, protein, and porphyrin. It is also involved in the synthesis of fatty acids, cholesterol, citrate, acetoacetate, and the neurotransmitter acetylcholine.(329,395,396)

Pantothenic acid is an essential component of the brain and must enter the brain and cerebrospinal fluid (CSF) from the blood. In the brain, as part of CoA, pantothenic acid is involved in many important reactions. In experiments with humans, Hodges et al. (1959) (397) and Fry et al. (1976) (398) have produced many of the symptoms identified with pantothenic acid deficiency such as fatigue, headache, insomnia, nausea, abdominal cramps, occasional vomiting, paresthesias of the hands and feet (burning foot syndrome), muscle cramps, and impaired coordination. Eosinopenic (abnormal deficiency of eosinophilic leukocytes in the blood) response to adrenocorticotrophic hormone (ACTH) was impaired, although other tests of the adrenal glands indicated function remained with in normal limits.(396-399)

Pantothenic acid is required for the synthesis of cholesterol precursors for sterol hormones in the adrenal cortex, and a pantothenic deficiency can produce cortical necrosis.(329)Conversely, pantothenic acid stimulates the adrenal glands and increases production of adrenal hormones.(400) There is data indicating that mercury can inhibit production of adrenal hormones and cause adrenal overgrowth.(2,401) In a recent 1986 study Veltman and Maines indicate that mercury caused a direct defect in adrenal steroid biosynthesis with apparent physiological consequences being lowered plasma levels of corticosterone and elevated concentrations of progesterone and dehydroepiandrosterone, all abnormal steroid hormone profiles. (178)

Mercury's affinity for thiols, sulfhydryl groups and the sulfur molecule, wherever they are biochemically available in the body, gives it the potential to affect countless metabolic functions. It is extremely interesting to note that symptoms produced by a pantothenic deficiency are all also documented as effects produced by mercury toxicity.

VITAMIN B$_6$ (PYRIDOXINE)

Vitamin B$_6$ participates in the metabolism of protein, carbohydrates, and lipids, and is a coenzyme constituent in the formation of erythrocytes and in amino acid metabolism. Our concern in relation to mercury centers on B$_6$'s involvement in the biochemical processes related to the sulfur-containing amino acids. For example, the conversion of methionine to cysteine is dependent on vitamin B$_6$.(396,402)

The three forms of vitamin B$_6$ that occur in foods are pyridoxine, pyridoxal phosphate, pyridoxmine phosphate.

The physiologically active forms of vitamin B_6 are pyridoxal phosphate and pyridoxamine phosphate. All three forms are converted in the body to pyridoxal phosphate.(396,403) Pyridoxal phosphate is involved with a number of enzymes in catalyzing reactions of amino acids. The most common of these are called transaminations, in which an amino group is transferred to a carbon atom. In these reactions, pyridoxal phosphate serves as a transient carrier of the amino group from its donor to the amino group acceptor. The derivative of this intermediate action is pyridoxamine phosphate which then donates its amino group to the carbon atom of alpha-keto acid, after which it reverts to its pyridoxal phosphate form.(366,403)

In the biochemical reactions related to conversion of methionine to cysteine, there is a need to transfer a sulfur component, and a amino component, which would make the process doubly vulnerable to mercury because its highest binding affinity is for the sulfhydryl group and then the amino group.(298,404) Further, mercury can bind to phosphate groups, which gives it a total of three possible mechanisms to affect the metabolism of pyridoxal phosphate, the biologically active form of vitamin B_6.

One of the functions of vitamin B_6 is called transsulfuration. This is the process whereby one sulfur molecule can replace another and represents an important biochemical function for utilization of sulfur. For example, when pyridoxine is deficient in the body, methionine metabolism is altered.(405) In vitamin B_6-deficient rats, there is a greatly decreased ability to form cysteine from cystathionine due to a decrease in the enzymes required. It was also determined that during conditions of vitamin B_6 deficiency there was a large accumulation of cystathionine in the pancreas, an organ which is very active in transsulfuration, and is known to have a rapid uptake of methionine.(406) These particular reactions suggest that mercury could possibly be involved in pancreatic dysfunctions.

What is so interesting about the foregoing data is that cystathionine is a major constituent of the pool of free amino acids in the brain. This fact raises the question of neurochemical involvement. Spector (1978) brings out the fact that although vitamin B6 is not synthesized in the brain, it readily enters the cerebral spinal fluid (CSF) and brain from the plasma. Once within the CSF, B6 can enter brain cells.(407) The holoenzyme needed to convert cystathionine to cysteine contains B6 in its pyridoxal phosphate form.(408) Data derived from animal studies indicate that it is relatively easy to deplete brain B6. (409)

It is evident from the above data that any substance that impedes or inhibits the metabolic functions of vitamin B6 in humans could have some very serious consequences. Symptoms of vitamin B6 deficiency, like those of micromercurialism, can be nonspecific and hard to pinpoint. They include weakness, mental confusion, irritability and nervousness, insomnia, poor coordination in walking, hyperactivity, convulsions, abnormal electroencephalogram, declining blood lymphocytes and white blood cells, anemia, and skin lesions.(410)

Mercury has the biochemical capability of reducing the availability of, or inhibiting the function of vitamin B6. For example, recently published research has demonstrated a positive correlation between brain mercury levels and the numbers and surfaces of amalgam fillings.(63) Is the mercury accumulating in the brain affecting the metabolic ability of the body to create cystathionine from methionine or the enzymatic process of reducing cystathionine to cysteine, or does it impact by inhibiting many of the critical functions required of vitamin B6? Consequently, in a patient presenting with a galaxy of vague symptomatology, is the clinician remiss if possible mercury toxicity has not been considered in the diagnosis?

VITAMIN B₁ (THIAMINE)

Thiamine is one of two vitamins in the body that contains a sulfur entity; the other is biotin. The high binding affinity that mercury has for the sulfur-containing molecule gives it the biochemical potential to affect the functions of this critical vitamin. Moreover, it is important for the reader to understand that, out of about two dozen substances produced by the metabolism of thiamine in the body and excreted in the urine, science has only identified the function of six of them thus far.(411) This means that there are a lot of things going on metabolically with vitamin B₁ that mercury could affect that haven't even been perceived as a potential problem because the complete biochemical function of the vitamin has not been identified.

A deficiency of vitamin B₁ produces a form of neuritis known as beriberi, a disease that became widespread during the nineteenth century in East Asia after the introduction of steam-powered rice mills, which produced polished rice lacking the vitamin-rich husk. Two forms of beriberi have been identified-- dry beriberi, which is related to the nervous system, and wet beriberi, which involves primarily the cardiovascular system.

Here again, the early symptoms of thiamine deficiency, which are intriguingly similar to mercury toxicity, are non-specific and hard to pinpoint: fatigue, anorexia, weight loss, gradual loss of muscle strength, peripheral neuritis (numbness or increased sensitivity, tingling in the extremities, loss of reflexes), irritability, confusion, depression, lack of initiative, poor memory, gastrointestinal problems (including constipation), and low body temperature. Cardiovascular symptoms can include edema of the ankles, feet and legs, palpitation, tachycardia, abnormal electrocardiograms, decreased blood pressure, and difficulty in breathing after exertion. (329,396,410)

Science has subsequently determined that thiamine is involved in many enzyme reactions in the body. In a series of complicated actions, thiamine is a critical factor in the whole process leading to the formation of acetyl CoA which is then involved in the formation of citrate, the first step in the citric acid cycle. The citric acid cycle is a system within the cells by which carbohydrate, fat, and protein are metabolized to produce energy. The product of the first step in the metabolic process is transferred to one of the sulfur atoms of the cyclic disulfide group of lipoic acid. Throughout the other enzymatic metabolic steps, the transfer is through thiol groups.(412) According to Lonsdale, "Thiamine is, therefore, one of the critical cofactors which have to be derived from the diet in mammalian systems and which stand astride the fundamental function of cellular energy production."(412)

What is so interesting about these biochemical pathways is the fact that not only does thiamine have a sulfur atom in its structure to start with, but its involvement as a coenzyme in critical biochemical processes is connected through transfers involving sulfur molecules. Consequently, it can be easily visualized how mercury, with its great affinity for binding to thiols, sulfur, and disulfides, could affect the availability of thiamine and effect critical energy processes in the body.

Another point that Lonsdale brings out is that thiamine participates in the metabolism of tryptophan to form nicotinic acid. He theorizes that because of this, a deficiency of thiamine could also cause a deficiency of vitamin B6, which is also required in the metabolic pathway of tryptophan.(412)

Axelrod (1953) evaluated the role of vitamins in the immune system. In this particular paper he discusses the role of various vitamins in the synthesis of antibodies. Deficiencies of pantothenic acid, pyridoxine, and folic acid caused a severe impairment of antibody synthesis, while only a moderate impairment was associated with a deficiency of thiamine and biotin. (413) As you probably surmise, all of the vitamins mentioned as impairing the production of antibody can be affected by the presence of mercury.

Thiamine is a cofactor in steroid hydroxylation, fatty acid synthesis, and glucose metabolism in the pentose phosphate cycle, which is another energy system. (Remember, mercury inhibits glucose-6-phosphatase, a key enzyme in the glucose cycle.) Although the pentose phosphate cycle appears to be relatively unimportant as a source of energy, the proportion of glucose metabolized by this route is high in the lactating mammary gland, the adrenal cortex, leukocytes and erythrocytes."(412) Each one of the entities mentioned also are effected by mercury in other ways than glucose metabolism.

It is evident that vitamins do not perform independently in the biochemical sense. There is an overlap of symptoms which can be produced by deficiencies. This seems to be especially true of the B vitamins. Perhaps more important clinically, there has been very little scientific exploration on investigating or evaluating the effect of concurrent multiple-vitamin deficiencies, where a latent insufficiency of one vitamin exists in the presence of a clinically identifiable insufficiency of another. This particular point is of major concern because of the ability of not only mercury but arsenic and lead (readily available through the food chain or environment) to impact on the biochemical pathways of these vitamins and minerals.

FOLIC ACID (293,414,415)

Folic acid deficiency is one of the most common vitamin deficiencies. Many of the symptoms are similar to those of B_{12} deficiency. As much as 100% may be lost if foods are improperly stored, cooking water is discarded, or foods are reheated or overcooked. Many medications, including aspirin and anticonvulsants, may also interfere with folacin absorption and metabolism, further decreasing its availability .

Folic acid is involved in the metabolism of pantothenic acid and is required for its utilization. It is through this participation that it is involved in antibody production of the immune system. Folic acid also has a relationship with other vitamins including vitamin C and E.(329) In the body, folic acid is rapidly converted to the biologically active form tetrahydrofolic acid (THFA) in the presence of NADPH (niacin's coenzyme form) and ascorbic acid. In conjunction with vitamin B_{12}, THFA participates in amino acid conversions and the methylation of choline, methionine, serine (also requiring pyridoxal phosphate, B6), and histidine.

Folates carry out their metabolic function as a carrier of one-carbon units in the tetra-hydro form (*tetra* meaning 4 and *hydro* meaning a combining form denoting a relationship to water or to hydrogen). It is this capability to accept one-carbon units, which synthesize various coenzymes, that makes folates so important and involves them in so many metabolic functions.

The liver actively reduces and methylates folates which are then transported into the bile for reabsorption by the gut and subsequent delivery to the tissues. This important path-

way may provide as much as 200 micrograms or more of folate each day for recirculation to tissues. The folates are a
family of coenzymes and function in association with their
respective enzymes to accomplish many intracellular metabolic functions. For example, Methyl-THFA is required as
the methyl donor in the conversion of homocysteine to
methionine (methyl methionine). This reaction utilizes
vitamin B_{12} as a cofactor and also requires vitamin B_6. Folates are also involved the conversion of the amino acid serine
to glycine, and histidine to glutamic acid. It is also necessary in the synthesis of glucose, and DNA. DNA has a universal function in all cells in the body as it is the storage or
repository of genetic information. Folic acid and vitamin B_{12}
are both involved in this vital process of synthesizing DNA.
In megaloblastic anemia (folate deficiency), certain steps in
this vital process of DNA synthesis are reduced, causing an
arresting of the synthesis of red blood cell replication.

The form of folacin most commonly found in the liver and
serum is methyl-THFA. There is some difference of opinion
that presently exists in the scientific community regarding
the biochemical recycling of methyl-THFA. The experiments
of several researchers have indicated that methyl-THFA can
only recycle through a B_{12}-dependent pathway. If a B_{12}
deficiency exists, folic acid is trapped as methyl-THFA and
is useless to the body. Consequently, a deficiency of either
vitamin B_{12} or folic acid will result in identical hematologi-
cal symptoms.

However, other researchers question the folate trap
hypothesis. For example, Chanarin et al. (1980) were not
able to demonstrate the methylfolate trap. They felt, instead,
that the primary control of folate metabolism was in the
vitamin B_{12} methionine pathway, with a B_{12} deficiency being
the prime defect impairing the homocysteine to methionine
reaction. The enzyme methionine synthetase requires vitamin

B_{12}. Therefore, it was suggested that failure of methionine synthesis leads to inadequate formulation of THFA, which as we stated earlier, is the biologically active form of folate from which all the other actions derive.(416) The efficacy of methionine in overcoming many of the effects of B_{12} deficiency in animals has been documented by Stokstad et al. (417) and Krebs et al. (418). Indeed, methionine deficiency has been equated with B_{12} deficiency.

The scientific community is providing additional data on deficiencies of folic acid affecting the immune system. Youinou et al. (1982), in a study involving ninety-two malnourished patients found that there was some impairment of their immune status. These researchers, in attempting to determine the linkage between malnutrition and immunologic status, determined that the phagocytic function of polymorphonuclear leukocytes (PMNs), and to a lesser degree bactericidal function, seemed to be adversely affected by folic acid deprivation. Because of their malnutrition status, many of the patients in the study had low folate levels. However, serum levels of vitamin B_{12} were normal in all of the patients and therefore was not considered as being implicated. Correction of the folic acid deficiency was accompanied by recovery of phagocytic function. For the pregnant woman, this aspect can become very important as folic acid requirements increase during pregnancy, so much so that low tissue-folate levels are suspected of being a predisposing factor in the bacteriuria (bacteria in the urine) of pregnancy.(419)

The potential for mercury to be involved in folate deficiency certainly exists. This is also true for lead. A report by Rader et al. (1982) clearly demonstrated that administration of lead to animals for seven weeks caused a marked decrease in serum erythrocyte folate values and a reduction in liver folate stores.(420)

There also is a relationship between folate, mercury, and the thyroid that we consider very intriguing. In 1980, Stokstad et al. did some experiments with rats that had either received a thyroidectomy (surgical removal of the thyroid gland), which created a hypothyroid condition (low levels of thyroid hormone), or received thyroid powder in their food, simulating a hyperthyroid condition of excess thyroid hormones.(421) The authors concluded that the thyroidectomy decreased the level of the enzyme needed in the metabolic steps leading to methyl-THFA, which, as stated previously, is required for the conversion of homocysteine to methionine. They also found that thyroidectomy increased the oxidation of histidine, which also mimics the action of methionine.(421) Conversely, they found that in the hyperthyroid situation, metabolic actions occurred that lead to increased liver levels of methyl-THFA, which could be a partial explanation for the symptoms of pseudo-B12 deficiency that appears in thyroidtoxicosis.(421) Aside from the fact that the study showed that thyroxine (a thyroid hormone) was involved in the biochemical pathways, what we find intriguing is visualizing the effects of mercury on the thyroid when superimposed on these findings.

For example, Trahktenberg (1969) reported that mercury first stimulates the thyroid and then suppresses thyroid function.(2) If exposure to mercury is allowed to continue, the damage to the thyroid gland was permanent and irreversible.(240) Also, there is a report that shows iodine causes an increased uptake of mercury by the thyroid.(237,422) Additionally, Goldman and Blackburn (1979) reported that short-term injection of mercury caused an accelerated release of iodine from the thyroid, but that chronic administration of mercury initially caused an increased uptake of iodine by the thyroid.(240) Suzuki et al. also indicated that previously published data had shown that mercury and lead chronically administered induced hyperfunction of the thyroid.(237)

Iodine is the primary element used by the thyroid in the production of hormones. Consequently, it is conceivable that the involvement of chronic inhalation of mercury vapor from mercury amalgam dental fillings could be an etiological factor in thyroid dysfunction involving folic acid, B_{12}, and thyroxine production.

VITAMIN B_{12} (293,414,415)

Normally, most people only think of vitamin B_{12} as the vitamin needed to prevent pernicious anemia. Although it functions in this capacity, that is but the tip of the iceberg. It has the most complex structure of all vitamins and is also unique in that it is the only vitamin containing a metal ion. Cobalamin is the generic name of the vitamin because of the presence of the metal ion cobalt in its structure.

The major functions of B_{12} is as an essential coenzyme for the normal metabolism of all cells, including those of the gastrointestinal tract, bone marrow, and nervous tissue. It also is a coenzyme in the synthesis of red blood cells and in the maintenance of nerve cells, and is involved with protein, lipid and nucleic acid synthesis. It is considered necessary for growth. The coenzyme of vitamin B_{12} is a carrier of methyl groups and hydrogen and is necessary for protein, fat, and carbohydrate metabolism.(329,414,423)

Vitamin B_{12} is a coenzyme in two important reactions. Coenzyme B_{12} methylcobalamin functions as a methyl-group donor to form methionine from homocysteine.(424) Vitamin B_{12} coenzyme deoxyadenosylcobalamin functions in the conversion of methylmalonic acid to succinic acid.(424,425)

Vitamin B_{12} and folic acid have an intimate and essential relationship in humans. Further, it appears that methionine and vitamin B_{12} coordinate in the regulation of folate metabolism. Hillman stated, "A deficiency of either vitamin results in defective synthesis of DNA in any cell that attempts chromosomal replication and division."(414)

The relationship between vitamin B_{12} and folic acid is very complex and controversy exists regarding certain metabolic aspects. Everybody agrees there is an impairment of folate function when a deficiency of vitamin B_{12} exists. The controversy concerns the mechanism by which folate metabolism is impaired.(see the discussion of the methyfolate trap hypotheses in the Folic Acid section)

Chronic mercury inhalation from mercury amalgam dental fillings, with its great affinity to bind to methionine and cysteine has the potential to decrease the availability of these amino acids and affect the metabolism of both vitamin B_{12} and folate in man.

Methionine is needed in choline synthesis, which means that vitamin B_{12} plays a secondary role in this lipid pathway. A choline deficiency that causes fatty liver can be prevented by vitamin B_{12} or the other methyl donors--betaine, methionine, and folic acid.

Impaired fatty acid synthesis, observed in vitamin B_{12} deficiency conditions, can result in impairment of brain and nerve tissue. The insulation around nerve cells, the myelin sheath, is misformed in a vitamin B_{12} deficiency, and this contributes to faulty nerve transmission. Ultimately, neurological disturbances result from prolonged vitamin B_{12} deficiency. Lesions of the peripheral nerves occur more frequently and earlier than lesions of the central nervous system. However, the biochemical basis for the defective myelin synthesis in unknown. (293)

Nakazawa et al. (1972) showed that the phosphatidyl-choline synthesis in the nervous tissue of B_{12}-deficient rats was increased by the administration of methyl-B_{12}, indicating that vitamin B_{12} is related to the lipid metabolism of nervous tissues and prevents neuropathy.(426)

Kasuya (1980) demonstrated that inorganic mercury inhibited outgrowth of nerve fibers and the development of glial cells, and also depressed the outgrowth of fibroblasts. Organic mercury produced similar effects, but required much higher concentrations of mercury. What is extremely interesting about this study is that methyl-B_{12} was able to inhibit the neurotoxic effects of organic mercury but not those caused by inorganic mercury.(427) Mercury vapor released from dental amalgam fillings is considered to be inorganic mercury.

Windebank (1986), in experiments with rats, also demonstrated that very low concentrations of mercury and arsenic were able to inhibit nerve outgrowth, and that lead directly interfered with the process of myelination.(428)

Proper DNA replication is dependent on the function of coenzyme vitamin B_{12} as a methyl-group carrier. Improper cell replication and inadequate DNA translation cause the large cells observed in megaloblastic anemia.(293)

There have been recent studies evaluating the effects of methyl-B_{12}, that suggested the possibility that it may play an important role in immune regulation. In a 1982 in vitro study by Sakane et al. (429), it was demonstrated that concentrations of methyl-B_{12} sufficient to enhance cellular proliferation were able to enhance the activity of helper T-cells for immunoglobulin synthesis of B cells. Furthermore, the presence of methyl-B_{12} significantly potentiated the induction of suppressor cells. The authors felt that their results suggested that methyl-B_{12} could modulate lymphocyte function through augmenting regulatory T-cell activities.

There is another aspect of lymphocyte function and the immune system, related to both vitamin B_{12} and mercury, that requires some discussion. Polymorphonuclear leukocytes (PMNs) are one form of white blood cells that functions in a phagocytic capacity (cells that are capable of destroying foreign substances). The initial immune response of PMNs to a foreign substance in the blood (certain foreign proteins, chemicals, and ions) is a metabolic reaction called the respiratory burst. Without this initial reaction, the PMNs cannot carry out their immune system function of destroying the foreign substance.(185)

Chanarin et al. (1985) found that PMNs from patients with severe vitamin B_{12} deficiency had an impaired oxidative burst (part of the respiratory burst), which resulted in a defect in bacterial killing. In other words, the deficiency caused an impairment of their immune systems.(430) In 1985, Malamud and his associates at the University of Pennsylvania demonstrated that low levels of mercury would inhibit the respiratory burst in human PMNs. (183) In an extension of these original studies, Lammey and Malamud (1987) concluded: "Most significant was the observation that human PMNs are sensitive to relatively low concentrations of mercury (1 ug/ml or less) as demonstrated by all of the assessments."(184)

SUMMARY

The biochemical pathways outlined in this chapter provide the basis for our hypothesis regarding the ultimate pathological action of mercury. The noted similarities between the pathology and symptoms of mercury poisoning compared to those of certain key nutrients provides additional confirmation. Biochemically, the evidence is clear and unmistakable. Mercury acts as an interference to normal biological functions involving the formation and/or function of sulfur containing proteins in cells, enzymes, and hormones. It does this by direct alteration of the protein and/or critical biochemical action related to utilization of essential nutrients. It is also obvious that biological damage will occur long before the appearance of any clinically observable signs and symptoms of mercurialism.

We fully realize that in some instances our proposed biochemical pathways depicting mercurial interference is based solely on our interpretation of existing scientific data. However, we feel that our interpretations are fundamentally sound and based on logical and defensible rationale. Regardless of interpretation, we hope that this book will stimulate the scientific and professional communities to address immediate concern and attention to the subtle but potentially devastating influence mercury vapor released from amalgam dental fillings can have on the human organism.

12

THE DIAGNOSIS OF MERCURY STATUS

Should you find the information presented in this book to be of more than casual interest and you decide to try to determine the influence of the mercury amalgam fillings on your life, you will discover the confusion and frustration encountered in the diagnosis of mercury poisoning. Dentists are not trained to recognize or consider chronic mercury poisoning. Physicians and scientists have not been made aware of the chronic exposure to mercury vapor from dental amalgam fillings and therefore have not seen the need to develop valid diagnostic protocols.

The diagnosis of medical ailments is accomplished whenever possible by conducting laboratory tests that will specifically identify the cause and condition. Unfortunately, as you will see, this is not yet possible for the identification of chronic mercury poisoning. There are no laboratory tests yet available that will specifically establish the diagnosis of chronic mercury poisoning, let alone determine the degree of damage.

Currently, medical diagnostic references emphasize the history of exposure to mercury and the appearance of clinically observable signs and symptoms of mercury poisoning to establish the diagnosis. The critical factor is finding health professionals who acknowledge patient exposure to mercury vapor from dental amalgam fillings and who have taken the trouble to learn the signs and symptoms of chronic mercury poisoning as well as the values and shortcomings of the various available tests.

MERCURY LEVELS IN BLOOD AND URINE

In recent years, the value of measurements of mercury in blood and urine has been subjected to a great deal of attention and controversy. Defenders of the use of dental mercury fillings claim that low urine and blood mercury values prove that the fillings are harmless, even though the ADA and NIDR have publicly admitted that there is no correlation between the toxic effects of mercury and the levels of mercury found in the urine and blood.(95,431) As early as 1964, Goldwater and associates stated that "those investigators who have studied the subject are in almost unanimous agreement that there is poor correlation between the urinary excretion of mercury and the occurrence of demonstrable evidence of poisoning".(432) This position has been thoroughly reinforced through the years with documentation and expert opinion.

The same can be said for blood mercury levels related to exposure to mercury vapor, although there is some validity related to recent exposure to ingested organic and inorganic mercury compounds. Magos, summarizing the research done by himself and a number of others, pointed out that inhaled mercury vapor passes from the blood into body tissues very rapidly after exposure.(55) Blood mercury measurements would therefore have to be performed immediately after exposure to reflect increased levels resulting from inhalation of mercury vapor.

In 1984, the U.S. Environmental Protection Agency (EPA) reviewed the scientific literature and concluded "no threshold air concentration and concentration in urine or blood have been identified".(18) The EPA also pointed out that the rapid evaporation of mercury vapor affects the validity of measuring the mercury levels in blood and urine.(18)

In 1981, Satoh and associates conducted research on the evaporation of mercury from samples of blood and urine and made the following recommendations to ensure the accuracy of analysis:

1.blood should be mixed with chilled ethanol solution immediately after collection;

2. the mixture should be stored at zero degrees centigrade;

3. mercury vapor content should be determined within 60 minutes and preferably within 30 minutes;

4. urine should be chilled; and

5. mercury vapor content should be determined as soon as possible, probably within 10 minutes.(433)

Relation of measured levels of mercury in the urine and blood to "normal" values presents another fallacy, since the so-called "normal" values were derived from population groups heavily infested with mercury dental fillings. Valid comparisons would require relating to control groups not possessing the influencing factor being investigated. The only "experts" that advocate diagnostic use of urine and blood mercury measurements are the same "experts" claiming the harmlessness of mercury vapor released from dental mercury fillings.

HAIR ANALYSIS

The analysis of hair for mercury levels is another story. Although the ADA and the NIDR place little value on hair mercury analysis (431), the EPA offers a different position. In a document reviewing over 130 references, the EPA states "human hair is a meaningful and representative tissue for antimony, arsenic, cadmium, chromium, copper, lead, mercury..."(434) The EPA also stated that "for measurement of levels of toxic metals for long periods or especially of exposure to a dangerously high level during a past period, hair appears to be superior to blood and urine for certain toxic elements concentrated in the hair."(434) In another EPA document, Jenkins reported that "of the 14 trace elements considered in this report, human hair is excellent for biological monitoring of arsenic, cadmium, chromium, lead and mercury."(435)

In 1983, Airey reviewed 113 references and concluded, "Mercury is deposited in the hair as it grows, and the amount deposited reflects the body burden of mercury."(436) Airey also stated. "This increased concern about the health of persons exposed to very low environmental mercury concentrations is because mercury causes subclinical effects at low concentrations. The symptoms are difficult to detect and measure. For example, slightly increased levels of mercury in hair have been associated with decreases in academic ability. Also, reduced productivity and development of asthenic vegetative syndrome, a subtle behavior change, can occur."(436)

Manson and Zlotkin, in a 1985 article printed in the *Canadian Medical Association Journal*, stated that "the analysis of hair for trace elements is potentially a safe, non-invasive and extremely useful diagnostic tool, but it has not yet been proven to be reliable or to reflect the status of trace elements elsewhere in the body. As well, little is known about the normal ranges of concentrations of elements in the hair or about the physiologic and pharmacologic factors that affect the concentrations."(437)

The opinion of Manson and Zlotkin differs from that of Airey and the EPA, so examination of the available data may be helpful towards resolution of the dilemma.

LABORATORY ANALYSIS

In 1985, Barrett sent hair samples from two healthy teenagers to thirteen commercial laboratories performing multimineral hair analysis.(438) The reported levels of most minerals varied considerably between identical samples sent to the same laboratory and from laboratory to laboratory. Barrett concluded that "commercial use of hair analysis in this manner is unscientific, economically wasteful, and probably illegal."

Although Barrett's findings are certainly worthy of consideration, his conclusions are overly dramatic, if not downright inflammatory. Schoenthaler capably addressed Barrett's data and conclusions.(439) Schoenthaler pointed out that the results were severely biased by the obvious ineptitude of a few of the labs, an unfortunate circumstance that has been demonstrated in the analysis performance on other widely accepted medical tests. The majority of labs were in statistical agreement on the analysis.

What Dr. Barrett failed to do was to draw some relationship of the validity of hair analysis in relation to the validity of the millions of blood tests ordered by physicians annually. Accordingly, and to place "the other side of the coin" in proper perspective, let's look at an astounding example.

The College of American Pathologists (CAP) conducts inter-laboratory comparisons of laboratories that do analysis (blood, urine, etc.) for hospitals and physicians. In their 1985 survey, 5000 laboratories were given identical blood samples to analyze; nearly 50% produced unacceptable results.(440) How many erroneous diagnostic decisions, possibly resulting in unnecessary treatment, are based on flawed and incorrect blood analysis? Does Dr. Barrett consider these analyses "unscientific, economically wasteful, and probably illegal"? It appears that Dr. Barrett is recommending throwing out the baby with the bath water. A reasonable recommendation, better serving the patient, would be to exercise prudent care in the selection of an analysis facility.

It is widely acknowledged that hair samples may be contaminated with minerals from sources outside of the body (exogenous contamination), such as shampoos and hair rinses or airborne contaminants. As Gibson pointed out (441), investigators have shown that by employing careful, standardized washing procedures, the effects of these exogenous materials can be minimized, if not completely eliminated. A wide variety of washing procedures using water, organic solvents, detergents and shampoos have been shown to be effective in removing exogenous contaminants from hair.

This position was disputed by Chittleborough (442), who claimed that pre-analysis treatment of hair clearly removed significant amounts of endogenous (from within the body) elements along with the exogenous elements, thereby altering the significance of the obtained results. Chittleborough advocated a holistic, no-wash policy for hair analysis.

Gibson also pointed out the necessity for standardization of the collection procedures for hair samples. Gibson recommends that only hair strands 1-2 centimeters in length, cut close to the occipital region (high nape of the neck) of the scalp be used for analysis.(441)

Atomic Absorption Spectrophotometry (AAS): The most widely used procedure for determining the most abundant trace elements in human hair is AAS. This procedure is rapid, simple, inexpensive, and widely available. Unfortunately, this method requires relatively large samples of hair, at least 200 milligrams, which severely hampers its use in infants. Moreover, AAS analysis results in destruction of the sample, thereby limiting its usefulness in measuring concentrations of more than a few select elements.

Neutron Activation Analysis (NAA): This method is specific, nondestructive, and can be used for the determination of several elements at the same time. Large samples are not required, so it is much more useful for analysis of infants' hair. Unfortunately, this technique is more expensive and less readily obtainable.

Proton (or Particle) Induced X-ray Emission (PIXE): This is a relatively new technique that is reliable and nondestructive. The absolute concentrations of elements in a single hair can be determined, as well as the distribution of these elements along the length and across the diameter of the hair. This technique is not readily available as yet.

AVERAGE (NORMAL) HAIR MERCURY LEVELS

The term *normal* is actually a misnomer when used by the medical and dental professions to describe health as determined by accepted parameters of diagnosis and testing. The so-called "normal" levels of ingredients found in the human body and tissues are determined by surveying a large number of subjects to establish ranges and averages for these ingredients in the general population.

It has been estimated that 70-80% of the adult population of the United States has one or more mercury dental fillings. It has been scientifically demonstrated that these people are chronically exposed to mercury vapor released throughout the lifetime of these fillings. It has also been scientifically demonstrated that even small amounts of mercury vapor have a detrimental effect on numerous aspects of metabolism.

Since a large percentage of the subject sample is environmentally contaminated by a metabolic poison (mercury), medical test parameters must be considered only "average," not "normal" or "healthy." Hair mercury concentrations must also be viewed in this manner, since no studies have been conducted to determine concentrations of mercury in the hair of subjects with and without dental mercury fillings.

Friberg and Vostal reported on "normal" concentrations of mercury in human hair.(60) The authors stated that the subjects were not exposed occupationally to mercury, and that data on their fish consumption was not available. Data from the following studies was presented:

COUNTRY	NUMBER	MEAN MERCURY LEVEL (mcg/g)	REFERENCE
Canada	776	1.8	Perkons & Jervis, 1965
England	840	5.1 (males)	
		6.9 (females)	Coleman et al, 1967
Japan	94	4.2	Yamaguchi & Matsumoto, 1966
	73	6.0	Hoshino et al., 1966
New Zealand	33	2.2	Bate & Dyer, 1965
	33	1.8	

Scotland	26	8.8	Nixon & Smith, 1965
	70	5.5	Howie & Smith, 1967
U.S.	33	7.6	Bate & Dyer, 1965

Samples from the two Japanese studies were analyzed with the chemical Dithizone Method; all of the rest used NAA.

Friberg and Vostal also reported on two Japanese studies investigating levels of methylmercury in hair:

	37	2.8 (males)	Sumino, 1968b
	26	1.7 (females)	
	21	2.4	Ueda & Aoki, 1969
	6	7.0 *	

* Subjects who ate only unpolished rice; 44% was methylmercury.

Since the 1972 Friberg and Vostal document, there have been several investigations that provide data on general population hair mercury levels. Gonzalez and associates measured mercury in the hair of residents of Madrid, Spain, utilizing AAS.(443) They found a mean concentration of 7.96 microgram per gram in the general population and 12.7 microgram per gram in occupationally exposed workers. The authors also noted that in 1971, a "Swedish Expert Group" had established an upper limit for hair mercury of 6.0 microgram per gram.

In 1983, Airey (444) analyzed the hair mercury levels in 559 samples of human hair from thirty-two locations in thirteen countries, reporting the following mean hair mercury concentrations for subjects who ate fish 1-4 times each month.

[Note: Micrograms per gram (mcg/g) is the same as parts per million (ppm).]

Australia	= 2.5 ppm	Canada	= 1.2 ppm
China	= 0.9 ppm	West Germany	= 0.5 ppm
Hong Kong	= 3.0 ppm	Italy	= 1.5 ppm
Japan	= 3.9 ppm	Monaco	= 1.7 ppm
New Zealand	= 1.3 ppm	Papua, New Guinea	= 1.8 ppm
South Africa	= 1.9 ppm	United Kingdom	= 1.6 ppm
U.S.A	= 2.4 ppm		

Airey subjected the samples to meticulous and stringent washing and preparation procedures, and analyzed them by laminar flow clean-room syringe injection AAS technique, which might explain the lower levels than reported in other studies.

In summary, it would seem that average hair mercury levels in general population groups fall in the range of 0.5-8.8 ppm, with the bulk being in the 1.2-4.2 ppm range. It should also be noted that an expert committee in Sweden has established an upper limit of 6.0 ppm (mcg/g) for hair mercury.

HAIR MERCURY CORRELATIONS

To establish the validity of measurements of hair mercury, it is necessary to determine if these measurements correlate with exposure to mercury and/or mercury levels within the body. As previously stated, extensive reviews by Airey and the EPA led to conclusions that hair mercury levels do represent body burden of mercury. These conclusions are supported by more recent documentation.

RELATION TO BLOOD MERCURY

Citing studies by Sexton and associates in 1978 and Kershaw and associates in 1980, Airey pointed out that the mercury concentrations in new growth of hair indicates blood mercury concentrations or body burden of mercury at the time of growth.(444) Airey also emphasized that mercury is excreted from blood into hair in both organic and inorganic forms. Hair mercury levels, therefore, will be reflective of blood levels of both forms of mercury.

In 1985, Gonzalez and associates stated "once mercury has been incorporated into the hair, its concentration does not change significantly, while mercury analysis of blood and urine can only reliably detect very recent exposures. Therefore, mercury analysis of sequential segments of human hair can provide an accurate representation of previous blood mercury levels." (443)

Gibson noted that trace element levels in hair are more concentrated than in blood and urine, thus facilitating analysis. (441) It may also be said that hair analysis, being noninvasive, would be more acceptable to patients and, most likely, less expensive.

In 1980, Phelps and associates analyzed samples of blood and head hair for organic and inorganic mercury from a population that consumed large amounts of fish contaminated with methylmercury.(445) Mercury levels in newly formed hair were found to reflect those in blood, with the concentrations in hair being approximately 300 times those in blood. There was a direct, linear relationship of organic and inorganic mercury levels in both blood and hair. In addition, the total mercury concentration and inorganic/organic ratio in hair remained constant with time. This important study demonstrated that both blood and hair mercury levels reflect an intake of methylmercury from food. It also suggests that a portion of the ingested methylmercury is converted within the body to inorganic mercury, or that there is some other nonoccupational factor that causes a temporal increase in the body burden of inorganic mercury (dental mercury fillings, perhaps?).

RELATION TO DIET

If hair mercury levels are shown to correlate with dietary intake of mercury, then problems with laboratory analysis notwithstanding, hair mercury analysis would have to be considered a valid diagnostic technique, at least for the evaluation of body burden from ingested mercury. Care and prudence in the analysis performance would obviate opposition to the procedure.

The previously cited Phelps study (445) demonstrates the correlation between hair mercury levels and dietary mercury intake. Other studies firmly support this correlation. Kyle and Ghani compared mean hair methylmercury levels in controls to fish eaters, finding almost two and one half times as much mercury in the hair of the fish eaters.(446) Inasmasu and associates demonstrated a correlation between hair mercury levels and consumption of canned tuna fish. The authors also cited four earlier studies that showed a correlation between hair mercury levels and fish intake.(447) In 1977, Harada and associates (448) examined the hair mercury content in seventy-one subjects in Ontario, Canada, and found a positive correlation between the mercury values in the hair and the quantity of fish in the diet. The highest hair mercury content was 80.3 ppm, with forty-four of the seventy-one

subjects showing more than 20 ppm and twenty-three subjects more than 30 ppm.

RELATION TO MERCURY VAPOR EXPOSURE

The early studies on occupational exposure to mercury vapor
did not, unfortunately, include investigation of hair mercury
levels. The investigators focused their attention on mercury
levels in blood and, particularly, urine. The only occupational group routinely exposed to mercury vapor that has been
evaluated for hair mercury levels is dental personnel.

An International Conference on Mercury Hazards in Dental Practice was held in 1981 in Glasgow, Scotland.(449)
Several presentations addressed hair mercury levels in dental personnel.

Paper 9, by Dale and associates, compared dental personnel to the unexposed population, citing a mean of 0.75 ppm
for the control group. Dental workers in general practice had
a mean of 3.31 ppm and those in health service clinics had a
mean of 1.54 ppm. Over 600 dental workers were surveyed
and 20-25% exhibited hair mercury levels above normal.
Levels of mercury in pubic hair were found to be significantly lower but still slightly higher than normal, suggesting that
most of the hair contamination was exogenous.

Paper 15, by Sairenji and associates in Japan, surveyed
fifty-eight male dentists employed at a dental school and
fifty male dentists engaged in private practice in Tokyo. The
hair mercury levels were found to be the same as in "normal
Japanese," which the authors placed at a mean of 5.26 ppm.
The authors cited three previous studies of hair mercury in
dental personnel to be means of 10.8 ppm, 11.5 ppm, and
12.3 ppm. Of special interest was their finding that fully 30%

of the mercury was lost from hair samples analyzed by NAA compared to samples that were treated with thioacetamide.

Paper 28, by Nishimura and Yamanaka, surveyed ninety-nine dentists in Japan by AAS. The mean hair-mercury level in the dentists was 8.64 ppm, compared to their citations of normal Japanese of 3.5 to 6.4 ppm. The authors further investigated the ability of hair to absorb mercury from the air and found this capability to be extremely low at the levels found in the air of the dental offices. They concluded that the higher levels of mercury found in the hair of dental personnel came from within the body or from touching the hair with hands contaminated with mercury. The authors also found that the waste water from almost all dental offices exceeded allowable limits, and further found that mercury levels in the soil around dental offices, and even around adjacent buildings, exceeded control sites.

In 1979, Lee and Sohn measured the mercury content in the head hair of eighty-seven Korean dental personnel and 210 control subjects with the following results: (1) The mean value of mercury content in dentists (8.57 ppm) was 3.3 times that of Seoul male citizens (2.57 ppm). The median of the former (5.92 ppm) was higher than that of the latter (2.39 ppm) by approximately 2.5 times. (2) The mean value of mercury content in dental nurses (5.79 ppm) was 2.8 times that of Seoul female citizens (2.11 ppm). The median of the former (4.62 ppm) was about 2.5 times that of the controls (1.86 ppm). (3) The mean value of mercury content in Seoul citizens was 2.29 ppm and the median was 1.98 ppm. (4) There was no correlation between the mercury content in the head hair of dentists and the length of dental surgery experience or the frequency of amalgam fillings per day. (5) The mercury content of Seoul citizens was higher in the male than in the female. (6) It appears more meaningful to employ median values than mean values when environmental pollution is considered.(450)

In 1982, Francis and associates analyzed the inorganic mercury content of hair from dental and nondental subjects in central Kentucky. They found no significant difference between the two groups.(451) Sinclair and associates used NAA to measure the mercury in head hair from sixty-one dental students and dental faculty members and found "significant" increases. They attributed this to increased pressure of work, which might have resulted in decreased standards of mercury hygiene.(452)

In 1986, Sikorski and associates analyzed fifteen women subjects exposed to metallic mercury at dental offices and eleven nonexposed control subjects. They found that the total mercury was significantly higher in both the scalp and pubic hair of the exposed women compared to the controls.(453)

RELATION TO DENTAL MERCURY FILLINGS

Only one study can be found that investigates the relationship between hair mercury levels and the presence of dental mercury fillings, that of Gonzalez and associates in 1985. (443) The authors concluded that "no relationship exists between mercury levels and number of dental fillings." However, examination of the data provided by the study casts considerable doubt on the validity of that conclusion. Of the ninety-six subjects included in the study, sixty-two (64.6%) had no dental fillings at all. Of the remaining thirty-four subjects, eight (8.3%) had only one filling, nine (9.4%) had only two fillings, and seventeen (17.7%) had three fillings. None of the subjects had more than three fillings. Moreover, no information was provided as to the location of the fillings. Dental mercury fillings that are on the chewing (occlusal) surface of teeth will release more mercury than those not on chewing surfaces. The authors' conclusion is hardly justified by the data provided. The existence of high numbers of large dental mercury fillings in subjects is not an uncommon occurrence; the relationship of this situation to hair mercury levels remains uninvestigated and unanswered.

RELATION TO PATHOLOGY

Studies investigating the relationship between hair mercury levels and pathologic conditions are very sparse. This unfortunate circumstance is quite amazing in view of the strong evidence that hair mercury levels do correlate to the body burden of mercury, the knowledge of the severe toxicity of mercury, and the lack of other diagnostic tests for mercury poisoning, especially chronic mercury poisoning. Gonzalez and associates stated "perhaps what is more important than the possibility of a few people showing definite signs of mercury poisoning is the likelihood that a large proportion may be at risk from subclinical effects of mercury with regard to behavior, learning ability, fertility, and immunologic response, etc., which may result from prolonged exposure to low levels of mercury."(443)

Airey said "it is now well known that methylmercury is deposited in and irreversibly destroys brain and nerve cells. It is less well known that subclinical accumulations may effect intelligence. People who are employed in buildings where mercury is used often show clinical and subclinical effects of mercury absorption, e.g. dentists; industrial workers; miners; and laboratory workers."(444)

An example of how hair mercury analysis can be applied to Airey's point may be found in the papers from the Glasgow Conference.(449) Paper 21, by Symington, is entitled "Clinical Features of Mercury Absorption." Symington reports on three dentists who were found to be occupationally poisoned by mercury where the office mercury vapor levels were well below the established standards. One of the dentists was treated with a daily dose of D-penicillamine for two weeks, which resulted in considerable clinical and biochemical improvement. During the period of treatment, mercury levels in daily beard shavings fluctuated between 38 and 124 ppm, which reflected the release of the high body burden. The diagnosis of mercury poisoning was suggested by the dentist himself while being tested for other possible causes for his illness. This reported case illustrates a very important application of post-challenge hair mercury analysis for the diagnosis and treatment of chronic mercury poisoning.

The previously cited study by Harada and associates in Ontario, Canada found fifteen of the seventy-one subjects with sensory neurologic disturbances and nine cases with visual disturbance. The cases with neurological symptoms showed higher mercury values in the hair than those subjects without symptoms, and were suspected of having mild methylmercury poisoning.(448)

In 1976, Clarkson and Amin-Zaki and associates reported the results of investigations of the methylmercury poisoning outbreak in Iraq. They found that hair and blood mercury levels correlated to exposure and were reflected by signs of mercury poisoning in mothers and severe brain damage in infants from prenatal exposure.(67,454)

The previously mentioned Sikorski study on fifteen women occupationally exposed to metallic mercury compared to eleven control women found a correlation between higher levels of mercury in scalp and pubic hair and lower blood serum levels of the IgG antibody.(453)

Considering the dynamic inference derived from these very few investigations, it is astounding that more attention and study has not been directed to this area. Moreover, low hair-zinc levels have been determined in mothers of infants born with spina bifida (455), in preschool children exhibiting anorexia and poor growth (456), and with the occurrence of diaper rash and hair loss in infants (457). Mercury is known to interfere with zinc and its metabolism.

HAIR MERCURY LEVELS OF MOTHER AND INFANT DURING PREGNANCY

This paper examines the high incidence of birth defects that still occur in the UK and suggests that it might be possible to reduce this by preparing prospective mothers for parenthood prior to conception. One test in particular is suggested as having a part to play in this preconception screening -- that being the hair metal analysis. Such a screening test is useful in identifying both excesses of toxic metals and deficiencies of essential metals.(458)

This dynamic statement by Barlow and associates dramatizes an important consideration for all prospective parents. Our children are very dear to us. Can a simple, inexpensive, and noninvasive test help reduce risks to our offspring and enhance their chance for a better life? The price of this insurance policy is certainly infinitesimal, especially compared to the price of potential consequences. Will hair mercury analysis be a valid part of this consideration?

As previously discussed, Clarkson and Amin-Zaki and associates have demonstrated that hair mercury levels correlate with brain damage found in infants of mothers exposed to methylmercury.(67,454) Other sections of this book establish that exposure to both methylmercury and mercury vapor present a definite threat to the fetus. Other investigations have determined that mercury in the blood of pregnant women will actually concentrate to higher levels in the fetal blood, resulting in even a greater exposure and threat to the fetus.

In 1976, Creason and associates wrote, "There have been numerous reports of abortion or fetal malformation due to excessive exposures of the expectant mother to mercury and other trace elements."(459) Their study investigated the levels of sixteen trace elements in maternal venous blood, cord blood, placenta, and maternal scalp and pubic hair. The maternal scalp hair sample and geometric means were 2.2 ppm and 1.4 ppm, and the maternal pubic hair sample and geometric means were 3.8 ppm and 0.7 ppm. The levels of mercury in the cord blood were higher than in the maternal blood and even higher in the placenta.

Fujita and Takabatake, in 1977, sampled blood and hair of mother-neonate pairs and mothers' breast milk of thirty-four subjects.(460) They found that the maternal samples showed generally lower total mercury levels than those of the babies. A significant correlation was found in the concentration of total mercury between the newborn babies' hair and maternal blood, and also between the neonatal hair and neonatal blood. In their investigation of the methylmercury poisoning outbreak in Iraq, Amin-Zaki and associates found that mercury in the milk of nursing mothers averaged 8.6% of the simultaneous blood level. (67) Gonzalez and associates measured the hair mercury levels of nursing infants and their mothers and found the correlation to be extremely significant.(443)

SUMMARY

Barlow and associates probably said it best in their 1985 study: "The technique of hair analysis has received a good deal of criticism by many people. Perhaps one of the main reasons for this is that the significance of the analysis has not been fully appreciated." The authors suggested that "the analysis of hair for its metal content is a useful technique for the primary screening of individuals and selected populations for the assessment of body burdens of metals." They pointed out that often in reported work relating to hair analysis the concept of "normal ranges" is used and that this concept is rather artificial because the actual levels of metal found will depend on the method of sample preparation and the analysis technique used. Further, Barlow and his colleagues felt that with the majority of biological variables there is no well defined boundary between what is normal and what is abnormal and concluded: "Thus, it is perhaps better to make use of 'reference levels' and then it can be said with more confidence that if a particular value falls within the reference range the subject under investigation is more likely not to be abnormal than normal whilst the converse applies to a value outside the reference range."(458)

These comments, of course, refer to the evaluation of all trace minerals found in hair analysis. The existence of contrary opinions such as that of Barrett (438) notwithstanding, it is quite apparent that the vast weight of scientific evidence favors the validity of hair analysis for trace mineral evaluation. The utilization of this procedure can certainly be supported with scientific documentation, providing that judicious care is exercised regarding technique and laboratory procedures.

Regarding analysis for mercury specifically, the cited documentation clearly indicates that hair mercury levels do reflect exposure to and body burden of all forms of mercury. It should be emphasized that consideration should be given to the exclusion of mercury contamination of the hair from sources outside of the body, without the elimination of that mercury within the hair in the process. Although a correlation between mercury levels in hair and exposure to mercury has been established, no correlation to the degree of pathological damage has been determined.

What is the significance of the mercury levels found in human hair? There can be no doubt that mercury is hazardous to human health, and most particularly to the developing child. Moreover, it is well established that the effects of mercury on the embryo/fetus are neurological and developmental and therefore not recognizable by mere visual observation at birth. The EPA states that the minimal amount of exposure to mercury vapor that humans can be exposed to without incurring harm is unknown.(18) Since the significant exposure to mercury from dental amalgam fillings is from the vapor form, and since mercury has no known beneficial biologic function, it may be argued that hair mercury levels should not exceed a reference range derived from subjects without dental amalgam fillings or exogenous exposure to mercury. Unfortunately, no such reference range has been established at this time. It is our hope that this book might stimulate efforts from reputable scientists to establish valid parameters for biological references derived from subjects free of chronic exposure to mercury from dental amalgam fillings. These parameters should cover the entire range of tests and not be limited to only mercury levels in hair, blood, and urine.

Finally, we would like to refer once more to statements from the 1985 study by Barlow and associates.(458) That group pointed out that in 1977 in the United Kingdom a total of 10,892 malformed babies were born alive. (This is not including babies born with developmental or neurological defects that would not be recognizable until a later time.) "This figure represents 20 per 1000 live births. Various reports suggest that between six and ten per cent of all children born have some degree of handicap by the age of five years and that possibly 20-50 per cent of such handicaps arose in the peri-natal period. In addition it has been suggested that many of these handicaps, be they mental or physical, might be preventable." If the utilization of the simple, inexpensive, and noninvasive hair analysis, along with the elimination of chronic mercury exposure from dental amalgam fillings, prevents even a fraction of these handicaps, the service to mankind would be inestimable.

CONCLUSIONS

It should be obvious from the preceding information that measurements of mercury in the blood and urine are not valid indicators of the body burden or toxic effects of mercury. Currently, medical diagnostic references are emphasizing the signs and symptoms and history of exposure as the key determinants in the diagnosis of chronic mercury poisoning. However, recent awareness and attention directed to exposure to mercury vapor from mercury amalgam fillings will hopefully result in the establishment of more specific protocols. Some areas of promise include specific enzyme testing, magnetic resonance imaging (MRI), post-challenge urine mercury measurement, and direct measurement of intra-oral mercury vapor exposure.

If you have been under a physician's care for any health problems for which no cause could be identified, and you have mercury amalgam dental fillings in your mouth, then you might wish to consider taking some of the following actions.

1. Return to your physician and discuss the possibility that mercury hypersensitivity or intoxication may be a possible cause. You should ask that lead determinations also be made

because of the synergistic effect with mercury. Hopefully, your physician will be aware of the chronic exposure to mercury vapor from your dental amalgam fillings and will be familiar with the signs and symptoms of chronic mercury poisoning.

2. The great metal diagnostic capabilities of magnetic resonance imaging (MRI) are beginning to appear with regularity in the scientific literature. If you have a health problem of unknown etiology, your physician should be able to order a magnetic resonance evaluation of your body burden of heavy metals. This could provide categorical scientific proof if mercury and lead are involved. If MRI is not feasible, you could have a hair analysis done to see what levels of mercury and lead it reveals. If the levels are above normal and you have had no exogenous exposure to mercury, it would be a positive finding warranting further evaluation of mercury or lead intoxication.

You could also have mercury blood and urine tests done. However, you should be fully aware that mercury blood and urine tests have no relationship to chronic exposure, tissue burden, or toxicity. Such tests are valid only for recent acute exposures. Some recent scientific data indicates that evaluation of mercury content of red blood cells may have a much greater diagnostic significance.

With regard to lead, your physician can order evaluations of your blood and urine for the enzyme d-aminolevulinic acid dehydrogenase (ALA-D). The changes in enzyme activities, particularly ALA-D in peripheral blood and excretion of ALA in urine, correlate very closely with actual blood lead levels and serve as early biochemical indices of lead effect.(461)

3. Ask your physician to read Chapters 5-9 and Chapter 11 of this book. If he or she is skeptical and derisive of the

idea, look for another physician who is at least willing to evaluate some of the data presented here. The reason we have cited almost 500 scientific references is to demonstrate to the most skeptical member of the medical profession that there is a sound scientific basis for consideration of the potential toxicity of dental mercury in any differential diagnosis related to health problems of unknown etiology.

4. Within the medical community, there are a group of physicians who are very knowledgeable about the adverse role of heavy metals in the human body. Most belong to the American College of Advancement in Medicine (ACAM), are highly trained in the administration of chelation therapy, and have been board certified by the American Board of Chelation Therapy. In addition, most have some knowledge of the mercury amalgam dental filling problem. Therefore, if you are looking for another physician or just another opinion, we suggest you contact the ACAM office to see if they can refer you to one of their physician members in your vicinity. Their phone number and address are listed in Appendix 2.

5. An allergist or clinical ecologist may be able to determine if you are hypersensitive to mercury, or some of the other metals contained in the amalgam. However, there are some problems associated with skin tests for mercury allergy. If you are already sensitized to mercury, the application of a mercury patch or the subcutaneous injection of mercury may aggravate your sensitivity. The use of this testing procedure is contraindicated in health conditions where anecdotal and/or scientific evidence indicates mercury toxicity may be a viable etiological consideration.

6. There are analytical instruments currently available that can be used to measure the intra-oral levels of mercury vapor. Some dentists and physicians may have them available. Use

of a mercury vapor analyzer is a simple, noninvasive test to determine how much mercury vapor is being released from your mercury amalgam dental fillings. Readings are taken in your mouth before and after chewing gum for 10 minutes. High readings would indicate that your dental fillings are releasing excessive amounts of mercury vapor whenever stimulated by normal functions such as chewing, drinking hot fluids, brushing your teeth, and so on. This would also mean that the chronic inhalation of mercury vapor from this source is contributing to your total body burden of mercury. However, the mercury vapor readings are not diagnostic of mercury toxicity. Occupational mercury vapor exposure standards, such as those established by OSHA and NIOSH, are limited to 40 hour per week exposures and therefore not valid for constant intra-oral exposure. The EPA exposure standard of one microgram per cubic meter and intake standard of twenty micrograms per day of all mercury from all sources other than food are the only valid comparisons.

7. Your dentist may have a device for measuring electrical current or potentials being generated by the dissimilar metals in your mouth. Again, this is of no value in diagnosing mercury toxicity or hypersensitivity, and only serves to demonstrate that the dissimilar metals in your teeth are creating electrogalvanic energy. It would, however, be an indication of metal corrosion, which would be a factor in the increased release of mercury vapor and ionized particles.

8. One of the three classic symptoms of mercury toxicity has always been gingivitis. Although there are many other factors that may cause periodontal disease, oral pathology textbooks and the scientific literature establish that mercury and/or amalgam fillings can pathologically damage periodontal tissue. Therefore, if you have been having recurring periodontal problems, your dentist and physician should con-

sider this as another possible indication that mercury may be an etiological factor in your health problems.

9. One test that has been used by many clinicians is called diagnostic chelation. In this type of testing protocol, you are given one of the compounds or substances that are known to bind or chelate mercury. Urine samples are then collected periodically and analyzed for mercury (or lead). Increased urinary excretion of the particular metal being investigated is usually an indication of excessive body burden. By ridding your body of large amounts of the offending metal, the procedure could also result in an amelioration of some of your health problems or symptoms. The increased excretion and abatement of symptoms would be additional diagnostic factors implicating mercury and/or lead.

10. Scientists around the world have been looking for more accurate diagnostic indicators of mercury biochemical effects. Much of this work is centered around evaluating various enzymes for either inhibition or impaired metabolic function in the presence of mercury. One of the major problems in this area of endeavor is that there are many chemicals in our environment that may depress, inhibit, or stimulate the same enzyme. However, much progress has been made. It is now known that mercury will affect the following enzymes or coenzymes:

glucose-6-phosphatase (294,298,466)

alkaline phosphatase (294,298,462)

acid phosphohydrolase (294)

acid phosphatase (466)

Mg, Ca, Na, K, adenosinetriphosphatase (298,465,466)

succinic dehydrogenase (298,466)

delta-amino-levulinic acid dehydrogenase (298)

acetylcholinesterase (335,470)

choline acetyl transferase (472)

coenzyme A (CoA or CoA-SH) (2,178,401)

sorbitol dehydrogenase (462)

alanine aminotransferase (462)

aspartate aminotransferase (294,462)

glutathione peroxidase (467,469)

3b-hydroxy-delta^5-steroid dehydrogenase (463)

RNA-polymerase (464)

adenylate cyclase (181)

cytochrome c oxidase (294,471)

cytochrome P-450 (178)

glutaminase (294)

ascorbic acid oxidase (239)

lactic dehydrogenase (294)

fatty acid synthetase (468)

ornithine decarboxylase (473)

21a-hydroxylase (178)

isocitric dehydrogenase (78)

Utilizing clinical laboratory tests for some of these enzymes may assist your physician in arriving at a valid differential diagnosis of mercury intoxication.

In the final analysis, current scientific research has clearly demonstrated that mercury amalgam dental fillings release mercury vapor that enters the subject's body and slowly builds up in the body with time. It is further evident that there are no scientific guarantees that any amount of exposure to mercury vapor can be considered harmless. Given this established information, you may decide to eliminate the source of the exposure on that basis alone. If you seek additional encouragement, we hope that the information provided in this chapter will be of some assistance to you.

13

HELPING YOURSELF

Many of you may still not believe in the information, or its applications, that we have advanced in relation to the ever increasing incidence of infertility and birth defects. Many of you may even be skeptical enough to say there have been millions of normal babies born to parents who have had mercury amalgam fillings, so there really isn't any basis for concern. Those of you who may feel that way are certainly entitled to your own opinion and beliefs. However, we urge you to keep an open mind, especially if you are a woman and of childbearing age. Remember, the effects of mercury on the fetus are not usually detectable by mere physical observation. We feel we have presented an overwhelming array of scientific data that warrants the most serious consideration by any couple who is presently infertile and those couples actively planning on having children.

For those of you who have taken the information in this book seriously and are planning a family, the first thing you have to do is make an individual and personal decision related to the presence of mercury amalgam dental fillings and other metals that may have been implanted in your teeth. For many people with a mouthful of mercury and other metals, the cost of replacing these with nonmetal-containing materials can be costly. Consequently, we feel this particular budgetary decision may be one of the first you will have to make other than the costs related to pregnancy and birth. You must also keep in mind that nonmetal dental filling materials are not as hard and may not last as long in the back teeth.

One aspect of the decision process can be to attempt to determine if there is any relationship between your health status and metal dental materials in your teeth. Take a sheet of paper and begin listing the approximate dates of the onset of any particular health problem. For example, if you started having episodes of mental depression, approximately when did they start? Or, if you have been feeling tired or fatigued, when did it start? In fact, you may wish to review the list of symptoms in Chapter 2. If you have any of the symptoms, list the symptom and the approximate date that it appeared.

Next, to the best of your knowledge, jot down the ap- proximate dates when you first had any dental fillings or res- toration work done, and all subsequent dates when additional work was done. The list should not be restricted to just fill- ings. It should include any metal placed in your mouth, in- cluding orthodontic devices.

Lastly, line up the two sets of dates and see if there is any relationship between the onset of symptoms and the dates of dental treatment. If some of the events seem to correlate, this could indicate that your own particular biochemical in- dividuality is not tolerating the presence of these foreign substances. This should also help you in making the final judgement as to whether or not you should have the offend- ing materials replaced.

If you are presently infertile, without any obvious pathologic cause identified by your physician, the above self- investigation could be very enlightening. More importantly, the investigation of whether mercury or lead, as well as other metals in the oral environment, might be the primary etiological cause assumes much greater importance, especially when viewed in context with some of the costs of fertility programs and the heartache and anguish that accompany many of the difficult decisions with which you could be confronted.

The realities of life being what they are, most of us have to be concerned with costs. Consequently, we think it important that the reader understand the current situation regarding health insurance policies defraying the dental costs of total metal replacement. Most will only cover costs of replacing individual fillings where there is evidence that the filling is no longer serviceable. The insurance carriers are primarily following the advice of the ADA. The ADA maintains, quite vociferously, that the implantation of a poison in your body, in most instances without your knowledge or consent, is correct and proper. In fact, for whatever the irrational and totally unsupportable reasons may be, the ADA has recently mounted a nationwide effort to place in jeopardy any dentist who advocates the removal of an amalgam restoration solely to substitute a material that does not contain mercury. Further, the ADA has stated publicly that they will take an increased role in stimulating active enforcement of that policy, including providing scientific personnel as expert witnesses to any state dental board that wishes to initiate action against a dentist replacing serviceable amalgam fillings.

IT IS AMAZING TO US, THAT AT THE SAME TIME THE ADA IS EXTOLLING THE SAFETY OF AMALGAM, THE SWEDISH GOVERNMENT HAS DECLARED AMALGAM TO BE TOXIC AND UNSUITABLE AS A DENTAL FILLING MATERIAL BASED ON AN EVALUATION OF THE SCIENTIFIC LITERATURE BY THAT COUNTRY'S LEADING MEDICAL AUTHORITY.

Consequently, if you make the decision to have your mercury amalgam fillings replaced with nonmetallic fillings, we suggest you inquire if your dentist would be willing to replace your amalgams with a nonmercury material. If not, find a dentist who operates a mercury-free practice, or one who is open-minded enough to honor your request of amalgam removal and replacement. Remember, they are *your* teeth and it is *your* health, so if you have made the decision to rid yourself of mercury amalgam fillings, then it is your right to do so. Don't be discouraged; keep looking until you find a dentist with whom you are comfortable and who will honor your feelings.

As most of you are aware, the threat of malpractice legal suits has forced most health care providers to practice defensively. In this regard, most dentists today, as with most physicians, may require you to sign an informed consent form. This procedure can work to your benefit as much as the dentist's. Before you sign any informed consent agreement, make sure your dentist has satisfactorily answered any questions you may have.

As was done in Sweden, we hope the U.S. Department of Health and Human Services will appoint an expert commission composed of physician neurologists and toxicologists to resolve the issue in this country. It is imperative that the medical profession of this country be made aware of, and understand, the wide spectrum of potential toxicity that may be attributable to mercury amalgam dental fillings, and that the "dental experts" whom they have relied on for the correct information on this subject have been poorly informed in their advice to physicians and dentists alike.

The objective of all of the above is to ultimately have your physician write a prescription directing the dentist to remove and replace mercury amalgam dental fillings with nonmetallic materials. The probability of having your health and/or dental insurance plan cover the costs of complete replacement therapy are much greater if your physician is actively involved in the decision. If, even under these conditions, the insurance carrier disapproves the pre-work approval request, then you should have your attorney write a letter to the insurance carrier demanding that their legal department respond in writing indicating that they assume full responsibility for any health problems you may experience from chronic mercury exposure from your mercury amalgam dental fillings.

WAYS TO HELP YOURSELF

If you are not presently able to accommodate the financial burden associated with complete removal and replacement of your mercury amalgam dental fillings, there are still some options available to you. First, do not permit any dentist to ever again implant any mercury in your teeth. If you require subsequent dental work, request that your dentist use only nonmetallic materials if at all possible. If he or she refuses to honor your request and you are determined to have the mercury amalgam fillings replaced with healthier materials, find another dentist.

Second, set up some time frame and goals that will permit you to have your mercury amalgam dental fillings replaced on a budget based-schedule. Remember, each mercury amalgam filling you have replaced with a nonmercury-containing material will reduce your exposure level to this insidious poison.

Finally, you can initiate actions to help reduce your total body burden of mercury and lead.

SUPPLEMENTS

Chapter 11 contained information on the nutrients that will tend to offset some of the damaging effects of mercury and lead. Many of the nutrients also have an ability to bind with mercury and lead, which would then tend to help your body excrete these toxic metals, thereby reducing your total body burden. You should be aware, however, that as long as you have mercury amalgam dental fillings, you will be inhaling micro amounts of mercury vapor 24 hours a day, 7 days a week, 365 days a year. Consequently, it is irrational to assume that augmentation of your nutritional status alone is all that is necessary. There is no question that it will help, but until the source of this implanted poison is eliminated, you will not be able to purge this particular poison effectively. With regard to removal or reduction of lead, the task is much easier because you do not have a constant source of lead implanted in your body.

There are several nutrient manufacturers in this country that have recognized the necessity of providing products that will assist in reducing body burdens of heavy metals and/or environmental pollutants. Most health food stores throughout the country carry some of these products, and store personnel are usually able to advise you of the manufacturers' technical information evolved from testing or the scientific literature related to formulation of the product.

The information that follows on supplements is not intended as medical advice. Rather, it is an interpretation of some of the scientific information contained in Chapter 11. Ideally, your effort to improve your nutritional status should be under the direction of a physician or health care professional familiar with nutritional therapy. This is especially true for those individuals who are presently allergic to a variety of substances and such individuals electing to self-experiment should do so with caution.

As a general caution with regard to embarking on a nutritional supplementation program--don't be in a hurry. The body has a very delicate balance mechanism and unless you are well read on nutrition and are presently supplementing, proceed slowly, giving your body a chance to adjust as you add new nutrients.

In some people the addition of some of the key nutrients that mercury and lead affect may produce some beneficial health effects through the amelioration of some symptomatology related to existing health problems. Although this does not constitute scientific proof that mercury from your mercury amalgam dental fillings is the culprit, it does tend to indicate that you may be on the right track. The following represents a simple program that you may wish to initially try

1. Those individuals with occlusal mercury amalgam fillings should stop chewing gum. The chewing forces involved will continually stimulate the release of mercury vapor from the fillings adding substantially to your body burden of mercury.

2. Glutathione. The reason for starting with glutathione, beyond those contained in Chapter 11, is that when any type of chelation activity is undertaken, there is usually a tissue redistribution of heavy metals within the body. This can result in additional mercury being taken up by the brain which could aggravate some of your symptoms. If you have actually been experiencing toxic effects of mercury, your available supply of glutathione should also be reduced. Therefore, the first nutrient you should supplement is glutathione which will help replenish your supply and should also minimize any effects related to redistribution. It usually comes in a 50

milligram tablet or capsule and you should start out taking 50 milligram three times a day on an empty stomach. (Amino acids are best taken on an empty stomach so as not to compete with those contained in your food.) You can take it between meals, before going to bed, or upon awakening in the morning. Take only glutathione for the first 3-4 days before you add the next nutrient.

3. Zinc is the next nutrient to be added. Zinc stimulates the production of metallothionein in the body, which is one way the body detoxifies the effects of mercury. There are several different kinds of zinc available, all with different potencies. It is suggested that you take one zinc tablet per day with a meal and the potency can be 15-30 Milligrams. After you have been taking the glutathione for 3-4 days, add the one zinc tablet per day to your regimen. Continue the two items for an additional 3-4 days, closely observing any changes.

4. Selenium is the next nutrient to be added. Selenium binds with mercury and will start to cause a redistribution of tissue mercury. It should also precipitate some excretion of mercury from the body. Selenium is available in several forms and potencies. It is suggested that you start with a 50-microgram tablet and take one with each meal, for a total of 150 micrograms daily. For those who are allergic to yeast derived products, sodium selenite in tablet or liquid form is available. Individuals who are sensitive to petrochemicals sometimes react to small quantities of selenium and should either be under the guidance of a physician or initiate selenium supplementation very slowly. Do not take more than 50 micrograms per day until you have established that you are experiencing no adverse allergic reaction.

5. Vitamin B_1 is the last nutrient to be added 3-4 days after selenium. Use a 50-milligram tablet and take one tablet with each meal for a total of 150 milligrams per day.

Some people may have beneficial health effects, from the supplementation indicated, within 3-5 days; in others, it may take 60-90 days to notice any improvement. There is also the chance that you won't experience any benefit. However, it is a non-invasive cost effective way to do a little health-detective work.Improvements in sense of well-being, energy levels, and amelioration of any existing symptomatology are all positive indications that your nutriture of glutathione, zinc, selenium and thiamine had been impaired. This does not mean, categorically, that mercury and lead were the cause. However, it does indicate that serious consideration should be given to that possibility.

DIETARY CHANGES

Assuming you have achieved some beneficial effects from your supplementation program, what else can you do to help your body more effectively cope with the stress of heavy metal exposure?

First and foremost is the consideration of dietary changes that might help in the overall goal of reducing intake and increasing excretion. The largest dietary source of mercury comes from fish and fish products. You should become very selective about the amount and type of fish you eat. Using the information in Chapter 3 will assist you in selecting types of fish to eat that are lower in mercury content. Intake of shell fish should be eliminated or greatly reduced as shell fish are scavengers and normally contain high levels of heavy metals. Anecdotal evidence indicates that individuals who are sensitive to mercury usually have some type of adverse reaction from shell fish.

You can also ensure that you routinely eat a high-fiber diet. This will tend to decrease fecal transit time, reducing the amount of time that liquids containing heavy metals remain in the colon. This will reduce the quantity reabsorbed from the colon that passes through the portal vein into the liver and is then recirculated throughout the body. A recent study by Rowland et al. in 1986 demonstrated the significance of fiber. Utilizing mice that had been exposed to methylmercury, the study set out to determine if fiber made any difference in the whole-body retention of mercury. The incorporation of 30% wheat bran in the diet of the mice significantly decreased the total mercury concentration in the brain, blood, and small intestine. The authors felt that wheat bran exerted its effects on mercury retention and brain level via a modification of the metabolic activity of the gut microflora.(474) For anyone taking supplementary fiber it is important that an adequate amount of water be consumed. Additionally, routine intakes of 6-8 glasses of water daily will also assist your body in getting rid of toxins.

The status of your intestinal flora also plays a significant role in the excretion of methylmercury in your feces. Stress and use of antibiotics can reduce viable strains of intestinal bacteria and cause overgrowth of undesirable strains, in essence reducing the quality of the intestinal flora. One way the body rids itself of mercury is via the bile which empties into your intestine. If your intestinal flora is impaired, then mercury, and for that matter other heavy metals that would have been excreted in your feces, are recirculated back to the liver. Including items in your diet that are rich in favorable bacteria, such as unsweetened yogurt with live cultures, acidophilus supplements, buttermilk and other clabbered milk products, will assist in the maintenance of your intestinal flora.

DIETARY SOURCES OF PARTICULAR NUTRIENTS

Foods are listed in decreasing order of content

1. Selenium: Butter, smoked herring, Brazil nuts, cashew nuts, wheat germ and bran, scallops, barley, whole wheat bread, milk, brown rice, brewers yeast, oats, garlic, cheddar cheese, and molasses.

2. Zinc: Herring, sunflower seeds, pumpkin seeds, ground round steak, lamb chops, pecans, brazil nuts, beef liver, egg yolk, whole wheat bread, oats, almonds, sardines, and chicken.

3. Thiamine: Wheat germ, rice bran, yeast, ham, dried raisins and prunes, asparagus, beans, broccoli, cauliflower, corn, lentils, brown rice, almonds, cashews, and eggs.

4. Methionine and Cysteine: NOTE: The determination of sulfur-amino acid content of various foods is not readily available. As a general rule recommendations as good food sources of sulfur-containing amino acids have been eggs, beans, brussels sprouts, onions, garlic, cabbage, cottage cheese, brown rice, sesame seeds, and pumpkin seeds.

Dietary intake of refined carbohydrates, sugars, and saturated fats should be reduced. These types of foods have high energy requirements for metabolism and may well reduce the availability of essential enzymes and nutrients required for more beneficial purposes.

PHARMACEUTICALS AND OTHER CONSIDERATIONS

You should also become very critical of every pharmaceutical product you use, prescription or over-the-counter, with regard to whether it contains mercury in any form. The same can be said for cosmetic products, many of which still contain some forms of mercury. It used to be that a great many ophthalmic solutions contained mercury as an antibacterial agent. However, a recent check of solutions for contact lenses revealed that the number containing mercury had been greatly reduced. Substitutes should be used for merthiolate or mercurochrome. There are several over-the-counter ointments as well as some ophthalmic ointments or eye salves that contain yellow mercuric oxide, or ammoniated mercury. There are also other ointments that contain calomel (mercurous chloride). Some cathartic pills also contain calomel. You will find antiseptic creams or lotions that contain ammoniated mercury. Many skin bleaching preparations contain ammoniated mercury. Some long acting nasal sprays may contain mercury in the form of thimerosal (merthiolate). As you can see from the range of products, it is important that you start reading labels and asking questions.(475)

If you are attempting to achieve pregnancy or are presently pregnant, you should also give serious consideration to either stopping or greatly curtailing smoking and the consumption of alcoholic beverages. We have touched on some aspects of alcohol previously, but we have made no previous mention of the possible effects of smoking. Let it suffice to say that there is some scientific evidence indicating that smoking can have an affect.

REPLACEMENT PROTOCOLS

WHAT TO DO IF PRESENTLY PREGNANT

If you are presently pregnant, the most important question to arise will be, What should I do about dental work or the replacement of mercury amalgam dental fillings? This is also the most difficult decision confronting your dentist or physician. There is no scientific evidence that provides a definitive answer to the question. Consequently, there are differing views.

One view is that mercury amalgam fillings should not be replaced during pregnancy because of the potential temporary increased mercury body burden that might result. This might increase the potential of toxic effects occurring to the embryo or fetus. Therefore, as has been stated as the position of the Swedish government, comprehensive amalgam work on pregnant women should not be performed. In effect, only dental care deemed absolutely essential should be provided, and amalgam is not to be used for any of the work that must be done.

The differing view is that elimination of the mercury source at the outset of pregnancy is the lesser of two evils. This view holds that the continuous release and inhalation of mercury from mercury amalgam dental fillings for the entire term of the pregnancy and nursing can present a greater hazard to the mother, fetus, and child, than the amount of exposure resulting from replacement.

As you can easily see, it is not an easy decision or one that can be taken lightly. Sadly, there is no scientific data upon which to make a decision. No studies have ever been done to determine what the potential body burdens of mercury are that would accrue from replacement done at the beginning of pregnancy compared to calculations of total mercury accrual during the nine months of pregnancy and approximately nine months of nursing.

There is, however, some scientific data that weighs heavily on the decision process. These were brought out in the chapter on birth defects and relate to the critical periods of development during the reproductive cycle. It would appear from the data available that any additional unnecessary mercury exposure during these critical periods of embryonic or fetal growth could have devastating results.

Consequently, we share the position taken by the Swedish government and the World Health Organization that mercury exposure during pregnancy should be avoided. Within that frame of reference, and until scientific research is available to the contrary, we believe that dental work during pregnancy should be confined to only that which is absolutely essential.

Having taken that position does not mean that there is nothing further to be done about the mercury problem. Quite the contrary should be the rule, as every effort should be made to reduce or control you mercury body burden during pregnancy. As discussed previously, stop chewing gum, eat a diet rich in sulfur-containing foods, discuss with your physician which supplements you can take and in what quantities, and finally, if acceptable with your physician, take periodic steam baths or saunas. The reason for taking steam baths or saunas is to induce sweating. Sweat is one of the body's mechanisms for getting rid of toxins including some heavy metals. In fact, induced sweating is the therapeutic regime used to detoxify workers employed at the mercury mines in Spain who have suffered excessive exposure.

WHAT TO DO IF PLANNING A FAMILY

What actions should be taken if you are planning a pregnancy? Here we feel the decision is much simpler, assuming that you have made the decision to have your mercury amalgam dental fillings replaced. Based on the scientific data available, we would recommend that amalgam replacement for both the husband and wife should be completed six months prior to attempting conception. The six-month period following final amalgam replacement will permit your body burden of mercury to reduce and for your body chemistry to rebalance or adjust.

A question we frequently get asked concerns supplementation programs prior to as well as after amalgam replacement. To help your body in detoxifying or reducing any existing body burden of mercury and to also assist you in coping with any additional exposure that might result from amalgam removal, the following regimen provides the nutrients that, based on the scientific literature, may be of help.

PRE-AMALGAM REPLACEMENT

1. Glutathione. One 50-milligram tablet 1 hour before lunch and 1 hour before supper.

2. Cysteine. One 500-milligram capsule 1 hour before lunch.

3. Vitamin C. One 500-milligram tablet with each meal.

4. Zinc. One 15-30-milligram tablet after supper.

5. Selenium. One 50-microgram tablet (or liquid equivalent of sodium selenite) taken with each meal.

6. Vitamin B$_1$. One 50-milligram tablet with each meal.

7. B Complex. Should provide 15-25-milligrams of each of the various B vitamins. Take the number of tablets indicated to provide the desired amounts.

8. Magnesium. One tablet per day providing 100-milligrams of elemental magnesium. May be taken at bed time.

9. Acidophilus capsules, powder, or liquid. Take before going to bed and upon awakening. May also be taken between meals.

SPECIAL NOTE: As indicated earlier under the supplementation section of this chapter, if you have not been taking vitamin supplements, it is important that you phase slowly into the program, giving your body a chance to adjust and balance to the changes.

POST-AMALGAM REPLACEMENT

If after amalgam replacement you are not experiencing any problems, no change in supplementation is required. However, if there has been a worsening of any existing symptoms or you experience new symptoms, you can make the following changes to the program.

1. Increase the glutathione to three times per day.

2. Increase cysteine to one 500-milligram tablet 1 hour prior to each meal.

3. Increase vitamin C to 1,000-milligrams with each meal and 1,000-milligrams 1 hour after supper.

4. Add pantothenic acid. One 100-milligram tablet with breakfast and supper.

5. Add vitamin E. If you have previously taken vitamin E and experienced no blood pressure changes, then you can supplement with 200 IU capsules. One capsule with each meal. If, however, you have previously experienced adverse reactions with vitamin E, then you should start with the lowest potency available and take no more than 50-100 IU per day for the first 30 days. Discontinue taking vitamin E if at any time you experience adverse effects such as an increase in blood pressure.

Detoxification should be started two weeks before scheduled amalgam removal/replacement and continued throughout the treatment plan. After completion of your dental treatment plan, continue on the detoxification protocols for an additional 30-60 days. You will be the best judge, based on how you are feeling, as to when to reduce, modify, or stop the supplements.

As stated elsewhere in this chapter, detoxification is more than just taking supplements. Dietary and lifestyle modifications are an essential adjunct to supplementation. Give up chewing gum until all the mercury amalgam fillings have been replaced. If possible, weekly sweat therapy should be instituted at the same time as supplementation. Sweat therapy does not mandate steam baths or saunas. Any exercise or activity that causes sweating serves the desired purpose of inducing the excretion of toxins and heavy metals through the skin. Regardless of the modality used, the objective should be to participate in the sweat generating activity for at least 30 minutes per session.

Another important aspect of pregnancy planning deals with when you should stop using the pill. Based on the scientific studies that have been done, it appears that use of the pill should be stopped three months prior to attempting conception. Here again, the elapsed time is required to restore the proper hormonal balance of estrogen and progesterone that is normally affected by the pill. It is interesting to note in this regard that mercury has been shown to stimulate the release of progesterone.(178) Therefore, if you are undergoing amalgam replacement, it may also be wise to stop using the pill prior to completion of the dental treatment plan (substituting some other form of birth control, if needed). Stopping the intake of exogenous hormones during the detoxification program should be beneficial and assist in the primary goal of reducing body burdens of mercury and lead.

DENTAL OFFICE PROTOCOLS

The last point we would like to make concerns the proper protocols for the removal of mercury amalgam dental fillings.

There are special techniques utilized by your dentist to remove mercury amalgam fillings. If done properly, there is minimum exposure to increased levels of mercury vapor caused by the removal procedure. However, we feel it important that you should be aware of certain aspects related to removing mercury from the oral environment:

***The office and operatory should be well-ventilated.

***The dentist should have an assistant present to assist in minimizing their exposure and yours to any mercury vapor. The correct protocol requires the use of high volumes of cold water both from the drill and separate irrigation by the assistant, who should also be simultaneously using high volume suction evacuation of the vapor and particles resulting from the removal procedure.

***It is the volatility of mercury that necessitates all the precautions and correct techniques. Mercury vapor pressure doubles with every ten degree centigrade rise in temperature. One acceptable procedure that minimizes extensive grinding (which generates great temperature increases) involves sectioning the amalgam into chunks versus just grinding it out.

***In some dental offices the dentist may ask you to breathe through a nose piece that will permit you to draw air from another area of the operatory or office. If the dentist has nitrous oxide/oxygen available and you have elected to use it, this will accomplish the same thing.

***During the procedure, the dentist and his assistant are at greater risk to mercury vapor exposure than the patient. To protect themselves, they will probably put on special mercury trapping masks and rubber gloves to protect them during repeated removal operations.

Unless your physician or dentist has deemed it absolutely essential and critical to a diagnosis, do not permit x-rays of any kind to be taken during pregnancy. There is substantial scientific documentation demonstrating the toxic maternal and fetal effects from extremely low-dose radiation.(476,477)

LET YOUR VOICE BE HEARD

In democratic societies throughout the world, when the voices of the citizenry are raised in angry protest, the politicians and government usually respond in direct proportion to the degree of furor. It is a fact of life, pure and simple. It doesn't matter how long the problem or condition that provoked the people has been treated with benign neglect. When enough people express their concern, it is a clarion call to remedial action.

This is a round-about way of saying that dedicated individuals and small groups of health professionals have been vociferously denouncing the use of mercury amalgam as a dental filling material for years without much effect. This protest has essentially fallen on deaf ears. However, be assured that if enough voters protested the continued use of mercury amalgam to their elected state and national representatives, the appropriate responsible government agencies would ban its use tomorrow.

It is on that theme that we end this odyssey on mercury. You, the people, must now speak. Let your voices be heard by your elected representatives, dentists, and physicians. Demand answers as to how the professional associations and governmental agencies involved have permitted mercury, an insidious poison, to be implanted in your body without your knowledge or consent. Demand that the U.S. government ban the use of mercury in dentistry, all pharmaceuticals whether prescription or nonprescription, and its use in cosmetics, without further delay.

Also be assured, just as the sun rises every day, that the mercury amalgam advocates will say, "There isn't a suitable replacement." That statement has the same degree of truth as the one previously uttered for the past 150 years, "Amalgam is safe."

GLOSSARY

-ASE: A word termination (suffix) used in forming the names of enzymes.

ABSORPTION: The uptake of substances into or across tissues; such as the skin, intestine, and kidney tubules.

ALLERGY: A hypersensitive state acquired through exposure to a particular allergen, reexposure resulting in an altered capacity to react.

AMALGAM: An alloy of two or more metals, one of which is mercury.

AMINO (GROUP): A chemical combination of the elements nitrogen and hydrogen in the form of ' NH2', It is a very important biological substance. The prefix 'amino' indicates the presence of the group in a molecule or compound.

AMINO ACIDS: Chemical molecules that are the building blocks of proteins, which are the major constituents of the body's cells, enzymes and hormones. The chemical elements that make up amino acids are carbon (C), hydrogen (H), oxygen (O), nitrogen (N), and sometimes sulfur (S). An amino acid is a compound that contains an amino group (-NH2) and a carboxyl group (-COOH).

AMNION: The thin but tough extraembryonic membrane that lines the chorion and contains the fetus and the **AMNIOTIC FLUID** around it.

AMP, ADP, ATP: Adenosine monophosphate (AMP), adenosine diphosphate (ADP), and adenosine triphosphate (ATP). An important series of organic compounds occurring in all cells with the function of storage and utilization of energy for cell functions. This is accomplished with the loss or gain of phosphate groups, hence the designating tri-(three), di-(two), and mono-(one) phosphate names.

ANALOGUE: 1. A part or organ having the same function as another, but of a different evolutionary origin. 2. A chemical compound with a structure similar to that of another but differing from it in respect to a certain component; it may have a similar or opposite action metabolically.

ANOVULATION: Absence of the discharge of an egg cell (ovum) from the follicle of the ovary.

ANTAGONISM: Opposition or contrariety between similar things, as between muscles, medicines, or organisms.

ANTIOXIDANT: One of many important natural or synthetic substances that prevent damage from the action of oxidation. Important biochemical antioxidants include vitamin E, vitamin C, and the enzymes glutathione peroxidase (GSH-Px) and superoxide dismutase (SOD).

ATAXIA: Failure of muscular coordination; irregularity of muscular action.

BILE: A fluid secreted by the liver and poured into the small intestine via the bile ducts. Important constituents are bile salts, cholesterol, bilirubin and electrolytes.

BILIARY: Pertaining to the bile (see definition), to the bile ducts, or to the gall bladder.

BIOAVAILABILITY: The degree to which a drug or other substance becomes available to the target tissue after administration.

BIOSYNTHESIS: The building up of a chemical compound in the physiologic processes of a living organism.

BIVALENT (DIVALENT): Having a valency (combining capability) of two; the ability to replace or combine with two atoms of hydrogen or its equivalent.

CARBOHYDRATE: An organic compound which is a derivative of certain organic alcohols. They are so named because the hydrogen and oxygen are usually in the proportion to form water

(CH_2O). The most important carbohydrates are the sugars, starches, celluloses, and gums.

CATALYST: Any substance that increases the speed of a chemical reaction or process that is not consumed in the net chemical reaction or process.

CHELATE: To combine with a metal in complexes in which the metal is part of a ring. By extension, a chemical compound in which a metallic ion is sequestered and firmly bound into a ring within the chelating molecule. Chelates are used in chemotherapeutic treatments for metal poisoning.

CHELATION: Combination with a metal in complexes in which the metal is part of a ring.

CHOREA: The ceaseless occurrence of a wide variety of rapid, highly complex, jerky movements that appear be to well coordinated but are performed involuntarily.

CNS: Central nervous system. Consists of the brain and spinal cord.

COENZYME: An organic molecule, usually containing phosphorus and some vitamin, and sometimes separable from the enzyme protein. A coenzyme and an apoenzyme must unite to establish a functional enzyme (holoenzyme).

CORROSION: The action, process, or effect of corroding. A product of corroding. (To corrode is to wear away gradually usually by chemical action.)

COVALENT: The combining of an element with carbon by the sharing of electrons.

CYTOTOXIN: A toxin or antibody that has a specific toxic action upon cells of special organs. They are named according to the special variety of cell for which they are specific; for example, 'nephrotoxin' for kidney cells.

DENTAL AMALGAM (SILVER AMALGAM, "MERCURY AMALGAM"): A material used for filling cavities in teeth consisting of mercury, silver, and tin, with lower concentrations of copper and sometimes zinc. The mercury content of dental amalgam fillings is 43% - 55% when initially placed. The average dental amalgam filling initially contains approximately 780 milligrams of mercury and a like amount of the other metals.

DISULFIDE: A compound containing two attached atoms of sulfur (-S-S-).

DIURETIC: 1. Increasing the secretion of urine. 2. An agent that promotes the secretion of urine.

DYSARTHRIA: Imperfect articulation of speech due to disturbances of muscular control which result from damage to the central or peripheral nervous system.

DYSPNEA: Difficult or labored breathing.

EMBRYO: In humans, the period of development from about two weeks after fertilization to the end of the seventh or eight week.

ENDOGENOUS: 1. Growing from within. 2. Developing or originating within the organism, or arising from causes within the organism.

ENDOMETRIOSIS: A condition in which tissue more or less perfectly resembling the mucous membrane of the uterus (the endometrium) occurs aberrantly in various locations in the pelvic cavity.

ENZYME: A protein, capable of accelerating or producing by catalytic action some change in a substrate for which it is often specific.

EPIDEMIOLOGY: 1. The study of the relationships of the various factors determining the frequency and distribution of diseases in a human community. 2. The field of medicine concerned with the determination of the specific causes of localized outbreaks of infection, or toxic disorders, or any other disease of recognized etiology.

ERYTHROCYTE: Red blood cell.

ESTRUS: The recurrent, restricted period of sexual receptivity in female mammals other than human females.

ETIOLOGY: The study or theory of the factors that cause disease and the method of their introduction to the host; the sum of knowledge regarding causes.

EXOGENOUS: Growing by additions to the outside; developed or originating outside the organism.

EXTRACELLULAR: Outside a cell or cells.

EX VIVO: Outside of the living body.

FETUS: The unborn offspring in the postembryonic period, after major structures have been outlined. In humans, from seven or eight weeks after fertilization until birth.

FREE RADICAL: A group of atoms acting as a unit with an unpaired electron, therefore being very reactive chemically. They have a great potential for interfering with normal body chemical reactions.

GESTATION: The period of development from the time of fertilization of the egg until birth, in animals that bear living young.

GLUCOSE (DEXTROSE): A simple carbohydrate occurring in normal blood and certain foods, especially fruits. It is a principal source of energy for living organisms.

GLUCOSE -6- PHOSPHATASE: An enzyme that is essential for the active transport of glucose (body sugar) into body cells for use as energy for cell functions. It is responsible for forming Glucose -6- Phosphate.

GLUCOSE -6- PHOSPHATE: A chemical compound important in carbohydrate metabolism, which is the principal pathway for energy in humans.

GLUTATHIONE: A tripeptide composed of three amino acids--glutamic acid, cysteine, and aminoacetic acid, and found in animal and plant tissues. It is an important coenzyme, forming several key enzymes, and acts as a respiratory carrier of oxygen.

GRAM (gm): The basic unit of weight (mass) of the metric system. One gram is the equivalent of 15.432 grains, 0.035 ounces.

1 kilogram (kg)=1000 grams (gm)

1 gram　　　　=1000 milligrams (mg)

1 milligram　　=1000 micrograms (mcg)

1 microgram　　=1000 nanograms (ng)

GSH: Reduced glutathione; a tripeptide present in red blood cells. If deficient, the red blood cells are more susceptible to the harmful oxidizing and hemolytic effects of certain drugs. GSH works in association with glucose -6- phosphate dehydrogenase (G-6-PD) and reduced nicotinamide-adenine dinucleotide phosphate (NADPH) in maintaining the integrity of red blood cells.

GSSG: Oxidized glutathione, the precursor of the important reduced glutathione (GSH).

HEMATOLOGY (-ical): That branch of medical science dealing with the blood and blood-forming tissues.

HEMATOPOIETIC: 1. Pertaining to or affecting the formation of blood cells. 2. An agent that promotes the formation of blood cells.

HEMOLYSIS: The separation of hemoglobin from the red blood cells, with the appearance of the hemoglobin in the blood plasma. It may be caused by chemicals, by freezing or heating, or by distilled water.

HISTOCHEMICAL: The identification of chemical components in cells and tissues.

HOMEOSTASIS: A tendency to stability in the normal body states (internal environment) of the organism.

HORMONE: A chemical substance, produced in the body by an organ or cells of an organ, which has a specific regulatory effect on the activity of a certain organ.

HYDROLYSIS: The splitting of a compound into fragments by the addition of water (HOH), the hydroxyl (-OH) group being incorporated in one fragment and the hydrogen atom (H-) in the other.

HYPERPLASIA: The abnormal multiplication or increase in the number of normal cells in normal arrangement in a tissue.

HYPERSENSITIVITY: A state of altered reactivity in which the body reacts with an exaggerated response to a foreign agent. Hypersensitivity reactions are pathologic processes induced by immune responses and may be immediate or delayed.

HYPERTROPHY: The enlargement or overgrowth of an organ or part due to an increase in the size of its cells.

HYPOXIA: Low oxygen content or tension. A deficiency of oxygen.

ION: An atom or a group of atoms having an electrical charge of positive (cation) or negative (anion), and therefore very active chemically.

INTRACELLULAR: Situated or occurring within a cell or cells.

IN VITRO: Within a glass; observable in a test tube; in an artificial environment.

IN VIVO: Within the living body.

LACTATION: 1. The secretion of milk. 2. The period of the secretion of milk. 3. Suckling.

LATENCY: A state of seeming inactivity, as that occurring between the instant of stimulation and the beginning of response. Concealed; not manifest; potential.

LEUKOCYTE (LEUCOCYTE): White blood cell or corpuscle. The varieties of leukocytes may be classified into two main groups:

> ***Granular Leukocytes*** - Neutrophils (polymorphonuclear leukocyte, or PMN); eosinophils, basophils.
> ***Nongranular Leukocytes*** - Lymphocytes, monocytes.

LEUKOPENIA: A decrease in the number of white blood cells in the blood.

LIGAND: An organic molecule that donates the necessary electrons to combine with metallic ions. (Therefore, a molecule in the body that easily combines with metals.)

LIPID (FAT): Any of a group of organic substances which are not soluble in water, but soluble in alcohol, ether, chloroform, and other fat solvents and which have a greasy feel. The lipids, which are easily stored in the body, serve as a source of fuel and are an important constituent of cell structure.

MEIOSIS: A special method of cell division occurring in maturation of sex cells. Each daughter cell receives one half the number of chromosomes characteristic of the body cells of the species.

MERCAPTAN: Any chemical compound containing the sulfur-hydrogen (sulfhydryl, thiol) combination bound to a carbon atom.

MERCAPTIDE: A compound derived from a mercaptan, with a metal replacing the sulfur-hydrogen radical.

MERCURIAL: 1. Pertaining to mercury.   2. A preparation of mercury.

MERCURY (QUICKSILVER): A silvery colored metallic element that is liquid at ordinary temperatures and readily evaporates to a vapor form. Its symbol is Hg (from hydrargyrum); atomic number is 80; atomic weight is 200.59. Mercurials are absorbed by the skin and mucous membranes, causing chronic mercury poisoning. Because of toxicity, the use of mercurials is diminishing. Mercury may exist in element form, as inorganic compounds, or as organic compounds.

> *Elemental Mercury* - Metallic mercury, vapor, ions.
> *Inorganic Mercury* - Combined with other elements, such as chlorine, oxygen, etc., or body tissue groups (ligands) as monovalent mercurous or divalent mercuric compounds.
> *Organic Mercury* - Formed by covalent bonds with the carbon atoms of organic compounds.

MERCURY AMALGAM (DENTAL AMALGAM, SILVER AMALGAM): A term used in this book, and numerous other sources, to be more descriptive of the filling material used to fill cavities in teeth and called "Dental Amalgam" or "Silver Amalgam" by the dental profession. The major constituent (approximately 50%) of the material is mercury, not silver, which averages approximately 33% of the material. (See Dental Amalgam)

METABOLISM: The sum of all the physical and chemical processes by which living organized substance is produced and maintained (anabolism), and also the transformation by which energy is made available for the uses of the organism (catabolism).

MINERAL: A nonorganic homogenous solid substance, usually a constituent of the earth's crust. Some serve essential roles in body functions.

MITOSIS: The process of division of cells by which the body grows and replaces cells. Each of the daughter cells possesses the same number of chromosomes as the parent cell, which is the number characteristic of the body cells of the species.

MOLAR: 1. Containing one gram molecular weight of a dissolved substance per liter of solution. 2. A posterior tooth which is used for grinding food and which acts as a major jaw support in the dental arch.

MONOVALENT (UNIVALENT): Having a valency (combining capability) of one; the ability to replace or combine with one atom of hydrogen or its equivalent.

MORBIDITY: 1. The condition of being diseased. 2. The sick rate; the ratio of sick to well persons in a community.

MORTALITY: 1. The quality of being mortal. 2. The death rate.

MOTILITY: The ability to move spontaneously.

MUCOCUTANEOUS: Pertaining to or affecting the mucous membranes and the skin.

MUTAGENESIS: 1. The production of change. 2. The induction of genetic mutation.

NADP: Nicotinamide Adenine Dinucleotide Phosphate: A coenzyme required for a number of reactions in human metabolism.

NADPH: Nicotinamide Adenine Dinucleotide Phosphate (Reduced): A coenzyme functioning as a carrier of hydrogen atoms and electrons to be used as a source of energy required for chemical reactions in the body. When NADPH loses the hydrogen atom (becomes oxidized), energy is produced and the resulting compound is oxidized NADH.

NATAL: Pertaining to birth. (See definitions - Neonatal, Perinatal, Postnatal, and Prenatal)

NECROSIS: Death of tissue, usually as individual cells, groups of cells, or in small localized areas.

NEONATAL: Pertaining to the first four weeks after birth.

NEURITIS: Inflammation of a nerve; a condition attended by pain and tenderness over the nerves, anesthesia and paresthesia, paralysis, wasting, and disappearance of the reflexes.

NEUROPATHY: A general term denoting functional disturbances and/or pathological changes in the peripheral nervous system.

NEUROTOXIC: Poisonous or destructive to nerve tissue.

OCCLUSAL: Pertaining to closure; applied to the chewing surfaces of the molar and premolar teeth.

ONCOGENESIS: The production or causation of tumors.

OPTIMAL: The best; the most favorable.

ORGANIC:

1. Denoting chemical substances containing carbon.
2.. Pertaining to substances derived from living organisms.
3. Arising from an organism.
4. Having an organized structure.
5. Pertaining to an organ or the organs.

ORGANOGENESIS: The development or growth of organs.

OVULATION: The discharge of an egg cell (ovum) from the follicle of the ovary.

OXIDATION: The act of oxidizing or state of being oxidized. Chemically it consists in the increase of positive charges on an atom or the loss of negative charges. Most biological oxidations are accomplished by the removal of a pair of hydrogen atoms (dehydrogenation) from a molecule. Such oxidations must be accompanied by reduction of an acceptor molecule. *Univalent Oxidation* - Loss of one electron. *Divalent Oxidation* - Loss of two electrons.

PALLIATIVE: 1. Affording relief, but not cure. 2. An alleviating medicine.

PARESTHESIA: An abnormal sensation, such as burning, prickling, crawling sensation.

PATHOGENESIS: The development of morbid conditions or of disease. More specifically, the cellular events and reactions and other pathologic mechanisms occurring in the development of disease.

PEPTIDE: A constituent in the formation of proteins containing two or more amino acids.

PERINATAL: Pertaining to or occurring in the period shortly before and after birth. In medical statistics generally considered to begin with completion of 28 weeks of gestation and variously defined as ending one to four weeks after birth.

PEROXIDE: That oxide of any element which contains more oxygen than any other, such as hydrogen peroxide.

PHAGOCYTE: Any cell that ingests microorganisms or other cells and foreign particles.

POISON: Any substance which, when ingested, inhaled or absorbed, or when applied to, injected into, or developed within the body, in relatively small amounts, by its chemical action may cause damage to structure or disturbance of function.

POSTNATAL: Occurring after birth, with reference to the new-born.

POSTPARTUM: After childbirth, or after delivery.

PRENATAL: Existing or occurring before birth; with reference to the fetus.

PROTEIN: Any one of a group of complex organic compounds containing nitrogen, widely distributed in plants and animals. Proteins, which are the principal constituents of the cell protoplasm, are essentially combinations of amino acids.

RADICAL: A group of atoms which enters into and goes out of chemical combinations without change, and which forms one of the fundamental constituents of a molecule.

REDUCTANT: The electron donor in an oxidation - reduction (redox) reaction.

REDUCTION: In chemistry, the addition of hydrogen to a substance, or more generally, the gain of electrons.

REPLICATION: 1. A turning back of a part so as to form a duplication. 2. The repetition of an experiment to ensure accuracy. 3. The process of duplicating or reproducing.

RETROSPECT (-IVE): 1. To refer back. 2. Surveying the past.

SENSITIVITY: The state or quality of being sensitive (able to receive or respond to stimuli); often used to mean a state of abnormal responsiveness to stimulation, or of responding quickly and acutely.

SILVER AMALGAM: (See Dental Amalgam)

SOLUBILITY: Susceptibility of being dissolved.

SPERM/SPERMATOGONIA/SPERMATOCYTE/SPER-MATOZOA: The *spermatogonia* are cells of the male. They originate in the seminal tube and divide into two primary - *spermatocytes*, which then develope into the mature male germ cell - the *spermatozoa* (or simply, the sperm).

SPERMATOGENESIS: The process of formation of sperm.

SPERMICIDAL: Destructive to sperm.

SUBCLINICAL: Without clinical manifestations (readily observable signs or symptoms).

SUBOPTIMAL: Less than the best or most favorable.

SULFHYDRYL (THIOL): The combination of sulfur and hydrogen together (-SH).

SYNERGISM: The joint action of agents so that their combined effect is greater than the algebraic sum of their individual effects.

TERATOGEN: An agent or factor that causes the production of physical defects in the developing embryo.

THIOL (SULFHYDRYL): Any organic compound containing the -SH group (combination of sulfur and hydrogen).

TOXIC: Pertaining to, due to, or of the nature of a poison.

TOXIN: A poison; frequently used to refer specifically to a protein produced by some higher plants, certain animals, and pathogenic bacteria, which is highly toxic for other living organisms.

TRIPEPTIDE: A constituent of proteins that contains three amino acids.

VALENCE: The numerical measure of the capacity to combine. In chemistry, it is an expression of the number of atoms of hydrogen (or its equivalent) which one atom of a chemical element can hold in combination, if negative, or displace in a reaction, if positive. Substances may be monovalent (univalent), bivalent (divalent), or covalent. (See definitions)

VITAMIN: A general term for a number of unrelated organic substances that occur in many foods in small amounts and that are necessary for the normal metabolic functioning of the body. They may be water-soluble (B-complex, C) or fat soluble (A,D,E,K).

XENOBIOTIC: A chemical foreign to the biologic system.

APPENDIX 2

NIDR/ADA WORKSHOP RECOMMENDATIONS

Workshop on Biocompatibility of Metals in Dentistry
National Institute of Dental Research/American Dental
Association July 11-13, 1984

RECOMMENDATIONS FOR FUTURE RESEARCH

Diagnostic and analytical procedures should be investigated for documenting exposure to metals in alloys.

An evaluation should be made of nickel salts or other nickel compounds which may be formed during the fabrication and use of base-metal alloys.

Investigate the role of nickel, beryllium and chromium as potential carcinogens in dental laboratory technicians.

An assessment should be made of mercury loss from chewing on dental amalgams of different alloy compositions.

Studies should be initiated to determine whether methyl mercury can be formed in vivo.

Epidemiologic studies should be initiated to assess the prevalence of mercury allergy in the United States population.

Biological sampling procedures should be investigated to determine a reliable means of estimating body burden of mercury.

Studies should be initiated to accurately assess blood levels of mercury which may result from dental amalgam.

Research should be initiated to determine whether the effects of mercury on T-lymphocytes may be a means of early detection of sub-clinical manifestations of mercury toxicity.

Studies should be initiated to develop more definitive tests for determining the hypersensitivity to metals used in dentistry.

Studies should examine the potential that thyroid gland enlargement may be an early predictor of mercury intoxication.

Studies are encouraged to determine whether a relationship exists between maternal exposure to mercury and teratogenesis.

The effects of conditions which accelerate corrosion of dental materials on the release of metal ions should be studied in more detail.

The composition of corrosion products should be identified as well as the effect they may have on oral tissues.

Continued research is recommended on the development of alternative restorative materials.

RECOMMENDATIONS FOR CLINICAL IMPLEMENTATION

There is a need by dentists and physicians to recognize nickel as a common allergen.

Manufacturers, laboratories and dentists should be encouraged to identify alloys used in the fabrication of prosthetic devices in terms of contents which may affect a patient's health (nickel, chromium, cobalt, etc.).

Dentists and administrators of dental laboratories should be encouraged to inform employees who work as technicians regarding the need to avoid inhalation exposure to dusts from alloys.

Practitioners are encouraged to document in patient records content of alloys used in restorative materials.

Health histories should include documentation of individuals sensitive to metals.

Patch testing for sensitivity to metals is the responsibility of professionals trained in the administration and interpretation of the tests.

Practitioners are encouraged to become familiar with the symptoms of metal exposure.

Practitioners are encouraged to report case histories of adverse reactions to or effects from biomaterials to the American Dental Association.

DIRECTORY OF ORGANIZATIONS

American Academy of Biological Dentistry
P.O. Box 856
Carmel Valley, CA 93924
(1)

National Center for Homeopathy
1500 Massachusetts Ave. N.W.
Washington, D.C. 20005
(1) (2)

International Academy of Preventive Medicine
P.O. Box 5832
Lincoln, NE 68505
(1) (2)

International College of Applied Nutrition
(Referral Service)
312 E Las Tunas Dr.
San Gabriel, CA 91776
(1) (2)

American Academy of Environmental Medicine
P.O. Box 16106
Denver, CO 80216
(2)

American Holistic Medical Association
2727 Fairview East #G
Seattle, WA 98102
(2)

American College of Advancement in Medicine
23121 Verbugo Dr., Suite 204
Laguna Hills, CA 92653
714-583-7666
(3)

Bio-Probe, Inc.
P.O. Box 580160
Orlando, FL 32858-0160
(1)

Dr. Jerry Mittelman,
263 West End Ave., #2A
New York, NY 10023
(1)

International Academy of Oral Medicine and Toxicology
P.O. Box 458
Ortonville, MI 48462
(1) (2) United States and Canada

(1) May be able to provide the name of a dentist in your area who is familiar with the mercury amalgam toxicity issue and the correct protocols for replacement.

(2) May be able to provide the name of a physician in your area who is knowledgeable about mercury and other toxic metals.

(3) May be able to provide the name of a physician in your area who has certified skills in chelation therapy.

OTHER MATERIAL AVAILABLE FROM BIO-PROBE

BOOKS

Silver Dental Fillings - The Toxic Time Bomb by Sam Ziff covers the history of the amalgam controversy from 1819 to the present time. Fully referenced, 197 pages, ISBN: 0-943358-24-8. Price $10.95 each plus $1.50 postage and handling. Canadian orders $2.50 for postage and handling.

Mercury Poisoning from Dental Amalgam - A Hazard to Human Brain by Patrick Störtebecker, M.D., Ph.D. Formerly Assoicate Professor of Neurology, Karolinska Institute, Stockholm, Sweden. Dr. Störtebecker describes his "Priniciple of The Shortest Pathway" with scientific evidence that mercury vapor released from amalgam fillings can be transported directly to the brain through the valveless venous system and from the mucous membranes of the nasal cavity along the olfactory nerves to the brain. Fully referenced, 213 pages. ISBN: 0-941011-01-1. Price $20.00 each plus $1.50 postage and handling. Canadian orders $2.50 for postage and handling.

Dental Caries As A Cause of Nervous Disorders - Epilepsy - Schizophrenia - Multiple Sclerosis - Brain Cancer. Additional notes on Myasthenia Gravis - High Blood Pressure by Patrick Störtebecker, M.D., Ph.D. Fully referenced, 235 pages. Price $20.00 plus $1.50 postage and handling. Canadian orders $2.50 postage and handling.

The Hazards of Silver/Mercury Dental Fillings by Sam Ziff and Michael F. Ziff, D.D.S. An educational booklet on the release of mercury vapor from amalgam dental fillings. Provides an overview of the entire mercury/amalgam issue as well as a complete list of symptoms that can be caused by mercury vapor toxicity. Fully referenced, 32 pages. Price $1.95 plus 50 cents postage and handling.

NEWSLETTER

The Bio-Probe Newsletter is published bi-monthly. The easy way for the professional to stay abreast of the current scientific research related to the mercury/amalgam issue and the use of other heavy metals in the mouth; their potential toxicity and nutritional impact. One year subscription $65.00.

AUDIO TAPES

Dental Amalgam Toxicity - Fact or Fiction? Six audio tape cassettes of a seminar that provides an accurate in-depth scientific treatment of the entire mercury/amalgam controversy. The seminar speakers were Dr. Murray J. Vimy, D.M.D., F.A.G.D., President of the International Academy of Oral Medicine and Toxicology and Michael F. Ziff, D.D.S., Vice President of the International Academy of Oral Medicine and Toxicology. Price $49.00 for the six tape set including postage.

TO ORDER, SEND CHECK OR MONEY ORDER IN U.S. FUNDS TO:

BIO-PROBE, INC.

P.O. BOX 580160

ORLANDO, FL 32858-0160

REFERENCES

1. Stock A. The hazards of mercury vapor and amalgam. Zeitschrift fur angewandte Chemie. 39:984-989, 1926.

2. Trakhtenberg I.M. Chronic effects of mercury on organisms. USDHEW Public Health Service, NIH. DHEW Pub No. (NIH) 74-473, USGPO, Wash D.C., 1974.

3. Phillips R.W. and Swartz M.L. Mercury analysis of one hundred amalgam restorations. J Dent Res. 28:569-572, 1949.

4. Radics J, Schwander H., and Gasser F. Die kristallinen komponenten der silberamalgam- unterschungen mit der electonischen roentgenmikrosonde. Zahnartzl Welt. 79:1031-1036, 1970.

5. Vimy M.J. and Lorscheider F.L. Intra-oral air mercury released from dental amalgam. J Dent Res. 64(8):1069-1071, 1985a.

6. Vimy M.J. and Lorscheider F.L. Serial measurements of intra-oral air mercury: Estimation of daily dose from dental amalgam. J Dent Res. 64:1072-1075, 1985b.

7. Skare, I. Mercury exposure from amalgam. A background study. Presentation of the Swedish National Board of Occupational Safety and Health at the August 1987 Scandanavian Hygiene meeting held in Iceland.

8. Sugita M. The biological half-time of heavy metals. The existance of a third, "slowest" component. Int Arch Occup Health. 41:25-40, 1978.

9. Newton D. and Fry F.A. The retention and distribution of radioactive mercuric oxide following accidental inhalation. Ann Occup Hyg. 21:21-32, 1978.

10. Bernard S.R. and Purdue P. Metabolic models for methyl and inorganic mercury. Health Phys. 46(3):695-699, 1984.

11. Vimy M.J., Luft A.J. and Lorscheider F.L. Estimation of mercury body burden from dental amalgam: Computer simulation of a metabolic compartment model. J Dent Res. 65(12):1415-1419, Dec 1986.

12. Dumanoski, D. The Boston Globe. July 15, 1985.

13. Lehninger A.L. Principles of Biochemistry. page 54. Worth Publishers Inc., NY, 1982.

14. Socialstyrelsen (Swedish National Welfare and Health Administration) Expert Commission. Svenska Dagbladet. May 22, 1987.

15. Goldwater L.J. Mercury: A History of Quicksilver. York Press, Baltimore, 1972.

16. Stortebecker P. Mercury Poisoning from Dental Amalgam - A Hazard to Human Brain. Stortebecker Foundation for Research, Stockholm, Sweden, 1985 and Bio-Probe Inc. Orlando, FL, 1986.

17. Stock A. and Cucuel F. Die verbreitung des quecksilbers. Naturwissenschaften 22/24:390-393, 1934.

18. EPA. Mercury Health Effects Update Health Issue Assessment. Final Report. (1984) EPA-600/8-84-019F. United States Environmental Protection Agency, Office of Health and Environmental Assessment. Washington D.C. 20460.

19. Billings C.E. and Matson W.R. (1972) Mercury emission from coal. Combustion Science. 176:1232.

20. Berlin M. In: Handbook on the Toxicology of Metals. Editors Friberg L., Nordberg G.F. and Vouk V.B. Chapter 30:503-525. Elsevier/North Holland Biomedical Press, 1979.

21. Friberg L.T. (Chairman) Maximum allowable concentrations of mercury compounds. Report of an International Committee. Arch Environ Health. 19:891-905, 1969.

22. Klassen C.D. Heavy metals and heavy-metal antagonists. Chapter 69, pp 1615-1637. In, Goodman and Gillman's. The Pharmacological Basis of Therapeutics. (6th edition) Macmillan Publishing Co. NY, page 1623, 1980.

23. DeBout B., Lauwreys R., Govaerts H., and Moulin D. Yellow mercuric oxide ointment and mercury intoxication. Eur J Pediatr. 145(3):217-218, 1986.

24. Bakir F. et al. and Clarkson T.W. et al. Methylmercury poisoning in Iraq. An interuniversity report. Science. 181:230-241, 1973.

25. Mercury toxicity in ear irrigation. FDA Drug Bulletin 13(1), 1983.

26. McAlpine D. and Shukure A. Minimata disease. An unusual neurological disorder caused by contaminated fish. Lancet. 2:629-631, 1958.

27. Nordberg G.F., Editor. Factors Influencing Metabolism and Toxicity of Metals. A Consensus Report by The Task Group on Metal Interaction. Environ Heath Perspect. 25:3-41, 1978.

28. Kling L.J. and Soares J.H., Jr. The effect of mercury and vitamin E on the tissue glutathione peroxidase activity and thiobarbituric acid values. Poultry Sci. 61(8):1762-1765, 1978.

29 . Nelson N. (Chairman) Expert committee: Hazards of Mercury. Special report to the secretary's pesticide advisory committee. Dept of Health Education and Welfare. Environ Res. 4:1-69, 1971.

30. Podrebarac D.S. Pesticide, metal and other chemical residues in adult diet samples.(XIV). October 1977 - September 1978. J Assoc Off Anal Chem. 67(1):176-185, 1984.

31. Podrebarac D.S. Pesticide, heavy metal, and other chemical residues in infant and toddler Total Diet Samples. (IV). October 1977 - September 1978. J Assoc Off Anal Chem. 67(1):167-175, 1984.

32. Johnson R.D. et al. Pesticide, heavy metal and other chemical residues in infant and toddler Total Diet Samples. (III). August 1976-September 1977. J Assoc Off Anal Chem. 67(1):145-154, 1984.

33. Johnson R.D. et al. Pesticide, metal, and other chemical residues in adult Total Diet Samples. (XIII). August 1976-September 1977. J Assoc Off Anal Chem. 67(1):154-166, 1984.

34. Buchet J.P. et al. Oral daily intake of cadmium, lead, manganese, copper, chromium, mercury, calcium, zinc and arsenic in Belgium: A duplicate meal study. Fd Chem Toxic. 21(1):19-24, 1983.

35. Mykkanen H. et al. Dietary intakes of mercury, lead, cadmium and arsenic. Hum Nutr Appl Nutr. 40(1):32-39, 1986.

36. Johnson P.E. and Shuber L.E. Accumulation of mercury and other elements by Spirulina (Cyanophyceal). Nutr Reports Intl. 34(6):1063-1070, 1986.

37. Schreiber W. Mercury content of fishery products: Data from the last decade. Sci Total Environ. 31(3):283-300, 1983.

38. ADA News. Jan 2, 1984. Editorial and accompanying patient handout on the safety of dental amalgam.

39. ADA patient pamphlet #W186. Dental Amalgam. Filling Dental Health Care Needs. 1985.

40. Gay D.D., Cox R.D., and Reinhardt J.W. Letter: Chewing releases mercury from fillings. Lancet. 1(8123):985-986, 1979.

41. Svare C.W. et al. The effect of dental amalgams on mercury levels in expired air. J Dent Res. 60:1668-1671, 1981.

42. Emler B.F. and Cardone M. Sr. An assessment of mercury in mouth air. J Dent Res. 64:247, Abstract #652, 1985.

43. Patterson J.E., Weissberg B.G. and Dennison P.J. Mercury in human breath from dental amalgams. Bull Environ Contam Toxicol. 34:459-468, 1985.

44. Stock A. The chronic mercury and amalgam poisoning. Geiverbehyg 7:388-413, 1936.

45. Bio-Probe Newsletter, 4(4), September 1987.

46. Störtebecker, P. Dental Infectious Foci and Diseases of Nervous System. Acta Psych Neurol Scan, 36(suppl 157):62, 1961.

47. Störtebecker, P. Dental Caries as a Cause of Nervous Disorders. Störtebecker Foundation for Research, Stockholm, Sweden, 1982.

48. Fredin B. Studies on the mercury release from dental amalgam fillings. Personal communication (1985).

49. Chang L.W. Neurotoxic effects of mercury - A review. Environ Res. 14:329-373, 1977.

50. Clarkson T.W. The pharmacology of mercury compounds. Ann Rev Pharmacol 12:375-406, 1972.

51. Environmental Protection Agency. Reducing lead in drinking water. A benefit analysis. EPA 230/9-85-019, Washington D.C., 1986.

52. McClintic J.R. Physiology Of The Human Body. John Wiley & Sons, Inc. New York, 1975.

53. Spector R. Cerebrospinal fluid folate and the blood-brain barrier. Chapter 21, pp 187-194. In, Folic Acid in Neurology, Psychiatry, and Internal Medicine. Boetz M.E. and Reynold E.H., Editors. Raven Press, NY. 1979.

54. Berlin M., Jerksell G. and von Ubisch H. Uptake and retention of mercury in the mouse brain. Arch Environ Health. 12:33-42, 1966.

55. Magos L. Mercury-blood interaction and mercury uptake by the brain after vapor exposure. Environ Res. 1:323-337, 1967.

56. Cutright E.E., Miller R.A., Battistone G.C. and Millikan L.J. Systemic mercury level caused by inhaling mist during high-speed grinding. J Oral Med. 28(4):100-104, 1973.

57. Magos L. Uptake of mercury by the brain. Br J Ind Med. 25:315-318, 1968.

58. Clarkson T.W., Magos L. and Greenwood M. The transport of elemental mercury into fetal tissues. Biol Neonate. 21:239-244, 1972.

59. Stock A. The effects of mercury vapor on the upper airways. Naturwissenschaften. 23:453-456, 1935.

60. Friberg L. and Vostal J. Mercury in the Environment - An Epidemiological and Toxicological Appraisal. pp 109-112, CRC Press. Cleveland, 1972.

61. Gerstner H.B. and Huff J.E. Clinical toxiciology of mercury. J Toxicol Environ Health. 2(3):491-526, 1977.

62. Schiele R. et al. Studies on the mercury content in brain and kidney related to number and condition of amalgam fillings. Institute of Occupational and Social Medicine. University of Erlangen-Nurnberg. Symposium March 12, 1984, Cologne, Germany - Viewpoints From Medicine and Dental Medicine.

63. Friberg L., Jullman L., Birger L., and Nylander M. Mercury in the central nervous system in relation to amalgam fillings. Lakartidningen. 83(7):519-521, 1986.

64. Steinwall O. Chemotoxic blood-brain barrier damage with special regard to some mercurial effects. In, Neurotoxicology. Roizin L. et al., Editors. Raven Press, NY. pp 271-274, 1977.

65. Khayat A. and Dencker L. Organ and cellular distribution of inhaled metallic mercury in the rat and Marmoset monkey (Callithrix jacchus): Influence of ethyl alcohol pretreatment. Acta Pharmacol. 55(2):145-152, 1984.

66. Khayat A. and Dencker L. Whole body and liver distribution of inhaled mercury vapor in the mouse: Influence of ethanol and aminotriazole pretreatment. J Appl Toxicol. 3(2):66-73, 1983.

67. Amin-Zaki L. et al. Prenatal methylmercury poisoning. Am J Dis Child. 133:172-177, 1979.

68. Report of an International Committee. Maximum Allowable Conentrations of Mercury Compounds (MAC Values). Arch Environ Health. 19:891-905, 1969.

69. Ware R.A., Chang L.W. and Burkholder P.M. An ultrastructural study on the blood-brain barrier dysfunction following mercury intoxication. Acta Neuropath (Berlin). 30:211-224, 1974.

70. World Health Organization. Recommended Health-Based Limits in Occupational Exposure to Heavy Metals. Technical Report Series 647, WHO, Geneva, 1980.

71. Mercury: Environmental Health Criteria 1. WHO, Geneva, 1976.

72 . Ferm V.H. and Hanlon D.P. Metal-induced congenital malformations. pages 383-397. Clarkson, Nordberg, Sager Editors in: Reproduction and Developmental Toxicity of Metals. Plenum Press, New York, 1983.

73. Naeye R.L. Do placenta weights have clinical significance? Human Pathology. 18(4):387-391, 1987.

74 . Goodman D.R., Fant M.E. and Harbison R.D. Perturbation of a-Aminoisobutyric acid transport in human placental membranes: Direct effects of $HgCl_2$, Ch_3HgCl, and $CdCl_2$. Teratogen, Carcinogen Mutagen. 3(1):89-100, 1983.

75. Danielsson B.R.G., Dencker L. Khayat A. and Olsen I. Fetotoxicity of in-organic mercury in the mouse: distribution and effects of nutrient uptake by placenta and fetus. Biol Res Preg Perinatal. 5(3):102-109, 1984.

76 . Baglan R.J. et al. Utility of placental tissue as an indicator of trace element exposure to adult and fetus. Environ Res. 8:64-70, 1974.

77. Mansour M.M. et al. Maternal-fetal transfer of organic and inorganic mercury via placenta and milk. Environ Res. 6:479-484, 1973.

78. Karp W.B. and Robertson A.F. Correlation of human placental enzymatic activity with trace metal concentration in placentas from three geographical locations. Environ Res. 13:470-477, 1977.

79 . Lauwerys R. et al. Placental transfer of lead, mercury, cadmium, and carbon monoxide in women. 1. Comparison of the frequency distributions of the biological indices in maternal and umbilical cord blood. Environ Res. 15(2):278-289, 1978.

80. Orlando P. et al. Indagine sulla concentrazione di alcuni micorelementi nel tessuto placentare. G. Ig Med. Prev. 19:68-75, 1978. Italian with English summary.

81. Greenwood M.R., Clarkson T.W. and Magos L. Transfer of metallic mercury into the foetus. Experientia. 28:1455-1456, 1972.

82. Suzuki T. et al. Placental transfer of mercuric chloride, phenyl mercury acetate, and methyl mercury acetate in mice. Ind. Health. 5:149-155, 1967.

83. Garrett N.E., Garrett R.B. and Archdeacon J.W. Placental transmission of mercury to the fetal rat. Toxicol Appl Pharmacol. 22:649-654, 1972.

84. Sasser L.B., Jarboe G.E. and Laprade J. The influence of selenium on the distribution of methyl mercury and mercury chloride in the pregnant rat. In Proceeding of the Fifteenth Annual Hanford Life Science Symposium, Richland Washington, Sept 29 to Oct 1, 1975.

85. Baltrukiewicz Z. Accumulation of mercury in genital organs and fetuses at different periods of pregnancy after intravenous administration of ^{203}Hg-neohydrin. Acta Physiol Pol. 21:645-651, 1970.

86. Kellman B.J. Inorganic mercury movements across the perfused guinea pig placenta in late gestation. Toxicol Appl Pharmacol. 41:659-665, 1977.

87. Satoh H. et al. Effects of sodium selenite on distribution and placental transfer of mercuric mercury in mice of late gestational period. J Pharm Dyn. 4(3):191-196, 1981.

88. Alexiou D. et al. Trace elements (zinc, cobalt, selenium, rubidium, bromine, gold) in human placenta and newborn liver at birth. Pediat Res. 11:646-648, 1977.

89. Windholz M. et al., Editors. In, The Merck Index (9th ed). An Encyclopedia of Chemicals and Drugs. Merck & Co., Inc. Rahway, NJ. Page 8045, 1976.

90. Tsuchiya H., Mitani K., Kodama K. and Nakata T. Placental transfer of heavy metals in normal pregnant Japanese women. Arch Environ Health. 39(1):11-17, 1984.

91. Nakano A. A study on the placental transfer of mercury in pregnant women. Japanese J Hygiene. 40(3):685-694, 1985. Japanese with English summary.

92. Suzuki T. et al. Normal organic and inorganic mercury levels in human feto-placental system. J Appl Toxicol. 4(5):249-252, 1984.

93. Khayat A. and Dencker L. Fetal uptake and distribution of metallic mercury vapor in the mouse: Influence of ethanol and aminotriazole. Int J Biol Res Pregnancy. 3(1):38-46,1982.

94. ADA. Council on Dental Materials, Instruments and Equipment, Council on Dental Therapeutics. Safety of Dental Amalgam. JADA, 106:519-520, 1983.

95. NIDR/ADA Workshop: Biocompatibility of metals in dentistry. JADA. 109(3):469-471, Sept 1984.

96. Djerassi E. and Berova N. The possibilities of allergic reactions from silver amalgam restorations. Int Dent J. 19(4):481-488, 1969.

97. North American Contact Dermatitis Group. Epidemiology of contact dermatitis in North America:1972. Arch Dermatol. 108:537-540, 1973.

98. Brun R. Epidemiology of contact dermatitis in Geneva (1000) cases. Contact Dermatitis. 1(4):214-217, 1975.

99. Nebenfuhrer L. et al. Mercury allergy in Budapest. Contact Dermatitis 10(2):121-122, 1984.

100. Mobacken H. et al. Oral lichen planus: Hypersensitivity to dental restoration material. Contact Dermatitis. 10:11-15, 1984.

101. Miller E.G., Perry W.L., and Wagner M.J. Prevalence of mercury hypersensitivity in dental students. J Dent Res. 64, Special Issue Abstracts, page 338, Abstract #1472, March 1985.

102. Berkow R. (Ed in chief). The Merck Manual of Diagnosis and Therapy. (14th ed), pp 1713-1715. Merck Sharp & Dohme Research Laboratories, Rahway, NJ, 1982.

103. Theofilopoulos A.N. Chapter 13, Autoimmunity. In, Basis & Clinical Immunology. (4th ed). Stites D.P., Stobo J.D., Fundenberg H.H. and Will J.V. (Eds). Lange Medical Publication, Los Altos, CA. 1982.

104. Caron G.A., Poutala S. and Provost T.T. Lymphocyte transformation induced by inorganic and organic mercury. Int Arch Allergy. 37:76-87, 1970.

105. Weening J.J. et al. Mercury induced immune complex glomerulopathy: An experimental study. Chapter 4: pp 36-66. VanDendergen, 1980.

106. Druet P. et al. Immunologically mediated glomerulonephritis induced by heavy metals. Arch Toxicol. 50:187-194, 1982.

107. Druet P. et al. Immune dysregulation and auto-immunity induced by toxic agents. Transplantation Proceedings Vol XIV(3):482-484, 1982.

108. Andres P. IgA-IgG disease in the intestine of Brown-Norway rats ingesting mercuric chloride. Clin Immun Immunopath. 30:488-494, 1984.

109. Robinson C.J.G., Balazs T. and Egorov I.K. Mercuric chloride-, gold sodium thiomalate-, and d-penicillamine-induced antinuclear antibodies in mice. Toxic Appl Pharmac. 86:159-169, 1986.

110. Hirsch F. et al. Autoimmunity induced by $HgCl_2$ in Brown-Norway rats: I. J Immun. 136(9):3272-3276, 1986.

111. Lymberi P. et al. Autoimmunity induced by $HgCl_2$ in Brown-Norway rats: II. J Immun. 136(9):3277-3281, 1986.

112. Pelletier L. et al. Autoreactive T cells in mercury-induced autoimmune disease: in vitro demonstration. J Immunol. 137(8):2548-2554, 1986.

113. Verschaeve L. et al. Genetic damage induced by occupational low mercury exposure. Environ Res. 12:306-316, 1976.

114. Eggleston D.W. Effect of dental amalgam and nickel alloys on T-lymphocytes: Preliminary report. J Prosthet Dent. 51(5):617-623, 1984.

115. Friberg L. Skaraborgs Lans Allehande. October 10, 1986.

116. Hughes W.L. A physiochemical rationale for the biological activity of mercury and its compounds. Ann NY Acad Sci. 65(5):454-460, 1957.

117. Suzuki T., Takemoto T., Shishido S. and Kani K. Mercury in human amniotic fluid. Scand J Work Environ & Health. 3:32-35, 1977.

118. Magos L. Selective atomic-absorption determination of inorganic mercury and methylmercury in undigested biological samples. Analyst 96:847-853, 1971.

119. Burk M., Guiet-Bara A. and Durlach J. Comparison of the effects of taurine and magnesium on electrical characteristics of artificial and natural membranes. V. A study of the human amnion of the antagonism between magnesium, taurine and polluting metals. Magnesium. 4(5-6): 325-332, 1985.

120. Kuntz W.D. et al. Maternal and cord blood background mercury levels: A longitudinal surveillance. Am J Obstet Gynecol. 143(4): 440-443, 1982.

121. Abraham J.E., Svare C.W. and Frank C.W. The effect of dental amalgam restorations on blood mercury levels. J Dent Res. 63(1): 71-73, 1984.

122. Kroncke A. et al. Uber die guecksilberkonzentrationen in blut und urin von personen mit und ohne amalgemfullungen. Dtsch Zahnaerztl Z. 35:803-808, 1980.

123. Ott K. and Kroncke A. Mercury concentrations in blood and urine of patients with or without amalgam fillings. J Dent Res. 60(13):1210, Abstract 48, 1981.

124. Snapp K.R., Svare C.W. and Peterson L.D. Contribution of dental amalgams to blood mercury levels. J Dent Res. 65:311, Abstract #1276, Special Issue March 1986.

125. Olsted M.L., Holland R.I., Wandel N. and Pettersen A.H. Correlation between amalgam restorations and mercury concentration in urine. J Dent Res. 66(6):1179-1182, June 1987.

126. Nylander M. Letter: Mercury in pituitary glands of dentists. Lancet. Feb 8, 1986.

127. Lee I.P. Effects of environmental metals on male reproduction. pp 253-278. Clarkson, Nordberg, Sager Ed's in: Reproduction and Developmental Toxicity of Metals. Plenum Press, NY, 1983.

128. Kruczynski D. and Passia D. The distribution of heavy metals in human ejaculate. A histochemical study. Acta Histochem. 79(2): 187-192, 1986.

129. Skandhan K.P. and Abraham K.C. Presence of several elements in normal and pathological human semen samples and its origin. Andrologia. 16(6):587-588, 1984.

130. Lee I.P. and Dixon R.L. Effects of mercury on spermatogenesis studied by velocity sedimentation cell separation and serial mating. J Pharmacol Exp Ther. 194(1):171-181, 1975.

131. Baker, Ranson and Tynen. A new chemical contraceptive. Lancet.2:882, 1938.

132. Eastman N.J. and Scott A.B. Phenylmercuric acetate as a contraceptive. Human Fert. 9:33-42, 1944.

133. Rotschild, L. A new method of measuring activity of spermatozoa. J Exp Biol. 30:178-199, 1953.

134. Van Duijn C. Jr., Van Voorst C. and Freund M. Movement characteristics of human spermatazoa analysed from kinemicrograph. Eur J Obstet Gynaecol. 4:121-135, 1971.

135. Makler A. A new multiple exposure photography method for objective human spermatozoal motility determination. Fertil Steril. 30:192-199, 1978.

136. Mohamed M.K. et al. Laser light-scattering study of the toxic effects of methylmercury on sperm motility. J Androl. 7(1):11-15, 1986.

137. Sakai K. and Takeuchi T. Biological reaction of tissue cells to alkylmercury. In, Environmental Mercury Contamination, Ann Arbor, MI. Vol 74:280, 1972.

138. Takeuchi T. Biological reaction and pathological changes of human beings and animals under the condition of organic mercury contamination. International Conference on Environmental Mercury Contamination. Ann Arbor, MI, 1970.

139. Ramel C. and Magnusson J. Genetic effects of organic mercury compounds II. Chromosome segregation on Drosophila melanogaster. Hereditias. 61:231-254,1969.

140. Lancranjan I. et al. Reproductive ability of workmen occupationally exposed to lead. Arch Environ Health. 30:396-401, 1975.

141. Behne D. et al. Selenium in testis of the rat: Studies on its regulation and its importance for the organism. J Nutr. 102: 1682-1687, 1982.

142. We S.H. et al. Effect of selenium on reproduction. Proc West Sec Am Soc Anim Sci. 20:85-89, 1969.

143. Behne D., Duk M. and Elger W. Selenium content and glutathione peroxidase activity in the testis of the maturing rat. J Nutr. 116(8):1442-1447, 1986.

144. McFarland R.B. and Reigal H. Chronic mercury poisoning from a single brief exposure. J Occup Med. 20(8):532-534, 1978.

145. Rothstein A. and Hayes A.D. The metabolism of mercury in the rat studied by isotope techniques. J Pharm Exp Ther. 130(2):166-176, 1960.

146. Baranski B. and Scymczyk J. Effects of mercury vapours upon reproductive function on white female rats. Medycyna Pracy. 24(3):249-261, 1973.

147. Lamperti A.A. and Printz R.H. Effects of mercuric chloride on the reproductive cycle of the female hamster. Biol Reprod. 8:373-387, 1973.

148. Lamperti A.A. and Printz R.H. Localization, accumulation and toxic effects of mercuric chloride on the reproductive axis of the female hamster. Biol Reprod. 11:180-186, 1974.

149. Pohl C.R. and Knobil E. The role of the central nervous system in the control of ovarian function in higher primates. Ann Rev Physiol. 44:583-593, 1982.

150. Knobil E. The neuroendocrine control of gonadotropin secretion in the rhesus monkey. Recent Prog Horm Res. 36:53-88, 1980.

151. Mattison D.R.et al. Reproductive and developmental toxicity of metals: female reproductive system, pp 43-91. In: Reproduction and Developmental Toxicity of Metals. Clarkson, Nordberg, Sager Editors. Plenum Press, NY 1983.

152. Smith C.G. Reproductive toxicity: hypothalmic pituitary mechanisms. In, Reproductive Toxicology, D.R. Mattison Editor, pp 107-112, Alan R. Liss. NY. 1983.

153. Mikhailova L.M. et al. The influence of occupational factors on disease of the female reproductive organs. Pediatriya Akusherstvoi Ginekologiya. 33(6):56-58, 1971.

154. Dorland's Illustrated Medical Dictionary, 25th ed, W.B. Saunders, Philadelphia, 1974.

155. Marinova G., Cakarova O. and Kaneva Y. A study on the reproductive function in women working with mercury. Problemi na akuserstvoto i Ginekologiyata. 1:75-77, 1973.

156. Panova Z. and Dimitrov G. Ovarian function in women having professional contact with metallic mercury. Akusherstvoi Ginekologiya. 13(1):29-34, 1974.

157. Goncharuk G.A. Problems relating to occupational hygiene of women in production of mercury. Gigiena Truda i Professional nye Zabolevaniya. 5:17-20, 1977.

158. Yang S. Influence of lead on female reproductive function. Chung Hua Fu Chan Ko Tsa Chih. 21(4):208-210, Jul 1986. (English abstract on page 252)

159. Derobert L. and Tara S. Mercury intoxication in pregnant women. Ann Med Leg. 30:4, 1950.

160. Wiksztrajtis. 1967. Cited in: Baranski B and Szymczyk I. Effects of mercury vapor upon reproductive functions of female white rats. Med Pr. 24:248, 1973.

161. Mishanova V.N., Stepanova P.A. and Zarudio V.V. Characteristics of the course of pregnancy and labor in women coming in contact with low concentrations of metallic mercury vapors in manufacturing work places. Gig Tr Prof Zabol. 2:21-23, 1980.

162. Heidam L.Z. Spontaneous abortions among dental assistants, factory workers, painters, and gardening workers: a follow up study. J Epid Comm Health. 38:149-155, 1984.

163. Gordon H. Pregnancy in female dentists-A mercury hazard. In, Proceedings of International Conference on Mercury Hazards in Dental Practice. Glasgow Scotland, 2-4 Sept. 1981.

164. Brodsky J.G. et al. Occupational exposure to mercury in dentistry and pregnancy outcome. JADA 111:779-780, 1985.

165. Berkow R. (Ed in Chief) The Merck Manual of Diagnosis and Therapy, (14th ed). Merck Sharp & Dohme Research Laboratories, Rahway, NJ, PP 1652-1655, 1982.

166. Simpson J.L. et al. Heritable aspects of endometriosis. I. Genetic studies. Am J Obstet Gynecol. 137:327-331, 1980.

167. Williams R.H (Ed). Textbook of Endocrinology. W.B. Saunders Co., Philadelphia. 1981.

168. Lauersen N. and Stukane E. Listen to Your Body. Berkley Books, NY. 1982. page 134.

169. Dmowski W.P., Steele R.W. and Baker G.F. Deficient cellular immunity in endometriosis. Am J Obstet Gynecol. 141:377-383, 1981.

170. Sogor L. Chapter 58, pp 1-9: Immune aspects of infertility. In, Gynecology and Obstetrics. (Vol 5) Revised edition 1987. Harper & Row, Philadelphia.

171. Theofilopoulos A.N. and Dixon F.J. The biology and detection of immune complexes. Adv Immunol. 28:89, 1979.

172. Witkin S.S. et al. Sperm related antigens, antibodies and circulating immune complexes in sera of recently vasectomized men. J Clin Invest. 70, 1982.

173. Witkin S.S. et al. Detection and characterization of immune complexes and the circulation of infertile women. Fertil Steril. 42:384, 1984.

174. Gleicher N, El-Roeity A., Confino E. and Friber J. Is endometriosis an autoimmune disease? Obstet Gynecol 70:115-122, July 1987.

175. Lesser M. Nutrition and Vitamin Therapy. Grove Press, Inc., NY. pp 69-70, 1980.

176. Stone I. The Healing Factor "Vitamin C" Against Disease. Grosset & Dunlop, New York. Chapter 24-25, 1972.

177. Tarasov Y.A., Sheibak V.M. and Moiseenok A.G. Adrenocortical function under pantothenate deficiency and during administration of this vitamin and its derivatives. Vopr Pitan. 4:54, 1985. (English abstract)

178. Veltman J.C. and Maines M.D. Alterations of heme, cytochrome P-450, and steroid metabolism by mercury in rat adrenal. Arch Biochem Biophys. 248(2):467-478, 1986.

179. Abraham G.E. Management of the premenstrual tension syndromes; rationale for a nutritional approach. In, 1986 A Year in Nutritional Medicine (2nd ed), Bland J. (ed). Keats Publishing, New Canaan, CT. pp 126-166, 1986.

180. Grossman C.J. Interactions between gonadal steroids and the immune system. Science. 227:257-261, 1985.

181. Ewers V. and Erbe R. Effects of lead, cadmium and mercury on brain adenylate cyclase. Toxicology. 16:227-237, 1980.

182. Lehninger A.L. The Principles of Biochemistry. Chapter 25, pp 721-752. Worth Publishers, Inc. NY, 1982.

183. Malamud D., Dietrich S.A. and Shapiro I.M. Low levels of mercury inhibit the respiratory burst in human polymorphonuclear leukocytes. Biochem Biophys Res Comm. 128(3):1145-1151, 1985.

184. Lamney M. and Malamud D. Mercury inhibition of PMN and HL-60 metabolic activity. J Dent Res. Vol 66 (Spec Issue):page 66, Abstract 1706, 1987.

185. Pangborn J.B. Nutritional and inflammatory aspects of amino acids. In, 1984-1985 Yearbook of Nutritional Medicine. Keats Publishing, New Canaan, Ct. pp 153-178, 1985.

186. Murad F. and Haynes R.C., Jr. Chapter 61, estrogens and progestins. In, Goodman and Gillman's. The Pharmacological Basis of Therapeutics. (7th ed). Macmillan Publishing Co., Inc. Ny. 1985.

187. Siiteri P.K. et al. Progesterone and maintenance of pregnancy: Is progesterone nature's immune suppressant? Ann NY Acad Sci. 286:384-397, 1977.

188. Lamperti A. and Niewenhuis R. The effects of mercury on the structure and function of the hypothalamo-pituitary axis in the hamster. Cell Tiss Res. 170:315-324, 1976.

189. Mottet N.K. and Body R.L. Mercury burden of human autopsy organs and tissues. Arch Environ Health. 29:18-24, 1974.

190. Kussmaul A. Mercurialismus un sein verhalniss zur constitutionellen syphilis. Druck und Verlag der Stahel'schen Buck- und Kunsthandling. Wurzburg, Germany 1861.

191. Alfonso J.F. and de Alvarez R.R. Effects of mercury on human gestation. Am J Obstet Gynecol. 80(1):145-154, 1960.

192. Koos B.J. and Longo L.D. Mercury toxicity in the pregnant woman, fetus, and newborn infant. A review. Am J Obstet Gynecol. 126(3):390-409, 1976.

193. Kurland L., Faro S. and Siedler H. Minamata disease. The outbreak of a neurologic disorder in Minamata Japan and its relationship to the ingestion of seafood contaminated by mercury compounds. World Neurol. 1:370-395, 1960.

194. Murakami U. Embryo-fetotoxic effects of some organic mercury compounds. Ann Rep Res Inst Environ Med. Nagoya Univ 19:61-68, 1972.

195. Takeuchi T., Kambara T., and Morikawa N. Pathologic observations of the Minamata disease. Acta Pathol Jap. 9:769, 1950.

196. Pierce P. et al. Alkyl mercury poisoning in humans. Report of an outbreak. JAMA. 220:1439-1442, 1972.

197. Snyder R.D. Congenital mercury poisoning. N Eng J Med. 18:1014-1016, 1971.

198. Manson J.M. Chapter 7 -Teratogens. In, Caserett and Doull's Toxicology. 3rd ed. Macmillan Publishing Co. NY, 1986.

199. Roberts C.J. and Lowe C.R. Where have all the conceptions gone? Lancet i:498-99, 1975

200. National Center For Health Statistics (NCHS). Births, marriages, divorces and deaths for 1979. Monthly vital statistics report. U.S. Dept of Health Education and Welfare, 1980.

201. Environmental Protection Agency. Air quality criteria for lead. EPA Publication No. 600/8-77-017, Washington D.C., 1977.

202. National Foundation/March of Dimes: Facts 1980. The Foundation, NY, 1981a.

203. Steffek A.J. et al. Effects of elemental mercury-vapor exposure on pregnant Sprague-Dawley rats. J Dent Res. 66(Spec Issue):239, Abstract# 1063, 1987.

204. Clarkson T.W., Magos L. and Greenwood M.R. The transport of elemental mercury into fetal tissues. Biol Neonate. 21(3):239-244, 1985.

205. Harris S.B., Wilson J.B. and Prinz R.H. Embryotoxicity of methylmercuric chloride in golden hamsters. Teratology. 6:139-142, 1972.

206. Wilson J.G. Critique of current methods for teratogenicity testing in animals and suggestions for their improvement. In, Shepherd, Miller, Marois. Methods for Detection of Environmental Agents That Produce Congenital Defects. page 29, North-Holland/American Elsevier, NY, 1975.

207. Nishimura et al. Normal mercury level in human embryos and fetuses. Bilogia Neonat. 24:197, 1974.

208. Jaffe M. et al. Prevalence of gestational and perinatal insults in brain-damaged children. Israel J Med Sci. 21(12):940-944, 1985.

209. Becker R.O. and Selden G. The Body Electric. Electromagnetism and the foundation of life. William Morrow and Co., Inc. NY. 1985.

210. Bland J. Energy in Medicine. Complimentary Medicine 2(4) Mar-April, 1987.

211. Janerich D.T. and Polednak A.P. Epidemiology of birth defects. Epidemiologic Reviews. 5:16-37, 1983.

212. Langman J., Webster W. and Rodier P. Morphological and behavior abnormalities caused by insults to the CNS in the perinatal period. In, Berry, Poswillo. Teratology Trends and Applications. Springer, Berlin, 1975.

213. Spyker J.M. and Smithberg M. Effects of methylmercury on prenatal development in mice. Teratology. 5:181-190, 1972.

214. Su M. and Okita G.T. Embryocidal and teratogenic effects of methylmercury in mice. Toxicol Appl Pharmacol. 38:207-216, 1976b.

215. Olson F.C. and Massaro E.J. Effects of methylmercury on murine fetal amino acid uptake, protein synthesis and palate closure. Teratology. 16(2):187-194, 1977b.

216. Gilani S.H. Fine structural changes in embryonic chick heart ventricle induced by lead poisoning. Pathol Microbiol. (Basel). 42(3):188-195, 1975.

217. Ware R.A., Chang L.W. and Burkholder P.M. Ultra structural evidence for foetal injury induced by in utero exposure to small doses of methylmercury. Nature. (London). 251:236-237, 1974.

218. Chang L.W. and Sprecher J.A. Degenerative changes in the neonatal kidney following in utero exposure to methylmercury. Environ Res. 11(3):392-406, 1976a.

219. Chang L.W. and Sprecher J.A. Hyperplastic changes in the rat distal tubular epithelial cells following in utero exposure to methylmercury. Environ Res. 12(2):218-223, 1976b.

220. Rizzo A.M. and Furst A. Mercury teratogenesis in the rat. Proc West Pharmacol Soc. 15:52-54, 1972.

221. McLain R.M. and Becker B.A. Teratogenicity, fetal toxicity, and placental transfer of lead nitrate in rats. Toxicol Appl Pharmacol. 31(1):72-82, 1975.

222. Tondury G. and Smith D.W. Fetal rubella pathology. J Pediatr. 68:867-879, 1966.

223. Yeh T.-F. et al. Mercury poisoning from mercurochrome therapy of infected omphalocele. Lancet. 1:210, 1978.

224. Nakayama H. et al. Mercury exantham. Contact Dermatitis. 9:411-417, 1983.

225. Howard J.D. and Mottet N.K. Effects of methylmercury on the morphogenesis of the rat cerebellum. Teratology. 34:89-95, 1986.

226. Chen W.-J., Body R.L. and Mottet N.K. Some effects of low dose congenital exposure to methylmercury on organ growth in the rat fetus. Teratology. 20:31-36, 1979.

227. Clark A.R. Placental transfer of lead and its effects on the newborn. Postgrad Med J. 53(625):674-678, 1977.

228. Lin-Fu J.S. Vulnerability of children to lead exposure and toxicity. N Eng J Med. 289:1229-1233, 1289-1293, 1973.

229. Arana J.M. Poisoning - Toxicology - Symptoms Treatments (4th edition) page 111. Charles C. Thomas. Springfield, IL. 1979.

230. Hetzel B.X. and Potter B.J. Chapter 3:83-133, Iodine deficiency and the role of thyroid hormones in brain development. In, Neurobiology of the Trace Elements. Vol 1. Driosti J.E. and Smith R.M. (eds). Humana Press, Clifton, NJ. 1983.

231. Buttfield I.H. and Hetzel B.S. Endemic goitre in East New Guinea. Australasia Ann Med. 18:217-221, 1969.

232. Connolly K.J., Pharoah P.O.D. and Hetzel B.S. Fetal iodine deficiency and motor performance during childhood. Lancet. II(8153):1149-1151, Dec.,1979.

233. Pharoah P.O.D., Connoly K, Hetzel B.S. and Ekins R. Maternal thyroid function and motor competence in the child. Develop Med Child Neurol. 23:76-82, 1981.

234. Potter B.J. et al. Production of severe iodine deficiency in sheep using prepared low-iodine diet. Aust J Biol Sci. 33:53-61, 1980.

235. Potter B.J. et al. Retarded fetal brain development resulting from severe iodine deficiency in sheep. Neuropath Appl Neurobiol. 8:303-313, 1982.

236. Kosta L., Byrne A.R. and Zelenko V. Correlation between selenium and mercury in man following exposure to inorganic mercury. Nature (London), 254:238-239, 1975.

237. Suzuki T, Miyama T and Katsunuma H. Affinity of mercury to the thyroid. Ind Health. 4:69-75, 1966.

238. Schulte-Wisserman H., Straub E. and Funke P.J. Influence of L-thyroxine upon enzymatic activity in renal tubular epithelium of the rat under normal conditions and in mercury induced lesions. 1. Histochemical studies of alkaline phosphatase, acid phosphatase, adenosine-triphosphatase and leucine-aminopeptidase. Virchows Arch (Cell Pathol). 23:163-173, 1977.

239. Friden E. and Naile B. Interaction of phenylmercuric chloride with thyroxine and related compounds. Arch Biochem. 48:448-457, 1954.

240. Goldman M and Blackburn P. The effect of mercuric chloride on thyroid function in the rat. Toxicol Appl Pharmacol. 48:49-55, 1979.

241. Kawada J. et al. Comparative studies on acute and subacute effects of organic and inorganic mercurials on thyroidal function. J Phamacobio-Dynamics. 4(5):S-71, 1981. Proceeding of the 7th Symposium on Environmental Pollutants and Toxicology, Kobe.

242. Kostial K. and Kargacin B. Iodine in diet increases mercury absorption in rats. J Appl Toxicol. 2(4):215-216, 1982.

243. Sillen L.G. Electrometric investigation of equilibria between mercury and halogen ions. VII Survey and conclusions. Acta Chem Scand. 3:539-553, 1949.

244. Wada L. and King J.C. Effect of low zinc intake on basal metabolic rate, thyroid hormones and protein utilization in adult men. J Nutr. 116:1045-1053, 1986.

245. Shrader R.E. et al. Thyroid function in prenatally protein deprived rats. J Nutr. 107:221-229, 1977.

246. Snell K., Ashby S.L. and Barton S.J. Disturbances of perinatal carbodydrate metabolism in rats exposed to methylmercury in utero. Toxicology. 8:277-283, 1977.

247. Harada M. Congenital Minamata disease: Intrauterine methylmercury poisoning. Teratology. 18(2):285-288, 1978.

248. Brix K.A. Environmental and occupation hazards to the fetus. J Reproductive Med. 27(9):577-580, 1982.

249. Diewert V.M. and Juriloff D.M. Abnormal head posture associated with induction of cleft palate by methylmercury in C57BL/6J mice. Teratology. 28:437-447, 1983.

250. Su M. and Okita G.T. Behavioral effects on the progeny of mice treated with methylmercury. Toxicol Appl Pharmacol. 38:195-205, 1976a.

251. Null D.H., Gartside P.S. and Wei E. Methylmercury accumulation in brains of pregnant, non-pregnant and fetal rats. Life Sce. 12:65-72, 1973.

252. Kostial K. and Momcilovic B. Transport of lead 203 and calcium 47 from mothers to offspring. Arch Environ Health. 29:28-30, 1974.

253. Mansour M.M. et al. Maternal-fetal transfer of organic and inorganic mercury via placenta and milk. Environ Res. 6:478-484, 1973.

254. Yang M.G. et al. Mammary transfer of ^{203}Hg from mothers to brains of nursing rats. Prc Soc Exp Biol Med. 142(2):723-726, 1973.

255. Smith A.M., Picciano M.F. and Milner J.A. Selenium intakes and status of human milk and formula fed infants. Am J Clin Curt. 35:521-526, 1981.

256. Clarren S.A. and Smith D.W. Fetal alcohol syndrome. N Eng J Med. 298(19):1063-1067, 1978.

257. Halmesmaki E, Alfthan G. and Ylikorkala O. Selenium in pregnancy: Effect of maternal drinking. Obstet Gynecol. 68(5):602-605, 1986.

258. Nielson-Kudsk F. Factors influencing the in vitro uptake of mercury in blood. Acta Pharmacol et Toxicol. 27:161-172, 1969.

259. Roe D.A. Drug - Induced Nutritional Deficiencies. The AVI Publishing Co., Inc. Westport CT, 1976.

260. Arana E.M. Chapter 5 The nutritional foundation of orthopedic gnathology. In, Hockel J.L. Orthopedic Gnathology. Quintessence Books, Chicago, IL, 1983.

261. Miller R.W. Prenatal origins of cancer in man. Epidemiological evidence. In, Tomatis L. and Mohr E. (Eds): Transplacental Carcinogenesis. IARC Pub. #4, p 175, 1973.

262. American Cancer Society (ACS): Cancer Facts and Figures. ACS, NY, 1980.

263. Gainer J.H. Activation of the Rauscher leukemia virus by metals. J Natl Cancer Inst. 51:609-613, 1973.

264. Mangal P.C. and Sharma P. Effect of leukaemia on the concentration of some trace elements in whole human blood. Indian J. Med Res. 74:559-564, 1981.

265. Rizk S.L. and Sky-Peck H.H. Comparison between concentrations of trace elements in normal and neoplastic human breast tissue. Cancer Res. 44(11):5390-5394, 1984.

266. Brewer A.K. The high pH therapy for cancer. Tests on mice and humans. Pharmacol Biochem Behav. 21(Suppl 1):1-5, 1984.

267. Levesque P.C. and Atchison W.D. Interactions of mitochondrial inhibitors with methylmercury on spontaneous quantal release of acetylcholine. Toxicol Appl Pharmacol. 87:315-324, 1987.

268. Ikehara T. et al. Rb^+ influx in responses to changes in energy generation: Effect of the regulation of the ATP content of HeLa cells. J Cell Physiol. 119(3):273-282, 1984.

269. Null G. Medical Genocide, part fourteen: Eat to Live. Penthouse, pp 109-114, July 1987.

270. Jennette W. The role of metals in carcinogenesis: Biochemistry and metabolism. Environ Health Perspect. 40:233-252, 1981.

271. Ledergerber E. On deaths and diseases leading to death among workers producing detonators. Schweizerische Medizinische Wochenschrift. 79:263-267, 1949. English translation by Dr. Mats Hanson. (Available through Bio-Probe).

272. Schwarzkopf H. Dental materials and cancer. Erfahrungsheilkunde 10:489-493, 1959. German. English translation by Dr. Mats Hanson, Sweden. (Available through Bio-Probe).

273. Druckrey H., Hamperl H. and Schmahl D. Cancerogenic effects of metallic mercury after intraperitoneal injection in rats. Zeitschrift fur Krebsforschung. 64:511-519, 1957. Translation by Dr. Mats Hanson. (Available through Bio-Probe).

274. Copeland D.H. and Salmon W.D. The occurence of neoplasms in the liver, lungs and other tissues of rats as a result of prolonged choline deficiency. Am J Pathol. 22:1059-1079, 1946.

275. Ghoshal A.K. and Farber E. The induction of liver cancer by dietary deficiency of choline and methionine without added carcinogens. Carcinogenesis. 5(10):1367-1370, 1984.

276. Latta D.M. and Donaldson W.E. Lead toxicity in chicks: Interactions with dietary methionine and choline. J. Nutr. 116:1561-1568, 1986.

277. Hoffman R.M. Altered methionine metabolism and transmethylation in cancer. Anticancer Res. 5(1):1-30, 1985.

278. van der Westhuyzen J. Methionine metabolism and cancer. Nutr Cancer. 7(3):179-183, 1985.

279. Hoffman R.M. and Erbe R.W. Proc Natl Acad Sci. USA. 73:1523, 1976.

280. Wallwork J.C. and Duerre J.A. Effects of zinc deficiency on methionine metabolism, methylation reactions and protein synthesis in isolated perfused rat liver. J Nutr. 115(2):252-262, 1985.

281. Herbst A.L. et al. Age incidence and risk of Diethlstilbestrol-related clear cell adenocarcinoma of the vagina and cervix. Am J. Obstet Gynecol. 128:43-50, 1977.

282. Bibbs M. et al. A twenty-five year follow-up study of women exposed to Diethlstilbestrol during pregnancy. N Eng J Med. 298: 763-767, 1978.

283. Bibbs M. et al. Follow-up study of male and female offspring of DES-exposed mothers. J Obstet Gynecol. 49:1-8, 1977.

284. Wulf H.C. et al. Sister chromatid exchange (SCE) in Greenlandic eskimos. Dose-response relationship between SCE and seal diet, smoking, and blood cadmium and mercury concentations. Sci Tot Environ. 48(1-2):81-94, 1986.

285. Heimburger D.C. et al. Improvement in bronchial squamous metaplasia in smokers treated with folate and B_{12}.. Am J Clin Nutr. 45(4):866, 1987.

286. Benum S. Viruses: A nonmedical view. Complimentary Medicine. 2(5):26-27, 1987.

287. Shannon B. and Demos P. Influence of estrogen treatment on hepatic cystathione synthase and cystathionase of female rats fed varying levels of vitamin B6. J Nutr. 107:1255-1262, 1977.

288. Kazantzis G. Role of cobalt, iron, lead, manganese, mercury, platinum, selenium and titanium in carcinogenesis. Environ Health Perspect. 40:143-161, 1981.

289. Congiu L. et al. The effects of lead nitrate on tissue distribution of mercury in rats treated with methylmercury chloride. Toxicol Appl Pharmacol. 51:363-366, 1979.

290. Sin Y.M., Wong M.K. and Low L.K. Effect of lead on tissue deposition of mercury in mice. Bull Environ Contam Toxicol. 34(3):438-445, 1985.

291. Corman L.C. The relationship between nutrition, infection, and immunity. Med Clin North Am. 69(3):519-531, 1985.

292. Chang L. Neurotoxic effects of mercury - A review. Environ Res. 14:329-373, 1977.

293. Herbert V., Colman N. and Jacob E. Folic acid and vitamin B12. In, Modern Nutrition in Health and Disease (6th ed), Goodhart R.S. and Shils M.E. eds. Lea & Febiger, Philadelphia. pp 229-259, 1980.

294. Vallee B.L. and Ulmer D.D. Biochemical effects of mercury, cadmium and lead. Ann Rev Biochem. 41:91-127, 1972.

295. Hughes, W.L. A physiochemical rationale for the biological activity of mercury and its compounds. Ann NY Acad Sci, 65(5):454-460, 1957.

296. Lehninger A.L. Principles of Biochemistry. Worth Publishers Inc. NY. 1982. pp 618-619.

297. Krause M.V. and Hunscher M.A. Food, Nutrition and Diet Therapy, 5th ed. W.B. Saunders Co., Philadelphia. page 108, 1972.

298. Homburger F., Hayes J.A., Peliken E.W. (eds). A Guide to General Toxicology. page 233, S. Karger AG. Basel, Switzerland. 1983.

299. Margel S. and Hirsh J. Chelation of mercury by polymercaptic microspheres: New potential antidote for mercury poisoning. J Pharm Sci. 71(9):1030-1034, 1982.

300. Stricks W. and Kolthoff I.M. Reactions between mercuric mercury and cysteine and glutathione. J Am Chem Soc. 75(22):5673-5681, 1953.

301. Winship K.A. Toxicity of mercury and its inorganic salts. Adverse Drug React Acute Poisoning Rev. 4(3):129-160, 1985.

302. Alfonso J.F. and Alvarez R. Effects of mercury on human gestation. Am J Obstet Gynecol. 80(1):145-154, 1960.

303. Wannag A. and Skjaerasen J. Mercury in placenta and foetal membranes as an indication of low mercury pressure. Commission of the European Communities. (Rep) 3, (5360):1233-1238, 1975.

304. Sturman J.A. In, Amino Acids -Metabolism and Medical Applications. Eds: Blackburn G.L., Grant J.P., Young V.R. Chpt 3, pp 29-36, 1983.

305. Stipanuk M.H. Metabolism of sulfur-containing amino acids. Ann Rev Nutr. 6:179-209, 1986.

306. Sprince et al. Protectants against acetaldehyde toxicity: Sulfhydryl compounds and ascorbic acid. Fed Proc. 33(3), March 1974.

307. Aihara M. and Sharma R.P. Effects of endogenous and exogenous thiols on the distribution of mercurial compounds in mouse tissues. Arch Environ Contam Toxicol. 15(6):629-636, 1986.

308. Sturman J.A. et al. Absence of cystathionase in human fetal liver. Is cystine essential? Science. 169:74-76, 1970.

309. Ogawa M. et al. Decrease of plasma sulfur amino acids in essential hypertension. Jpn Circ J. 49(12):1217-1224, 1985.

310. Blackstone S., Hurley R.J. and Hughes R.E. Some inter-relationships between vitamin C (L Ascorbic Acid) and mercury in the guinea pig. Food Cosmet Toxicol. 12:511-516, 1974.

311. Huxtable R.J. Insights on function: metabolism and pharmacology of taurine in the brain. Prog Clin Biol Res. 68:53-97, 1981.

312. Martin D.W., Jr., Mayes P.A., Rodwell V.W. Harper's Review of Biochemistry (19th ed). Lange Medical Publications. Los Altos, CA, 1983.

313. Hayses K.C., Stephan Z.F. and Sturman J.A. Growth depression in taurine depleted infant monkeys. J Nutr. 110:2058-2064, 1980.

314. Gaull G.E. Taurine in human milk: growth modulator or conditionally essential amino acid? J Pediat Gastro Nutr. 2:S266-S271, 1983.

315. Sturman J.A., Rassin D.K. and Gaull G.E. Minireview. Taurine in development. Life Sci. 21:1-22, 1977.

316. Naismith D.J., Rana S.K. and Emery P.W. Metabolism of taurine during reproduction in women. Hum Nutr Clin Nutr. 40C:37-45, 1986.

317. Tateishi N. et al. The L-methionine-sparing effect of dietary glutathione in rats. J Nutr. 112(12):2217-2226, 1982.

318. Meister A. et al. Glutathione. Ann Rev Biochem. 52:711-760, 1983.

319. Cranton E. and Frackelton J. J. Treatment of free radical pathology in chronic degenerative diseases with EDTA chelation therapy. J Hol Med. 6(1), 1984.

320. Urabe A., Hamilton J., and Sassa S. Dexamethasone and erythroid colony formation: contrasting effects in mouse and human bone marrow cells in culture. Hematol. 43:479, 1973.

321. Droge W. et al. Glutathione augments activation of cytotoxic T lymphocytes in vivo. Immunobiol. 172(1-2):151-156, 1986.

322. Rothstein A. Mercurials and red cell membranes. In, The Function of Red Cells: Erythrocyte Pathobiology. Allan R. Liss, Inc., NY. pp 105-131, 1981.

323. Ansari K.A., Bigelow D. and Kaplan E. Glutathione peroxidase activity in surgical and autopsied human brains. Neurochem Res. 10(5):703-711, 1985.

324. Ridlington J.W. and Whanger P.D. Interactions of selenium and antioxidants with mercury, cadmium and silver. Funam Appl Toxicol. 1:368-375, 1981.

325. Ballatori N. and Clarkson T.W. Inorganic mercury secretion into bile as a low molecular weight complex. Biochem Pharmacol. 33:1087-1092, 1984a.

326. Ballatori N. and Clarkson T.W. Dependence of biliary secretion of inorganic mercury on the biliary transport of glutathione. Biochem Pharmacol. 33:1093-1098, 1984b.

327. Rowland I.R., Robinson R.D. and Doherty R.A. Effects of diet on mercury metabolism and excretion in mice given methylmercury: Role of gut flora. Arch Environ Health. 39(6):401-408, 1984.

328. Naganuma A, Koyama Y and Imura N. Behavior of methylmercury in mammalian erythrocytes. Toxicol Appl Pharmacol. Jul: 54(3):405-410. 1980.

329. Kutsky R.J. Handbook of Vitamins, and Minerals and Hormones. (2nd edition) Van Nostrand Reinhold Co. NY, 1981.

330. Frost D.V. The two faces of selenium - can selenophobia be cured? CRC Crit Rev Toxicol. 8(1):1, 1980.

331. Chmielnicki J., Brezeznicka E. and Sniady A. Kidney concentration and urinary excretion of mercury, zinc, copper, following the administration of mercuric chloride and sodium selenite to rats. Arch Toxicol. 59(1):16-20, 1986.

332. Burk R.F., Chapter 35: pp 519-527. In, Nutrition Reviews' Present Knowledge in Nutrition / Fifth Edition. The Nutrition Foundation, Inc. 1984.

333. Virtamo J. et al. Serum selenium and the risk of coronary heart disease and stroke. Am J Epidemiol. 122(2):276-282, 1985.

334. Stock A. and Cucuel F. Uptake and distribution of mercury in the organism. Zeitschr. angew Chem. 47:801, 1934.

335. Wada E. et al. Response to a low concentration of mercury vapor. Relation to human porphyrin metabolism. Arch Environ Health. 19(4):485-488, 1969.

336. Personal communication with Dr. Mats Hanson of Sweden, 1987.

337. Willet W.C. et al. Prediagnostic serum selenium and risk of cancer. Lancet. July 16, 1983, page 130.

338. Salonen J.R. et al. Association between cardiovascular death and myocardia infarction and serum selenium in a matched pair longitudinal study. Lancet. July 24:175-179, 1982.

339. Dworkin B.M et al. Selenium deficiency in the Acquired Immunodeficiency Syndrome. J Parenter Enteral Nutr. 10(4):405-407, 1986.

340. Guidi G. et al. Platelet glutathione peroxidase activity is impaired in patients with coronary heart disease. Scand J. Clin Lab Invest. 46(6):549-551, 1986.

341. Recommended Dietary Allowances. Food and Nutrition Board, National Academy of Sciences, Washington, D.C., 1980.

342. Inglett G.E. Editor. Nutritional Bioavailability of Zinc. ACS Symposium Series 210. American Chemical Society, Washington D.C., 1983.

343. Pearson R.B. Hard and soft acids and bases. HSAB, Part II. J Chem Educ. 45:643-648, 1968.

344. Williams D.R. An Introduction to Bio-organic Chemistry. Charles C. Thomas, Springfield IL, 1976.

345. Day F.Z. and Brady F.O. In vivo and ex vivo displacement of zinc from metallothionein by cadmium and mercury. Chem Biol Interact. 50(2):159-174, 1984.

346. Bunk M.J. et al. Dietary zinc deficiency impairs plasma transport of vitamin E. Am J Clin Nutr. 45(4):865-866, 1987.

347. Alexander J., Aaseth J., and Refsvik T. Excretion of zinc in rat bile - A role of glutathione. Acta Pharmacol Toxicol. 49:190-194, 1981.

348. Yonaha M., Itoh E., Ohbayashi Y. and Uchiyama M. Induction of lipid peroxidation in rats by mercuric chloride. Res Comm Chem Pathol Pharmacol. 28(1):105-112, 1980.

349. Fukino H. et al. Effect of zinc pretreatment on mercuric chloride induced lipid peroxidation in the rat kidney. Toxicol Appl Pharmacol. 73(3):395-401, 1984.

350. Gale T.F. The amelioration of mercury-induced embryotoxic effects by simultaneous treatment with zinc. Environ Res. 35(2):405-412, 1984.

351. Bjorksten B. et al. Zinc and immune function in Down's syndrome. Acta Paediatr Scand. 69:183-187, 1980.

352. Anneren B. et al. Selenium in plasma and erythrocytes in patients with Down's syndrome and healthy controls. (Variation in relation to age, sex and glutathione peroxidase activity in erythrocytes). Acta Paediatr Scand. 74(4):508-514, 1985.

353. Aaseth J. et al. In, Selenium in Biology and Medicine. Eds. Spallholz, Martin and Ganther. AVI Publ. Co., Inc. Connecticut. 1981, p 418.

354. Ahlroth-Westerlund B. et al. Altered distribution patterns of macro- and trace elements in human tissues of patients with decreased levels of blood selenium. Submitted for publication.

355. Carmignani M. and Boscolo P. Cardiovascular homeostasis in rats chronically exposed to mercuric chloride. Arch Toxicol. (Suppl 7):380-383, 1984.

356. Cherian M.G. and Goyer R.A. Minireview - Metallothioneins and their role in the metabolism and toxicity of metals. Life Sci. 23:1-9, 1978.

357. Tandon S.K., Magos L. and Cabral J.R.P. Protection against mercuric chloride by nephrotoxic agents which do not induce thionein. Toxicol Appl Pharmacol. 52:227-236, 1980.

358. Oleske J.M. et al. Plasma zinc and copper in primary and secondary immunodeficiency disorders. Biol Tr El Res. 5:189-194, 1983.

359. Edman J., Sobel J.D. and Taylor M.L. Zinc status in women with recurrent vulvovaginal condidiasis. Am J Obstet Gynecol. 155:1082-1085, 1986.

360. Zamm A.V. Candida albicans therapy. Is there ever an end to it: Dental mercury removal: an effective adjunct. J Orthomolec Med. 1(4):261-266, 1986.

361. Vallee B.L. and Ulmer D.D. Biochemical effects of mercury, cadmium, and lead. Ann Rev Biochem. 41:91-127, 1972.

362. Miyamoto M.D. Hg^{2+} causes neurotoxicity at an intracellular site following entry through Na and Ca channels. Brain Res. 267(2):375-379, 1983.

363. Shier W.T. and DuBourdieu D.J. Stimulation of phospholipid hydrolysis and cell death by mercuric chloride: Evidence for mercuric ion acting as a calcium-mimetic agent. Biochem Biophys Res Comm. 110(3):758-765, 1983.

364. Tomera J.F. and Harakal C. Mercury-and lead-induced contraction of aortic smooth muscle in vitro. Arch Int Pharacodyn Ther. 283(2):295-302, 1986.

365. Aikawa J.K. The Relationship of Magnesium to Disease in Domestic Animals and Humans. Charles C. Thomas, Springfield IL, 1971.

366. Lehninger A.L. Principles of Biochemistry. pp 258-259. Worth Publishing Co., Inc. NY, 1982.

367. Thompson J.D. and Nechay B.R. Inhibition by metals of a canine renal calcium, magnesium activated adenosine triphosphatase. J. Toxicol Environ Health. 7(6):901-908, 1981.

368. Mehra M. and Kanwar K.C. Enzyme changes in brain, liver and kidney following repeated administration of mercuric chloride. J Environ Pathol Toxicol Oncol. 7(1-2):65-71, 1986.

369. Basu T.K. and Schorah C.J. Vitamin C in Health and Disease. AVI Publishing Co. Westport Ct. 1982.

370. Ginter E. Chronic marginal vitamin C deficiency: Biochemistry and pathophysiology. Wld Rev Nutr Diet. 33:104-141, 1979a.

371. Turley S.P., West C.E. and Horton B.J. The role of ascorbic acid in the regulation of cholesterol metabolism and in the pathogenesis of artherosclerosis. Atherosclerosis. 24:1-18, 1976.

372. Vauthey M. Protective effects of vitamin C against poisons. Praxis. (Bern). 40:284-286, 1951.

373. Mavin J.V. Experimental treatment of acute mercury poisoning of guinea pigs with ascorbic acid. Revista de la Sociedad Argentian de Biologia. (Buenos Aires). 17:581-586, 1941.

374. Mokranjac M. and Petrovic C. Vitamin C as an antidote in poisoning by fatal doses of mercury. Comptes Rendus Hebdomadaires des Seances de l Academie des Sciences. 258:1341-1342, 1964.

375. Chapman D.W. and Shaffer C.F. Mercurial Diuretics. Archives of Int Med. 79:449-456, 1947.

376. Basu T.K. In, Clinical Implication of Drug Use. Ed: Basu T.K., Vol 1, page 11. CRC Press, Boca Raton, Fl, 1980.

377. Basu T.K. Possible toxicological aspects of megadoses of ascorbic acid. Chemico-Biol Interactions. 16:247-250, 1977.

378. Goldberg et al. Effect of heavy metals on human rheumatoid synovial cell proliferation and collagen synthesis. Biochem Pharmacol. 32(18):2763-2766, 1983.

379. Robins S.L., Cotran R.S. and Kumer V., Ed's. In, Pathologic Basis of Disease (3rd ed). W.B. Saunders Co. Philadelphia. Page 421, 1984.

380. Ziff S. Bio-Probe Newsletter. 3(1):8-10, 1986.

381. Bieri J.S. Chapter 16:226-240, In, Nutrition Review - Present Knowledge in Nutrition. Nutrition Foundation, Wash D.C., 1984.

382. Mitchell H.S., Rynbergen H.J., Anderson L. and Dibble M.V., Eds. In, Nutrition in Health and Disease. (16th ed). J.B. Lippincott Co., Philadelphia 1976, pp 86-88.

383. Kutsky R.J. Handbood of Vitamins, Minerals and Hormones (2nd ed). Chapter 24. Van Nostrand Reinhold Co. New York. 1981.

384. Fukino H. et al. Effect of zinc pretreatment on mercuric chloride induced lipid peroxidation in the rat kidney. Toxicol Appl Pharmacol. 73(3):395-401, 1984.

385. Seelig M.S. Auto-immune complications of D-penicillamine - A possible result of zinc and magnesium depletion and pyridoxine inactivation. J Am Coll Nutr. 1(2):207-214, 1982.

386. Hoffeld J.T. Agents which block membrane lipid peroxidation enhance mouse spleen cell immune activities in vitro: Relationship to the enhancing activity of 2-mercaptoethanol. Eur J Immunol. 11(5):371-376, 1981.

387. Marsh J.A. et al. Effect of selenium and vitamin E dietary deficiencies on chick lymphoid organ development. Proceedings of the Society for Experimental Biology and Medicine. 182(4):425-436, 1986.

388. Meekes H.C. et al. Antioxidant effects on cell-mediated immunity. J Leukocyte Biol. 38(4):451-458, 1985.

389. Addya S. et al. Effects of mercuric chloride on several scavenging enzymes in rat kidney and influence of vitamin E supplementation. Acta Vitaminol Enzymol. 6(2):103-107, 1984.

390. Oksi F.A. Vitamin E - A radical defense. N Eng J Med. 303:454-455, Aug 1980.

391. Dormandy T.L. Free-radical oxidation and antioxidants. Lancet. 1(8605):647-650, Mar 25, 1978.

392. Farrell P.M. et al. The occurrence and effects of human vitamin E deficiency. A study with cystic fibrosis. J Clin Invest. 60(1):233-241, 1977.

393. Sheetz M. In, Discussion: Schulman J.D. Moderator. Genetic disorders of glutathione and sulfur amino-acid metabolism. Ann Intern Med. 93:330-346, Aug 1980.

394. Corash et al. Reduced chronic hemolysis during high-dose vitamin E administration in Mediterranean type glucose-6-phosphate dehydrogenase deficiency. N Eng J Med. 303:416-420, Aug 21, 1980.

395. Nutrition Reviews Present Knowledge in Nutrition (5th ed). The Nutrition Foundation, Washington D.C., 1984. Chapter 26. Robert Olson, 377-382.

396. Danford C.E. and Munro H.N. Water Soluble Vitamins. In, Goodman and Gillman's The Pharmacological Basis of Therapeutics, (6th ed). Chpt 66, pp 1560-1582. Macmillan Publishing Co., Inc. 1980.

397. Hodges R.E. et al. Human pantothenic acid deficiency produced by omega-methyl pantothenic acid. J Clin Invest. 38:1421-1425, 1959.

398. Fry P.C., Fox H.M. and Tao H.G. Metabolic response to a pantothenic acid deficient diet in humans. J Nutr Sci Viatminol. (Tokyo). 22:339-346, 1976.

399. Robishaw J.D. and Neely J.R. Coenzyme A metabolism. Am J. Physiol. 248 (endocrine metab 11):E1-E9, 1985.

400. Kirschmann J.D. Nutrition Almanac. McGraw-Hill Book Co. New York, 1979.

401. Burton B.V. and Meikle A.W. Acute and chronic methyl mercury poisoning impairs rat adrenal and testicular function. J Toxicol Environ Health. 6:597-606, 1980.

402. Sturman J.A. Vitamin B6 and the metabolism of sulfur amino acids. In, Human Vitamin B6 Requirements. National Academy of Sciences. Wash D.C. pp 37-60, 1978.

403. Henderson L.M. Vitamin B6. In, Nutrition Reviews' Present Knowledge In Nutrition. Chapter 21. pp 303-317. The Nutrition Foundation, Inc. Wash D.C. 1984.

404. Wilson E.D., Fisher K.II. and Garcia P.A. Principles of Nutrition (4th ed), page 86. John Wiley & Sons, NY, 1979.

405. Leklem et al. Metabolism of methionine in oral contraceptive users and control women receiving controlled intakes of vitamin B6. Am J. Clin Nutr. 30:1122-1128, 1977.

406. Sturman J.A., Cohen P.A. and Gaull G.E. Effects of deficiency of vitamin B6 in transsulfuration. Biochem Med. 3:244-251, 1969.

407. Spector R. Vitamin B6 transport in the central nervous system: In vitro studies. J Neurochem. 30(4):889-897, 1978.

408. Stipanuck M.H. Metabolism of sulfur-containing amino acids. Annu Rev Nutr. 6:179-209, 1986.

409. Thiele V.F. and Brin M. Availability of vitamin B6 vitamers fed orally to Long-Evans rats as determined by tissue transaminase activity and vitamin B6 assay. J Nutr. 94:237-242, 1968.

410. Garrison R.H. Jr. and Somer E. The Nutrition Desk Reference. Keats Publishing. New Canaan, CT, 1985. page 48.

411. Neal R.A. and Sauberlich H.E. In, Modern Nutrition in Health and Disease (6th ed). Goodhart R.S. and Shils M.E., Ed's. Lea & Febiger, Philadelphia, 1980, pp 191-197.

412. Lonsdale D. Thiamine metabolism in disease. Crit Rev Clin Lab Sce. 5(3):289-313, 1975.

413. Axelerod A.E. Role of vitamins in antibody production. Metabolism 2:1-8, 1953.

414. Hillman R.S. Vitamin B12, Folic Acid and the treatment of megaloblastic anemia. In, Goodman and Gillman's The Pharmacological Basis of Therapeutics. Chpt 57. pp 1331-1346, 1980.

415. Das K.C. and Herbert V. Vitamin B12-folate interrelations. Clin Haematol. 5:697-725, 1976.

416. Chanarin I. et al. Vitamin B12 regulates folate metabolism by the supply of formate. Lancet. Sept 6:505-508, 1980.

417. Stokstad E.L.R. and Koch J. Folic acid metabolism. Physiol Rev. 47:83-116, 1967.

418. Krebs H.A., Hems R. and Tyler B. The regulation of folate and methionine metabolism. Biochem J. 158:341-353, 1976.

419. Youinou P.Y et al. Folic acid deficiency and neutrophil dysfunction. Am J. Med. 73(5):652-657, 1982.

420. Rader J.E. et al. Effect of lead acetate on rats fed diets containing low levels of folic acid. Drug Nutr Interact. 1(2):131-142, 1982.

421. Stokstad E.L.R. et al. Nutritional interactions of vitamin B12, folic acid and thyroxine. Ann NY Acad Sci. 355:119-129, 1980.

422. Kostial K and Kargacin B. Iodine increase mercury absorption in rats. J Appl Toxicol. 2(4):215-216, 1982.

423. Krause M.V. and Hunscher M.A. Food, Nutrion and Diet Therapy (5th ed). W.B. Saunders Co. Philadelphia. pp 140-144, 1972.

424. Weissbach H. and Taylor R.T. Metabolic role of vitamin B12. Vitam Horm. 26:395-412, 1968.

425. Huennekens F.M. Folate and B12 coenzymes. In, Biological Oxidation (Singer R.P., Ed). John Wiles & Sons, Inc. NY. pp 439-513, 1968.

426. Nakazawa T., Mizuno S, and Kanno T. Significance of phosphatidyl-choline synthesis pathway via stepwise methylation of phos-phatidylethanolamine depending on methylcobalamin. Vitamins. (Japan). 46:319-323, 1972.

427. Kasuya M. The effect of methylcobalamin on the toxicity of methylmer-cury and mercuric chloride on nervous tissue in culture. Toxicol Lett. 7(1):87-93, 1980.

428. Windebank A.J. Specific inhibition of myelination by lead in vitro; com-parison with arsenic, thallium, and mercury. Exp Neurol. 94(1):203-212, 1986.

429. Sakane T. et al. Effects of methyl-B12 on the in vitro immune functions of human T lymphocytes. J Clin Immunol. 2(2): 101-109, 1982.

430. Chanarin I. et al. Cobalamin-folate interrelations: A critical review. Blood. 66(3):479-489, 1985.

431. Workshop on Biocompatibility of Metals in Dentistry, July 11-13, 1984. Sponsored by the NIDR and hosted by ADA. Transcript provided by the ADA.

432. Goldwater L.J., Ladd A.C. and Jacobs M.B. Absorption and excretion of mercury in man: VII. Significance of mercury in blood. Arch Environ Health. 9:735-741, 1964.

433. Satoh H., Hursh J.B., and Clarkson T.W. Selective determination of elemental mercury in blood and urine exposed to mercury vapor in vitro. J Appl Toxicol. 1 (3): 177-181. 1981.

434. U.S. Environmental Protection Agency. 600/4-79-049. Aug 1979.

435. Jenkins D.W. U.S. Environmental Protection Agency. 600/3-80-089. Sept 1980.

436. Airey D. Mercury in human hair due to environment and diet: A review. Environ Health Perspectives. 52:303-316, 1983.

437. Manson P. and Zlotkin S. Hair analysis - A critical review. Can Med Assoc J. 133(3):186-188, 1985.

438. Barrett S. Commercial hair analysis. Science or scam? JAMA. 254(8):1041-1045, Aug 1985.

439. Schoenthaler S. Controversy Brews: An alternate view of the accuracy of hair analysis. Complementary Medicine. 2(2):42-44, Nov/Dec 1986.

440. Health Facts, Vol XII(97):2, June 1987. 237 Thompson St. NY, NY 10012.

441. Gibson R.S. Hair as a biopsey material for the assessment of trace element status in infancy - A review. J Hum Nutr. 34:405-416, 1980.

442. Chittleborough G. A chemist's view of the analysis of human hair for trace elements. Sci Tot Environ. 14(1):53-75, Jan 1980.

443. Gonzalez M.J. et al. Mercury in human hair: A study of residents in Madrid, Spain. Arch Environ Health. 40(4):225-228, 1985.

444. Airey D. Total mercury concentrations in human hair from 13 countries in relation to fish consumption and location. Sci Tot Environ. 31(2):157-180, Nov 1983.

445. Phelps R.W. et al. Interrelationships of blood and hair mercury concentrations in North American population exposed to methylmercury. Arch Environ Health. 35(3):161-168, 1980.

446. Kyle J.H. and Ghani N. Elevated mercury levels in people from Lake Murray, Western Province. Papua, New Guinea Med J. 25(2):81-88, June 1982.

447. Inasmasu T. et al. Mercury concentration in human hair after the ingestion of canned tuna fish. Bull Environ Contam Toxicol. 37:475-481, 1986.

448. Harada M. et al. Mercury contamination in human hair at indian reserves in canada. Kumamoto Med J. 30(2):57-64, 1977.

449. Internation Conference on Mercury Hazards in Dental Practice. Glasgow, Scotland. 2-4 Sept 1981. Proceedings. Dept of Clinical Physics and Bio-Engineering. West of Scotland Health Boards. 11 West Graham St. Glasgow G4 Scotland.

450. Lee T.S. and Sohn D.H. A study on the content of total mercury in the head hair of dental personnel. Yakhay Hoeji. 23(1):17-29, 1979.

451. Francis P.C. et al. Mercury content of human hair: A survey of dental personnel. J Toxicol Environ Health. 10(4-5):667-672, Nov 1982.

452. Sinclair P.M., Turner P.R. and Johns R.B. Mercury levels in dental students and faculty measured by neutron activation analysis. J Prosth Dent. 43(5):581-585, 1980.

453. Sikorski R. et al. An effect of an occupational exposure to metallic mercury on blood serum levels of the selected immune and transport proteins - A preliminary report. Pol Tyg Lekarski 41(27):855-857, July 1986.

454. Clarkson T.W., Amin-Zaki L. and Al-Tikriti S.K. An outbreak of methylmercury poisoning due to consumption of contaminated grain. Fed Proc. 35(12):2395-2399, 1976.

455. Bergmann K.E., Makosch G., and Tews K.H. Abnormalities of hair zinc concentrations in mothers of newborn infants with spina bifida. Am J Clin Nutr. 33(10):2145-2150, 1985.

456. Chen X.C. et al. Low levels of zinc in hair and blood, pica, anorexia and poor growth in chinese preschool children. Am J Clin Nutr. 42(4):694-700, 1985.

457. Collipp P.J. et al. Hair zinc, scalp hair quantity, and diaper rash in normal infants. Cutis. 35(1):66-70, 1985.

458. Barlow P.J., Sidani S.A. and Lyons M. Trace elements in hair in the U.K.: Results and interpretation in the preconception situation. Sci Tot Environ. 42(1-2):121-131, 1985.

459. Creason J.P et al. Maternal-fetal tissue levels of 16 trace elements in 8 selected continental United States communities. Trace Substances in Environ Health. 10:53-62, 1976.

460. Fujita M. and Takabatake M. Mercury levels in human maternal and neonatal blood, hair and milk. Bull Environ Contam Toxicol. 18:205-209, 1977.

461. Goyer R.A. Chapter 19: Toxic Effects of Metal. In: Caserett and Doull's Toxicology (3rd ed). Macmillan Publishing Co. NY. 1986.

462. Cholewa L. et al. The hepatoxicity of mercury vapors in the light of biochemical scintographic and morphological data. Mater Med Pol. 17(1):23-29, 1985.

463. Chowdhury A.R., Vachrajani K.D. and Chatterjee B.B. Inhibition of 3b-hydroxy-delta 5-steroid dehydrogenase in rat testicular tissue by mercuric chloride. Toxicol Lett. 27:45-49, 1985.

464. Bryan S.E. Chapter 3, pp 87-101. In, Eichorn G.L. and Marzilla L.G.(Eds). Metal Ions In Genetic Information Transfer. Elsevier/North Holland, 1981.

465. Berg C.G. and Miles E.F. Mechanisms of inhibition of active transport of ATPases by mercurials. Chem Biol Interact. 27(2-3): 199-219, 1979.

466. Mehra M. and Kanwar K.C. Enzyme changes in the brain, liver, and kidney following repeated administration of mercuric chloride. JEPTO. 7(1-2):65-72, 1986.

467. Chang L.W. and Suber R. Protection effect of selenium on methylmercury toxicity: A possible mechanism. Toxicol. 29:285-289, 1982.

468. Donaldson W.E. Mercury inhibition of avian fatty acid synthetase. Chem Biol Interact. 11:343-350, 1975.

469. Kling L.J. and Soares J.H., Jr. The effect of mercury and vitamin E on tissue glutathione peroxidase activity and thiobarbituric acid values. Poult Sci. 61(8):1762-1765, 1982.

470. Chao L.-P. and Wolfgran F. Activation inhibition and aggregation of choline acetyltransferase. J Neurochem. 23(4):697-701, 1974.

471. Kissane J.M., Ed. In, Anderson's Pathology. Volume One, page 196. C.V. Mosby Co. St. Louis, 1985.

472. Dwivedi C. et al. Effect of mercury compounds on choline acetyltransferase. Res Commun Chem Pathol Pharmacol. 30(2):381-384, 1980.

473. Bartonome J., Whitmore W.L. and Slotkin T.A. Effect of neonatal mercuric chloride administration on growth and biochemical development of neuronal and non-neuronal tissue in the rat: Comparison with methylmercury. Toxicol Lett. 22(1):101-111, 1984.

474. Rowland I.R. et al. The effect of various dietary fibers on tissue concentration and chemical form of mercury after methylmercury exposure in mice. Arch Toxicol. 59(2):94-8, 1986.

475. F.D.A. - Computer listing of products in the drug listing file containing mercury. Sept 1985. Obtained under the freedom of information act.

476. Hobbs C.H. and McClellan R.O. Chapter 21: Toxic effects of radiation and radioactive materials, pp 669-705. In, Caserett and Doull's Toxicology (3rd ed). Macmillan Publishing Co., NY, 1986.

477. Norwood C. At Highest Risk. Protecting Children From Environmental Injury. Chapter 6, pp 156-188, Penguin Books. 1981.

AUTHOR & SUBJECT INDEX

A

NOTE: Entries listed by chapter and page number

NOTE: Entries listed by chapter and page number

NOTE: Entries listed by chapter and page number

NOTE: Entries listed by chapter and page number

NOTE: Entries listed by chapter and page number

NOTE: Entries listed by chapter and page number

NOTE: Entries listed by chapter and page number

NOTE: Entries listed by chapter and page number

NOTE: Entries listed by chapter and page number

F

NOTE: Entries listed by chapter and page number

G

NOTE: Entries listed by chapter and page number

H

NOTE: Entries listed by chapter and page number

NOTE: Entries listed by chapter and page number

NOTE: Entries listed by chapter and page number

J

K

L

NOTE: Entries listed by chapter and page number

NOTE: Entries listed by chapter and page number

NOTE: Entries listed by chapter and page number

NOTE: Entries listed by chapter and page number

NOTE: Entries listed by chapter and page number

N

NOTE: Entries listed by chapter and page number

P

NOTE: Entries listed by chapter and page number

NOTE: Entries listed by chapter and page number

R

S

NOTE: Entries listed by chapter and page number

NOTE: Entries listed by chapter and page number

NOTE: Entries listed by chapter and page number

NOTE: Entries listed by chapter and page number

W

NOTE: Entries listed by chapter and page number

X

Y

Z